D1106168

Community Engagement, Organization, and Development for Public Health Practice

Frederick G. Murphy, MSHyg, MPIA, is currently the Executive Director of Life-long Health, Inc., a nonprofit 501 c 3 organization based in Atlanta, GA. For the past two decades he has served as an adjunct faculty member at Morehouse School of Medicine, Department of Community Health and Preventive Medicine, and since 1998 as an adjunct faculty member at Georgia State University, College of Health and Human Science. Murphy completed his undergraduate studies at Oak-wood University in Huntsville, Alabama and his graduate studies at the University of Pittsburgh, School of Public Health and School of Public and International Affairs. He also received postgraduate training with the World Health Organization, Jhi Chi Medical School (Japan), at Harvard University, the United States Public Health Service, the Centers for Disease Control, and Georgic State University. Mr. Murphy presently holds the rank of Captain in the United States Public Health Service (USPHS), where he has served (active and inactive reserve) as a Commissioned Corp Officer since 1978. Mr. Murphy, for more than 14 years, served as a Project Officer and Human Subject Contact at the Centers for Disease Control and Prevention in Atlanta Georgia, and has more than 30 years of experience in the area of community health. His previous positions include: Community Health Organizer at the Morehouse School of Medicine, Executive Director of the Southeastern Primary Care Consortium/Area Health Education Center. Murphy is also the author and coauthor of several book chapters and journal articles on public and community health.

DREXEL UNIVERSITY
HEALTH SCIENCES LIBRARIES
HAHNEMANN LIBRARY

Community Engagement, Organization, and Development for Public Health Practice

Frederick G. Murphy, MSHyg, MPIA

Editor

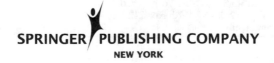

SPRINGER PUBLISHING COMPANY
NEW YORK

Copyright © 2013 Springer Publishing Company, LLC

All rights reserved.

No part of this publication may be reproduced, stored in a retrieval system, or transmitted in any form or by any means, electronic, mechanical, photocopying, recording, or otherwise, without the prior permission of Springer Publishing Company, LLC, or authorization through payment of the appropriate fees to the Copyright Clearance Center, Inc., 222 Rosewood Drive, Danvers, MA 01923, 978–750-8400, fax 978–646-8600, info@copyright.com or on the Web at www.copyright.com.

Springer Publishing Company, LLC
11 West 42nd Street
New York, NY 10036
www.springerpub.com

Acquisitions Editor: Sheri W. Sussman
Composition: Newgen Imaging

ISBN: 978-0-8261-0801-2
E-book ISBN: 978-0-8261-0802-9

Instructor's Manual ISBN: 978-0-8261-7088-0
Power Point Presentation ISBN: 978-0-8261-7087-3

(Available upon request from textbook@springerpub.com)

12 13/ 5 4 3 2 1

WA
546.1
C734
2013

The author and the publisher of this Work have made every effort to use sources believed to be reliable to provide information that is accurate and compatible with the standards generally accepted at the time of publication. The author and publisher shall not be liable for any special, consequential, or exemplary damages resulting, in whole or in part, from the readers' use of, or reliance on, the information contained in this book. The publisher has no responsibility for the persistence or accuracy of URLs for external or third-party Internet websites referred to in this publication and does not guarantee that any content on such websites is, or will remain, accurate or appropriate.

Library of Congress Cataloging-in-Publication Data
Community engagement, organization, and development for public health practice / Frederick G. Murphy, editor.
    p. ; cm.
Includes bibliographical references and index.
ISBN 978-0-8261-0801-2—ISBN 978-0-8261-0802-9 (e-book)—ISBN 978-0-8261-7088-0 (instructor's manual)—ISBN 978-0-8261-7087-3 (instructor's powerpoint presentation)
I. Murphy, Frederick.
[DNLM: 1. Community Health Services—methods. 2. Community Networks.
3. Community-Institutional Relations. 4. Consumer Participation.
5. Public Health Administration—methods. WA 546.1]
LC classification not assigned
362.12–dc23   2012021547

Special discounts on bulk quantities of our books are available to corporations, professional associations, pharmaceutical companies, health care organizations, and other qualifying groups.

If you are interested in a custom book, including chapters from more than one of our titles, we can provide that service as well.

For details, please contact:
Special Sales Department, Springer Publishing Company, LLC
11 West 42nd Street, 15th Floor, New York, NY 10036–8002s
Phone: 877–687-7476 or 212–431-4370; Fax: 212–941-7842
Email: sales@springerpub.com

Printed in the United States of America by Gasch Printing.

82105508

This textbook is dedicated to the many community leaders and public health practitioners living and working in diverse communities here in the United States
and throughout the Globe. We say thank you to these servant leaders who have
committed their life work to improving the quality of life for disparate and disenfranchised populations residing in communities and villages worldwide.

This work is also dedicated to all strata of quality leadership and stewardship, espe-
cially those unsung heroes, such as Terrell M. Bond, MD, MPH; Julia Smith and
Ms. Strickland (Joyland Community City of Atlanta NPU Y); Louis Sullivan,
MD, Former Secretary of Health and Human Services and Former President and
Founder of Morehouse School of Medicine; Ruth Goode-White, Former Director
of Sickle Cell Disease Center of Pittsburgh; Tom and Zora Murphy of Pittsburgh,
Pennsylvania, and many others.

9-28-12 Kitt 154.60

Contents

Contributors

Daniel S. Blumenthal, MD, MPH
Professor of Community Health
  and Preventive Medicine
Associate Dean for Community
  Health
Morehouse School of Medicine
Atlanta, GA

Karen E. Bouye, PhD, MPH, MS
Senior Advisor for Research
CDC/Office of the Director/Office
  of Minority Health and Health
  Equity
Atlanta, GA

Arletta T. Brinson, PhD
Education Consultant
LIN Associates
Atlanta, GA

Jessie Daniels, PhD
City University of New York
  (CUNY)
Associate Professor
Graduate Center and Hunter
  College
New York, NY

**Pamela V. Daniels, MBA,
  MPH, PhD**
Epidemiologist
Morehouse School of Medicine
Atlanta, GA

Stephen B. Fawcett, PhD
Director, KU Work Group for
  Community Health and
  Development
Lawrence, KS

Rafael Flores, MFA
Director
23rd and Union
Oakland, CA

**Lynda Murphy-Freeman,
  MPH, MBA**
Lifelong Health, Inc.
Nova Southeastern
  University Doctorate
  Student
Montgomery, AL

**Barbara Glickstein, RN,
  MPH, MS**
Hunter College
New York, NY

Christina M. Holt, MA
Associate Director, KU Work
  Group for Community Health
  and Development
University of Kansas
Lawrence, KS

Emanuel Joseph,
  MBBS, MPH
Atlanta, GA

Richard W. Klomp,
  MOB, MS, LPC, BCPC
Centers for Disease Control and
  Prevention
Atlanta, GA

Sandy D. Maclin, Jr., MDiv, DMin
Associate Director of the Institute
  for Faith-Health Leadership,
Adjunct Professor at the Inter-
  denominational Theological
  Center, and
Chief Operating Officer of the
  HEALing Community Center
Atlanta, GA

Noble Maseru, PhD, MPH
Cincinnati Health Department
Cincinnati, OH

Diana J. Mason, RN, PhD, FAAN
Hunter College
New York, NY

Robert M. Mayberry, MS,
  MPH, PhD
Professor of Epidemiology
Associate Director for Clinical
  Research and Community
  Engagement
Department of Community
  Health and Preventive
  Medicine
Morehouse School of Medicine
Atlanta, GA

Stephanie Miles-Richardson,
  DVM, PhD
Associate Professor, Department of
  Community Health and Preven-
  tive Medicine
Interim Director, Master of Public
  Health Program
Morehouse School of Medicine
Atlanta, GA

Ramal Moonesinghe, PhD, MS
Mathematical Statistician
CDC/Office of the Director/Office
  of Minority Health and Health
  Equity
Atlanta, GA

Rose L. Pfefferbaum, PhD, MPH
Phoenix Community College
Phoenix, AZ

Darryl Scriven, PhD
African American Family Enrich-
  ment Institute
Atlanta, GA

Jerry A. Shultz, PhD
Co-Director, KU Work Group for
  Community Health and Devel-
  opment
University of Kansas
Lawrence, KS

Adrienne C. Smith, MSHS
Consultant
Welmaker Data & Associates
Atlanta, GA

Winifred Smith, MPH
Morehouse School of Medicine
Atlanta, GA

Monica Taylor-Jones,
  PhD, MPH
Part-time Assistant Professor
Department of Health Policy and
  Management
University of Georgia
Athens, GA

Rueben C. Warren, DDS, MPH,
  DrPH, MDiv
Professor of Bioethics and
  Director of the Tuskegee
  University National Center
  for Bioethics in Research and
  Health Care
Tuskegee, AL

Roland Bernard Welmaker, Sr.,
  PhD, MSLS
Librarian/Archivist
Morehouse School of Medicine
Atlanta, GA

Robina Josiah Willock,
  MPH, PhD
Research Associate
Clinical Research Center
Research Instructor
Department of Community
  Health and Preventive
  Medicine
Morehouse School of Medicine
Atlanta, GA

Foreword

In the 21st century, it is well documented by the academic health science community and health care providers that only a small percentage of health can be directly attributed to health care. While that is true, those who are disproportionately experiencing excess disease, disability, dysfunction, and premature deaths desperately need health services that are more available, accessible, and acceptable. Also, the inequitable distribution of social, economic, and environmental resources demands new and renewed means of building strong community-based partnerships to address social determinants of health and health care inequities. However, successfully integrating what we know about effective health care delivery, the distinctive cultures of our communities, and what we know about public health theory and practice is an enormous task.

Throughout my career, I have been heavily involved in various sectors of public and community health ranging from providing direct patient care, overseeing the activities of an urban public health department, to directing one of the nation's largest federally qualified community health centers. It is from this perspective that I am convinced that unless the health professions community fully invests and assists in community empowerment, poor individual and population health status outcomes, excess spending, and overuse of health technology will continue. We can do better if we listen to the voices of our communities!

Community Engagement, Organization, and Development for Public Health Practice, edited by Frederick G. Murphy, MSHyg, MPIA, confronts the abovementioned challenges in novel and provocative ways. It emphasizes important nontraditional approaches and partnerships, and the need to readjust methods based on the 21st-century community changes. It calls for the reassessment of existing community partnerships, and the establishment of new partnerships to readily address pressing community needs, and for creation of new community-based translation strategies to address high-risk behaviors and events. Issues of community organization and development, boundaries, ethics, servanthood, cultural competency, partnership, faith, environmental health, equity and resilience, and evaluation are saliently and thought-provokingly discussed.

Murphy and the list of scholars solicited to write the contributing chapters in this book have captured the complex issues of community engagement, organization, and development that have mystified public health practice. While the challenges addressed in the chapters of this textbook have been previously identified, and proposed solutions have been previously published, there have been few texts that have gathered these issues and solutions under one umbrella. Not only has Murphy brought together a transdisciplinary group of public health theoreticians and practitioners, interestingly, he has also coauthored several of the chapters, which provides a uniquely consistant voice throughout the book.

This textbook provides valuable information, examples of strategies, and real-life community experiences and "lessons learned" that should be shared with all segments and sectors in the country. It identifies skills required to both analyze the health and health care delivery challenges of minority and underserved communities and to understand the social, cultural, environmental, and economic determinants of health and disease. Most importantly, this textbook provides a renewed translation of the "community engagement, organization and development process." It also speaks to the creation of partnership through "formal" coalition building, empowering grassroots communities to address social determinants of health, recognizing that no one group, be it health care providers, public health practitioners, or community members, can accomplish the many tasks required for changing social, economic, and environmental conditions that impact health.

Moreover, this book is a vital resource to a new generation of community health practitioners, educators and organizers working in "grassroots communities" as they try to stay relevant to, and in fact ahead of, the inevitable social, environmental, and public health changes taking place. It is also important to note that the skills and approaches discussed herein are critical elements of a bridge between local neighborhoods and the medical school that enables the creation of innovative programs of education, research, and service focused on the special health problems of minority and other underserved populations globally, including those in the developing world. Undergraduate and graduated students; junior and senior faculty in the liberal arts and physical and biological sciences, business and information science, engineering and technology and professional schools will benefit from the outstanding scholarly work contained in this book. Moreover, those who are actively engaged in the public and private sectors that provide goods and services to the general public, as well as targeted population groups, will also benefit from the information provided. I took forward to learning about how this book is used and the responses based on the experiences of its users.

John E. Maupin Jr., DDS, MBA
President
Morehouse School of Medicine

Preface

Community Engagement, Organization, and Development for Public Health Practice is first and foremost a textbook for 21st-century public health advocates who are coming of age in a global environment fraught with historic and ongoing tensions between privileged and less-privileged communities. Through this book, students who were born after the pioneering era in community organization and development will sit at the foot of the pioneers and learn, through reading their stories, the best practices those groundbreakers learned through hard-fought battles. The authors write from their long history of community development, in which principles have been forged, tested, and refined.

Through educating public health advocates of the future, these pioneers aspire to develop the leadership required to build effective networks of community leaders within the communities they serve. This book addresses the key competencies of an effective community leader in the 21st century: personally empowered, lifelong learner and educator, facilitator of the empowerment process who inspires others to achieve their highest potential, knowledgeable in ways to build effective community coalitions, steward of personal and environmental resources, a savvy and capable political strategist, and keenly aware of the interdependent nature of local, national, and global issues (Robinson & Green, 2011).

A practical, theory-based approach to dealing with community health issues, as-yet unknown, emerges from these chapters. The outstanding authors of this edited work make a strong claim for public health as the lynchpin of achieving social equity in an increasingly inequitable world. This is a departure from other textbooks on community organization and development, which tend to focus primarily on economic development issues (Robinson & Green, 2011). While other books have covered community empowerment and community development—important parts of a grassroots movement's engine—this book examines how that engine, placed in the right vehicle, can help transport a community from sickness to health.

A community development model is highly complex, beginning with the definition of community, which may be defined by its geographic boundaries or by common interests of a face-to-face organization or increasingly by a virtual group brought together in cyberspace. "Development" also has various meanings depending on who is defining the need and how to meet the identified need or how to solve the underlying problem that created the need. One could argue that the one who has the power to define development wields a powerful social determinant of health. For example, the need for "urban development" may be defined by some as "cleaning up blighted areas" with a solution that demolishes poor housing and replaces them with parking lots, as was done in Pittsburgh. Others would define the need to be reversing long years of neglect in which there was little to no economic investment or job development, as in those Pittsburgh neighborhoods, despite their community cohesion and desire for local opportunities. The huge, negative health and social impact on community residents in that Pittsburgh community when the first rather than the second need definition was enacted is graphically detailed in Fullilove's history of urban development (Fullilove, 2004).

There is a growing recognition that this definitional diversity reflects core differences in community development. Geoghegan and Powell (2008) identify three typologies: neoliberal, where civil society serves needs defined by economic developers; corporatist, where the state, market, and civil society partner define and resolve issues; and activist, where empowered communities provide an opposing voice to neoliberalism. The United Nations Environment Program (2007) characterizes four typologies depending on the priority, placed first among priorities for action are markets, policy, security, or sustainability. Scenarios for the 21st century related to which of these typologies is prioritized clearly show that sustainability trumps the others for increasing global health and welfare. The sustainability approach is characterized by a corporatist model, but one that further prioritizes improving the environment and human well-being, with a strong emphasis on equity, transparency, and legitimacy for all partners. And, this is the approach taught by this book.

One of the toughest parts of this approach is building and maintaining effective coalitions and partnerships. Frisch and Servon (2006) describe a community development system, including government entities at all levels; national intermediaries such as the Local Initiatives Support Corporation that provide a formal structure for community development with funding, investments, and other resources such as training and technical assistance, community development financial institutions such as microloan funders, community development corporations such as the Association for Enterprise Opportunity, which are nonprofit organizations that are designed to improve the community's quality of life through support of local efforts to develop services (like child care, early developmental education, as well as housing, etc.); community-based development organizations that tend to embrace the activist approach (e.g., ACORN); various nonprofit organizations, including faith-based organizations;

private foundations; for-profit organizations; professional associations; and educational institutions such as community colleges and universities. While this list can be daunting to even the most seasoned public health advocate, the real-world case studies in this book illustrate, by both precept and example, how to bring the disparate pieces together for effective public health action.

Changes come about through dedicated and long-term efforts. The 19th-century Progressive Movement bore fruit beginning early in the 20th century and continued for more than 70 years as a potent social determinant of health. We are now seeing the fruits of a backlash movement that began to coalesce in the 1970s and threatens to undo much of the improvement in the public's health engendered by the Progressive Movement. If actions in the 21st century are to reflect a new and sustainable approach to problem solving, the movement must be well organized and educated. The shared experiences of the authors of this book provides a guidebook that should serve now and in the future as a potent tool for the success of that endeavor.

There is an accompanying Instructor's Manual and PowerPoint slide presentation available from Springer Publishing Company upon request at textbook@springerpub.com. Dr. Sydney Freeman, Jr., PhD, director of the teaching Center College of Vetinary Medicine, Nursing, and Allied Health at Tuskegee University assisted with the Instructor's Manual.

Carol J. Rowland Hogue, PhD, MPH
Jules and Uldeen Terry Professor of Maternal
and Child Health, Professor of Epidemiology
Director of the Women's and Children's Center
Rollins School of Public Health, Emory University, Atlanta, GA
Frederick G. Murphy, MSHyg, MPIA (Editor)

REFERENCES

Frisch, M., & Servon, L. J. (2006). CDCs and the changing context for urban community development: A review of the field and the environment. *Community Development: Journal of the Community Development Society, 37*, 88–108.

Fullilove, M. T. (2004). *Root shock: How tearing up city neighborhoods hurts America, and what to do about it*. New York, NY: Random House Publishing Group.

Geoghegan, M., & Powell, F. (2008). Community development and the contested politics of the late modern *agora*: Of, alongside or against *neoliberalism? Community Development Journal, 44*, 430–447. Doi: 10.1093/cdj/bsn020

Jules and Uldeen Terry Professor of Maternal and Child Health, Professor of Epidemiology, Director of the Women's and Children's Center, Rollins School of Public Health, Emory University, Atlanta, GA.

Robinson, J. W., Jr., & Green G. P. (Eds.). (2011). *Introduction to community development: Theory, practice and service-learning*. Los Angeles, CA: Sage Publications.

United Nations Environment *Programme*. (2007). *Global environmental outlook (GEO-4): Environment for development*. Nairobi, Kenya: Author.

Acknowledgments

We would first like to acknowledge the many community residents, who live and work in communities of need and despair throughout the globe. Also, we acknowledge their perseverance, resilience, and ongoing edification of neighborhoods, communities, and cultures throughout the United States and abroad.

Second, we say a special thanks to public health practitioners of all stripes, that work in and alongside community residents to improve the communities health and reduce risk factors associated with the years of life lost in communities everywhere. We acknowledge and thank the faculty, professionals, and staff member contributors from institutions and organization such as: the Morehouse School of Medicine, Emory University, University of Pittsburgh, United States Naval War College, Price Waterhouse Cooper, Cincinnati Department of Public Health, Interdenominational Theological Center, Centers for Disease Control and Prevention, Phoenix Community College, City University of New York, and Georgia State University, University of California San Bernardino, Tuskegee University, Kansas University, and Rhode Island University. Also, to all the public and private business persons and community representatives that contributed to the text.

A special thanks goes out to the editorial and support staff at Springer Publishing Company for their professional assistance and consultation. We especially thank Sheri W. Sussman (Sergeant Major) and those that work alongside her including: Katie Corasaniti, Lindsay Claire, and Ashita Shah for their professional guidance, patience, and ongoing support into this most important work.

Lastly, thanks to the Almighty God for allowing such a publication to come to fruition, so that it can be used as an additional tool in edifying public health leadership, addressing the social determinants of health and improving the public health and well-being of disparate cultures and communities globally.

1

Fundamental Core Concepts in the Community Engagement, Organization, and Development Process

Frederick G. Murphy, Stephen B. Fawcett, Jerry A. Schultz, and Christina Holt

LEARNING OBJECTIVES

What you can learn by studying this chapter:

- How to define basic concepts in creating community profiles
- How to define basic concepts in establishing relationships with community gatekeepers
- How to define basic concepts in building credibility
- How to define basic concepts in developing a Community Coalition Board (CCB)
- Why it is important to work with the CCBs to conduct a health needs assessment
- Why it is important to collaborate with CCBs for development and implementation of community-based health programs
- How to compare the Transtheoretical Model (TTM) and stages of change with Community Engagement, Organization, and Development (CEOD) change strategies
- Why it is important to develop and sustain CCBs

The work of community health and development is both science and art. On the one hand, it grows from the lessons and experiences learned by community activists and professionals in trying to create public systems, programs, interventions, and policy that improve the lives and health of everyone in the communities targeted. On the other hand, it stems from the passion for social justice, equity, and fairness that can lead to the creation of truly healthy communities where all citizens, regardless of their backgrounds or circumstances, have what they need.

Commitment to community does not rise out of nowhere. It comes from and is guided by values, principles, and assumptions that spring from our backgrounds and cultures, from our experiences, and from our conscious decisions about what is right. These values, principles, and assumptions shape our vision of the world as it should be, and motivate us to try to make it so.

The purpose of this first chapter is to provide a practical framework for the CEOD process, and for the more concept-specific chapters that follow. The foundation of that framework is a set of values, principles, and assumptions that inform a view of community health and development for public health practitioners. Concepts expressed are drawn from "real-life" grassroots community experiences and from theoretical and policy developments at public health institutions including Morehouse School of Medicine, Georgia State University, Emory University, University of Pittsburgh, University of Kansas, and many others.

CREATING A COMMUNITY ECOLOGY

Learning and analyzing the community ecology (CE) should be viewed as the initial step in the CEOD process. This step will assist the community organizer or public health professional to gain preliminary knowledge about the community they are seeking to enter. This knowledge comes in the form of compiled data and information, which can, subsequently, assist in the selection and development of meaningful evidence-based health promotion and disease prevention programs.

Community Entry Planning: Before beginning to document the CE, one should make a list of the types of preliminary information/data that could be most beneficial in forming subsequent community entry strategies. In other words, first enter the community "on paper" or "electronically" by documenting clearly the community's geographic, demographic, economic, and political parameters. The Internet can be a vital source today for this discovery process. Community archives, if available, can also be a useful source. Although many communities are similar in their ecology, each one should be viewed as unique during the initial information-gathering process, so as to avoid predeterminations or community profiling. Communities are constantly changing these days, so ongoing information updates about them can be very useful. Some useful CE information that should be gathered initially includes the following:

- *Community Mapping:* Study an existing map of the community, or develop one, that lays out its geographic boundaries. The map should include as much detail as possible—not only street names but also the directions and distances of these streets (i.e., which ones dead-end, which ones run north, south, east, and west). Also, information should be compiled on the names and locations of churches, housing projects, community centers, hospitals, health centers, businesses or business districts, and so on, throughout the community. State, county, and city government offices and municipalities can provide much of this information.

■ *Population and Demography:* Demographic data should be collected including: age ranges, sex, racial/ethnic distributions, income levels, education levels, disease prevalence rates, and the like. Health departments, state, county, and city government offices and municipalities can provide much of this information.

■ *History of the Community:* How long in existence and why established (refer to the community archives).

■ *Formal Leadership:* Make note of exactly who the elected officials are that represent the community. If they have office space in the community, note the location on the map. Also, identify their political affiliation/party and their pet issues.

■ *Informal Leadership:* Note the names of key residents and community activists residing in the community (most times nonelected). These leaders may become more identifiable later as one mingles and becomes more involved in the community.

■ *Business Establishments:* Note names of business owners, types, and numbers of businesses in the community and where they are located.

■ *Transportation System:* Identify what types of public and private commuter systems run in and around the community, including their schedules and routes.

■ *Churches:* Note how many and the types of churches (i.e., denominations, name of leadership, etc.). Identification of church leadership will prove invaluable throughout the CEOD process.

■ *Community Centers:* Note how many, the schedules, and the types of services offered.

■ *Community Organizations:* These may be general neighborhood improvement organizations that any resident might join, or special interest organizations focused on education (e.g., parent teacher associations [PTAs]), recreation (e.g., sports teams, book clubs), business associations, or social clubs.

It should be noted that the CE does not, nor should not, stop with the collection of the above items, many of which are available in archived formats. Once the community organizer or public health professional physically enters the community, a whole new level of information gathering should emerge that provides even more in-depth knowledge concerning the community's ecology. This information comes from mingling in the community and having one's ear to the ground and immersing oneself in the community on an almost daily basis.

Examples of additional ongoing strategies for determining and documenting the CE in even more detail are as follows:

1. *Windshield/Observational Survey:* This involves riding or walking through the community at various time periods (morning, mid-day, evening), to "observe" who is doing what, when, and where. Notations

are made and added later to the notes previously taken during the pre-liminary descriptive CE phase.

2. ***Listening:*** This involves visiting business establishments and other community institutions (i.e., barbershops, beauty salons, churches, transportation system, etc.) to listen to what members of the community have to say about their community. It may involve riding public transportation through the community during different times of day to listen to conversations and watch behavior patterns. These observations provide "community awareness" like no other.

3. ***Informal Engagement:*** This involves taking proactive approaches to spontaneous conversation(s) with community residents about their community. This spontaneity can only occur if one is *in the community on an ongoing basis* and will almost always result in identification of *informal gatekeepers.* To show respect to the resident, one should only make mental notes during this engagement, to be written down later.

4. ***Formal Engagement:*** Involves formally contacting community leaders (gate keepers), respectfully seeking scheduled visits with them in their offices, places of business, residences, or in any other setting they designate. In some cases, telephone calls will suffice; however, *face to face contact* is always recommended, as it is the most effective method of engaging when *seeking to build trust.* Telephone contact can be the most practical and time-sensitive means of following up, after face-to-face contact has been made, or when this is the only method of engaging.

Note: To be "fully engaged" with a community, on a formal or informal level, calls for a preparation and involvement. Such engagement means working with communities to truly assist them in public health awareness and education. This can be done through a variety of methods, whether it be through town hall meetings, focus group sessions, one-on-one interpersonal dialogues, or a long-term community intervention project.

Any written account and analysis describing a community's ecology should, at a minimum, include information about each of the areas cited above. Such introductory descriptive information will serve as a foundation for choosing subsequent evidence-based intervention activities. The CE description serves as a prerequisite to community entry, and can be as lengthy as necessary depending on identified needs. In some cases, thorough CE documentation can take 1 year or even longer to complete.

Taking the time to develop a good CE description is as close as a community organizer or public health professional can come to getting a birds-eye view and/or prospective vision of the challenges and potential social capital awaiting them. A successfully composed and well-studied CE can serve as a priceless tool for planning in the short and long term. It could very well be the difference between success or failure when seeking to form relationships and to gain an initial trust with community members.

Again, CE documentation will prove extremely useful in the development of community health intervention programs.

A thorough study of the particular community that needs to be engaged and organized will disclose to the community organizers/public health practitioners whether they need to approach the community as a "virgin community" that must be organized from the ground up, or whether a modified approach is needed that takes into account the existing individuals and/or organizations with advanced levels of maturity and activity.

ESTABLISHING RELATIONSHIPS WITH COMMUNITY GATEKEEPERS

The CE phase of the CEOD process is inseparably linked to that of establishing and building relationships with community gatekeepers. In many cases, community organizers or public health practitioners are new, or outsiders to the communities they seek to enter. Therefore, having as much background information on the community as possible can help catapult one forward in the relationship-building process. Studying this preexisting information beforehand can help to spark dialogue with community leadership, especially when one is just starting out, creating instant comfort zones between parties. However, when the public health practitioner starts the process of seeking *long-term, established relationships* in the community the "community entry process" truly and formally begins.

Examples of some useful strategies for establishing relationships with community leaders include the following:

1. *Making Introductory Contact:* The public health practitioner's initial introductory contact with community leaders (formal and informal) many times may have to first occur via telephone. However, follow-up face-to-face meetings should be scheduled as soon as possible. Proactively reaching out to community leaders will inevitably serve as an "ice breaker" and the conduit through which tracks are laid for building trusting and credible relationships. This critical period of initial engagement can be a delicate time in the relationship-building process, and can serve as the platform from which "word of mouth" spreads concerning whether the community will "trust or distrust" the public health practitioner's efforts. Tact and respect are the ticket here.
2. *Sharing Talking Points:* Sharing specific talking points about the community, many of which can be drawn from the CE process, can lead to an increase in confidence, relaxation, and the genuineness needed to move toward building credibility and trust. Credibility and trust are the true catalysts of the building relationship process, and will only be realized with time, ongoing community involvement, and by showing tangible deliverables to community leadership. Public health

practitioners or health professionals should present themselves as "servant leaders" and clarify to community leaders their rationale for entering the community.

3. ***Relationship Listening:*** Listening in this context, different from that mentioned in the CE process, is of a more intense nature and may involve asking for permission to take notes while engaging. The listening that takes place during this initial step in relationship building involves prudent speaking intervals. This listening has a specific goal of building trust. Listening shows respect. It projects the perception that what is being said by the gatekeeper is valued and important. Also, by listening and making mental notations, one can further add to the information/data-collection inventory started during the CE process. So then, this intense listening is especially important when engaging with the informal gatekeepers such as community residents.

Examples of some key community gatekeepers with whom relationships should be established include the following:

- Elected officials
- School officials and PTA leaders
- Clergy
- Directors of community centers
- Leaders of clubs and organizations
- Social workers
- Health care providers
- Council persons
- Neighboring Planning Unit (NPU) ward, or precinct chairpersons
- Community activists
- School principals
- Church pastors
- Social workers
- Business owners

BUILDING TRUST AND CREDIBILITY

The public health practitioner should always show respect for the core values and beliefs of the community they are seeking to enter.

Credibility and trust are the essential factors in the relationship-building process, and should be seen as the glue that holds things together. Examples of key considerations when attempting to build credibility with community leaders/members include, but are not limited to, the following:

1. ***Respect, Credibility, and Trust:*** These are the most essential interwoven ingredients in the relationship-building process. These underpinning elements must be established before one can effectively proceed

toward developing a CCB. They can only be achieved, however, by *genuinely getting to know people*. These come with time and involvement, so quite frankly stated: "if no time, engagement and involvement is spent in the community…no respect, credibility or trust will ever be built."

2. **Building Interpersonal Relationships**: If credibility and trust are to occur, it will be important for the community organizer/health professional to have established interpersonal relationships with key individual community members and leaders. Again, this takes time to build, and will only happen with *ongoing tactful face-to-face engagement/ involvement*. Showing *genuine concern* about the individual's and community's well-being can be an invaluable first step toward building a trusting relationship. As mentioned previously, public health practitioners should present themselves as "servant leaders" and clarify their role in providing technical assistance in the CEOD process.

   Example: One must routinely visit community members' homes (when invited), offices, and places of business, and so on. Many times, community members become involved in a community group or organization just because they have a credible and trusting relationship with another person who asks them to participate.

Further, while seeking to establish relationships throughout the community, it will also be important for public health practitioners to express that *they are also there to learn*, as well as to share. This is where reciprocity (give-and-take) can be an important asset, as many times community leaders/residents will more readily accept help if they know that they too can share and educate in some fashion. The public health practitioner's role as "helpee" can prove very important to the trust-building process.

3. **Referrals:** As initial relationships are established, referrals will be made across the community from "one community leader to another community leader" (horizontal referral). This is a very important step in the process of building community credibility, as these types of referrals may open doors leading to *trust and credibility* that would otherwise remain locked to an outsider for indefinite periods. Such referrals can save days, months, even years in the credibility-building process.

   Example: To be able to name drop that: "Mr. Smith or Pastor John" recommended that I "call you or come see you" could add tremendous value to the initial contact. Many times, trust relationships are accelerated because of such "across community" referrals.

4. **Community Participation:** It is also important to "show up" and participate in scheduled and unscheduled community activities. This includes attending community activities that have nothing specifically

to do with health or the leading causes of death and was not initiated by the public health practitioner.

Examples: *attending worship services or Little League games, or working out once or twice a week in the community center, or attending a neighborhood meeting when invited, and so on.*

5. **Identifying Resources:** Credibility can be further enhanced by assisting the community to conduct some of its preplanned community activities. Many days, and even months, may have to be spent in this effort. A general principle applicable to both this and later stages of the CEOD process is: *It is essential to address the community's priorities first.*

   Example: *This may mean assisting the community to locate resources (i.e., individuals, materials, funding, etc.) that will help it to successfully hold a block party, or purchase jerseys for the Pee Wee League football or/basketball team, or sponsor a community-sponsored fashion show, and so on.*

6. **Initiating Community Activities:** The public health practitioner can volunteer to assist community members to plan and conduct a health-related activity. In doing so, the public health practitioner can identify and arrange for professionals (vertical referrals) that have specific skills and trades to participate. For example, they may recommend that the community hold a health fair or block party. Here, the public health practitioners can recommend and identify the health professionals and other resources for participation.

Lastly, it is worth repeating here that, in order for the CEOD process to have a chance, there must first be *trusting and credible relationships* formed. When trust is missing a Community Coalition Board will have little chance of coming to fruition, and even if it does, its members will have a difficult time functioning cooperatively over time. Conversely, if credibility and trust exist throughout the coalition-building process, they will serve as invaluable ingredients to the coalition's sustainability and resilience when or if conflict arises. If trusting relationships (vertical and horizontal) are already in place, all will be in a better position to help solve conflict and misunderstanding that will inevitably occur, over time.

DEVELOPING A CCB

One of the primary purposes of the CEOD model is the edification and sustaining of communities. Community edification should be defined as the building of communities through health education, training, and skill development. Further, to edify is building up and empowering of communities through community involvement and by demonstrating that one truly cares for those residing and working in the community.

A CCB is a group of individuals with a common interest who agree to work together toward a common goal. Further, a truly *empowered* or edified CCB is one that becomes a formally "incorporated" organization with a mission statement, bylaws, a governing body, community responsibilities, funding, and sustainability. The CCB may also, eventually, serve as a community employer when it has identified funding for specific health programs. Again, its primary purpose for existence is to create and/or support efforts to reach a particular set of common community goals.

Here are some key fundamentals used in the initial CCB development process. These steps may include the following:

1. **Start with people you know:** Make a list of those community leaders and gatekeepers with whom relationships and credibility have already been established (see previous section on CE process). Persons with whom there is an "established credibility and trust" are usually important to choose from for CCB membership, since they can be more easily persuaded to participate than individuals with whom there is no established relationship. In addition, they may have additional reliable referrals that can be pulled into the recruitment circle. This group of people can also serve as an informal "advisory committee or steering committee" and may play a key role, short and long run, in the unfolding of the CCB process. Beware, however; some of these same folks may opt *not* to stay on after the CCB is formed.
2. **Identify other important potential CCB members:** In almost every community there will be various other formal and informal leaders with whom you *have made no contact*. These individuals may already have ongoing programs and activities launched in the community. For example, The coach who is attempting to raise funds to purchase jerseys for the Pee Wee League team he has established, or the lady who has decided to pull together a block party to promote neighborhood clean-up, or the pastor who has planned to have a community benefit dinner in the basement of the church to raise awareness of HIV, drugs, or teen pregnancy prevention. These individuals are using the resources they already have at their disposal to improve the community, but each may fall under a different community umbrella as far as their community goals are concerned. The CEOD CCB concept seeks to bring these leaders under one formally structured umbrella to collectively partner, while reaching community goals. It will be important, therefore, to persistently seek them out. These persons, once on board ("buy-in"), tend to have staying power.
3. **Beginning the formal CCB recruitment process.** Once a well-thought-out list of potential CCB members has been formed, and thoroughly reviewed by the CCB, the formal recruitment process begins. Depending on the programs and activities proposed, there will be

persons or organizations identified as essential for membership recruitment to the CCB. Although it is important to start with the individuals and groups mentioned above, an open mind should be kept during the process, because new referrals and ideas will continually emerge. The core advisory group of community leaders can be very important to the recruitment process, as they may know many other potential members personally, and can make immediate contact with them. They may give the invitation to join much more credibility and may reduce recruitment time for the public health practitioner by hours, maybe even days. However, CCB recruitment efforts must be closely monitored, on an almost daily basis, to ensure that things do not get out of hand and that *inappropriate individuals* are not accidentally or unintentionally recruited.

Below are listed some of the key methods for contacting individuals and organizations for recruitment. These are listed in their approximate order of effectiveness. Face-to-face contact is the best approach; however, it also takes more time and effort and should be reserved for those individuals most important, or most difficult, to recruit.

The listing is as follows:

- Face-to-face meetings
- Phone calls
- E-mail
- Personal letters
- Mass mailings
- Public service announcements or ads in the media
- Flyers and posters

In almost every community a combination of these recruitment methods is recommended for use.

FORMALIZING THE CCB STRUCTURE

Without fail, communities will have preexisting landmark organizations, which have served as bedrocks to the community's history and culture. These could come in the form of tenant- or faith-based organization, or PTAs, and so on. For example, the church has served as the key to respect, justice, and beneficence, especially in many low-income and African American communities, the CCB may, however, be that new organization that brings about a renewed focus and structure for public health activities in the community.

Therefore, before formalizing the CCB, it is critical to capture whether or not there is "buy-in" to the overall CEOD CCB concept by the key gatekeepers/community leaders. This buy-in, in most instances, is usually a seriously expressed verbal commitment to becoming partners or members to a formalized structured CCB. A formal meeting should be called between the organizer/health practitioner and these leaders. This meeting should have a set agenda, which leaves room to lay out all intentions, and brings to the table a "full disclosure type atmosphere." Only after all participants have bought in, should a formalized development process of an incorporated 501(c) 3 CCB be pursued.

Reasons why it is important for a 501c (3) CCB to be developed include the following:

- A CCB provides a structured community health driven *"culture/environment"* for building cooperation and trust between its members. It can give *added value and identity* to individuals and organizations that join the group, as well as to the group itself.
- It provides a *"corporate structure"* and gives the group the opportunity to establish: (1) a community-based mission statement, (2) corporate bylaws, (3) organizational guidelines, (4) an arena for bringing together "community partners" under one umbrella to address community health concerns, (5) a structured environment for resolving community disagreements, and (6) the social capital needed to maintain and sustain community culture and investment.
- Sets *"roles and responsibilities"* so that all members are accountable to each other and to the activities they pursue. No one person and/or group will make decisions in a vacuum but in the best interests of the community and the CCB.
- Creates a structure where *"rules, bylaws, and oversight"* are established. Officers are elected, agendas are set, and *Robert's Rules of Order* is used to conduct meetings. Norms (checks and balances) emerge as part of the organized "CCB culture."

An Alternative Approach to Traditional Bottom-Up CEOD

"Top-Down Approach"

The 21st century has broadened and introduced many new public health challenges including natural disasters, pandemic outbreaks, record unemployment, increased numbered of uninsured and underinsured, as well as a rise in many other social determinants that impact health status. Emergency preparedness has become one of the top public health concerns. All of these have caused leaders to rethink how they approach public health issues at local, state, and global levels.

The complexity of these social determinants brings about the need for immediacy in organizing partnerships to readily address pressing community risk factors. These partnerships are determined by the institutions' service structure (the types of services they provide), their political position in the community (state vs. city government, etc.), and the degree to which all partners are currently engaged in the partnership's activities.

It is essential to *build partnerships* to address social determinants of health because no one group, be it health care providers, public health practitioners, or community members, can accomplish the many tasks required for changing social, economic, and environmental conditions that impact health. Tapping into existing partnerships provides instant knowledge and brings experience to the table concerning services that can realistically be addressed. However, although existing groups are important, they may not address all the social determinants of health or include people or organizations from the community who can inform initiatives to address social determinants. Therefore, it is important to invite others to join your efforts, particularly those who have insight into or experience harm from the political, social, economic, and environmental conditions in the community.

Listening to the voices of people who belong to organizations in the community who have previous experience in the equitable distribution of social, economic, and environmental resources can help to build a strong partnership to address social determinants of health inequities. Together with other members of the community, they can assist to identify important nontraditional partners, and to help make a list of the other relevant sectors of the community (e.g., government, education, business, public services, faith, funding agencies) and help ensure that your partnership includes representatives from each of these sectors, as well as other appropriate community members. To effectively identify those who may be interested in the work of your partnership, it may first be necessary to consider how your community is defined (see also CE section).

WORKING WITH THE CCB TO CONDUCT A HEALTH NEEDS ASSESSMENT

In many instances, CCB members may have preexisting knowledge, information, and experience in issues of health and wellness. They may already know the causes and risky behaviors existing in their community for diseases such as violence and HIV, and may have already participated in informational campaigns about specific health issues and their consequences. Many community residents may have already learned about many health issues from radio and TV commercials, the Internet, public service announcements, newspaper articles, and other sources. The information accessed through these campaigns, while useful, may not always be specific enough for use by a community group trying to solve health disparities specific to its target area.

The best way for the community to get relevant and updated health information is to develop and implement an organized "health needs assessment" that is community driven. This assessment can provide detailed information about the needs of its residents, and will identify resources available to the community to help solve those needs. Therefore, the public health practitioner should first provide an orientation to the CCB about the "value added" by conducting its own community needs assessment. This orientation should include, at a minimum, the importance of such things as:

- *Understanding the community environment:* Mapping the resources and limitations of the area. The previously developed CE tool can be a valuable start here.
- *Knowing what the community thinks and feels:* About health issues and what they think needs to be done about it.
- *Setting priorities for programs or system improvement:* It should be brought forward to the CCB how much easier it will be *to make informed decisions and set priorities* if a comprehensive identification of needs and resources has taken place. For example, an assessment can help more truly identify those community persons who are in most need. It will help to gain fresh data and information from the people who are directly experiencing the problem, allowing them to openly discuss their health needs.
- *Identification of health care/service providers:* Knowing the health care organizations and providers that serve, or could potentially serve, the community can be useful to the CCB in conducting evidence-based public health intervention programs.
- *Potential community health leaders:* Once the CCB has a complete picture of the health needs and resources of the community, they will have the knowledge base to become community leaders or "servant leaders" and to make informed health-related decisions, to explain actions, even to eventually write grants and lobby for the organization.

Choosing an Assessment Method—Preliminary Steps

- *Determining assessment feasibility:* Preliminary steps should be taken by the CCB to select an appropriate community assessment methodology, as this is not a "one size fits all" deal. Therefore, it is important for the CCB to evaluate thoroughly the amount of resources available to them, as this has much to do with which method can feasibly work. For example, "face-to-face interviews combined with telephone surveys" could be an excellent combination, if there is a large enough budget.
- Regardless of the method desired, it is important to first take into account some reality factors, such as:
  - The amount of time available
  - The number of people available to conduct the assessment
  - Available resources (i.e., funding, materials, etc.)
  - The size and characteristics of the target population(s)

Therefore, the public health practitioner can assist the CCB to first take some basic preliminary steps, prior to identifying and conducting a formal community assessment. Examples of these steps could include:

■ *Brainstorming with CCB members:* The public health practitioner can recommend the CCB to take a very practical first step: think and talk about what information really needs to be gathered during the assessment. Will the assessment seek to gather a panoramic/overall view of the health needs of the entire community, or only a snapshot of specific disease areas and/or services? Identifying the "specific data/information needed" is a key first step for the community.

■ *Reviewing of existing CE data/information:* After determining the specific data/information needed, the CCB should review the CE and other preexisting data sets (i.e., health departments, census data, etc.). This review can be a time-saver. It can also help highlight what data *do not exist.* This review will be very useful in subsequently determining what type questions need to be included when developing the assessment tool(s).

■ *Identification of the target population to be assessed:* After the brainstorming and existing data review are completed, the public health practitioner should sit down with CCB members to determine what are the purpose of the assessment and the method of the assessment. Also, this would include such ideas as: whether households will be assessed by randomly going to homes such as every other household, or only assessing so many households per block, and so on.

■ *Formulating appropriate assessment plan:* Once the preliminary steps have been completed, an assessment plan should be developed. This would include the when, the where, the how, the who, and so on for implementing the assessment. Appropriate questions and formats are developed, and strategies drawn up. In most cases, institutional partners on the CCB with expertise in conducting assessments should be called upon. The public health practitioner can help identify these experts if they are not already part of the CCB. It will be important that the questions are appropriately formulated (i.e., culturally sensitive, proper reading levels, etc.) for use with the group(s) to be assessed.

Potential Survey Methods

Other than the 501(c) 3 phases of the CEOD process, accomplishment of a community assessment can serve as first official "team act" of the CCB. The accomplishment of this most important, organized, team-oriented task can do wonders to boost the confidence and sustainability of the CCB. CCB team involvement in this process should range from planning, to training, to data analysis, and ultimately to compiling the health-related findings. They should be encouraged to feel that they are individuals involved in a specific project to yield a distinctive product.

The public health practitioner can bring to the CCB several alternative methods and strategies for conducting the community assessment. However, it should be noted again that institutional partners with expertise in conducting assessments (i.e., universities, health department staff, private agencies, etc.), some of which may be represented on the CCB, should be called upon to assist in this process. Survey methodology can be a complex science. Therefore, a compromise may need to be made between what is acceptable scientifically and what a small organization can afford. The assistance of a scientific professional with experience in conducting surveys can be very useful.

There are several assessment methods to choose from and there is no one perfect method. In some cases, depending on resources available, a combination of methods is better than just one. Here are a few standard methods a public health practitioner, or the experts, can bring to the CCB for consideration:

- *Community Forums:* This method can provide community residents of diverse backgrounds the opportunity to openly express their views. Keen listening and recording of minutes are essential during the implementation of this method. This form of assessment provides data and information that facilitates "learn first hand," the community's perspectives on health, as well as other community resources, concerns, and ideas. Forums may be the most appropriate method, particularly for communities where there may be some residents who have difficulty interacting and/or reading self-administered printed materials. This method could be most successful if conducted during a regularly scheduled community meeting at which groups gather routinely to discuss community issues. The CO, or CCB member, can ask permission to be placed on the agenda.
- *Face-to-Face Interviews:* The use of this method can be especially valuable in communities where disparate and low literacy rates are high. In communities where significant numbers of residents have difficulty reading printed materials, or where more in-depth answers are required, the face-to-face interview method can create the dialogue needed to gather information from these participants.
- *Phone Surveys:* Telephone surveys can have similar benefits to face-to-face interviews; however, for communities where there exist low-income populations, telephone access may be limited. This would mean very low encounters and could cause extreme frustration to the assessment process. Also, unless your "community" is represented by an entire area code, or phone numbers are assigned in such a way that they can be associated with your community (for instance, if all phone numbers in the community have the same first three digits), your needs assessment may be more far-ranging than you intend.

- *Self-Administered Questionnaires:* This method may be best utilized when dealing with respondents who can easily read the questions and write. It can be used when asking for information that does not require interpretation, or explanation charts, graphs, and so on.
- *Direct Mailings:* Direct-mailed surveys to people whose addresses are known is the most common strategy. However, in many communities, this method has a low rate of response. Direct-mailed surveys are, of course, self-administered, and so the rules relevant to self-administered questionnaires apply.
- *Convenience Sampling:* Taking surveys in a public place—setting up a booth or table in at a barber shop or beauty salon, a church or in a parking lot at a local discount store, on the sidewalk in the shopping district, and so on—provides an opportunity to get some exposure for your organization as well as a sample of public opinion.
- *Group Survey Administration:* This method, as with community forums, could be most successful if conducted at an organization or precinct meeting where there are large groups gathered. The public health practitioner, or a CCB member, can request the chairperson's permission to be placed on the agenda for one or more meetings, as needed. At the meeting, the assessment could be introduced, the purpose explained, and the survey instrument distributed and collected.

Training of Potential Interviewers

The public health practitioner should organize a formal interviewer training workshop. While such training is a must for potential interviewers, it also has a built-in weeding out process that will determine who can truly succeed as an interviewer. Everyone who participates in the training may not be appropriate for the task. Thus, the interviewer selection process must be handled delicately and tactfully, as hurt feelings and resentment can come into play here, subsequently causing serious damage, possibly even setting back the CEOD process.

Below are some examples of a few topics, which could potentially be covered during the CEOD interviewer training:

1. *Orientation:* Providing potential interviewers information about the survey, its purpose, and the overall mission and goals of the CCB. This can also ensure that the information they pass on to respondents concerning the CCB and the assessment is uniform and accurate.
2. *Safety:* The importance of interviewer safety while conducting interviews, especially for face-to-face household interviews, and so on.
3. *Importance of Etiquette:* Regardless of the method chosen, interviewer etiquette and respect should be emphasized. For example, the importance of simple gestures such as saying *please* and *thank you* cannot be overstated. Respect for the community and its residents should be emphasized during this section of the training workshop.

4. *Potential Termination of Interviewers:* Emphasis should be placed on the importance of confidentiality, accuracy in completing surveys, honesty and reliability in survey completion, and so on. However, interviewers should be made to understand that if one or any combination of these requirements is found to be lacking, they may be asked to withdraw from participation.
5. *How Surveys Will Be Gathered:* Indicating the when, where, how, and who, about collecting incoming surveys as they are completed.
6. *Review and Verification of Completed Surveys:* Indicating to potential interviewers how checking and verification will take place to ensure interviewer honesty, completion, and reliability.
7. *Data Analysis and Translation:* This will be an essential part of the assessment process and will require institutional experts to compile and analyze. However, information and data analysis must be done in a practical manner for ease in translation and interpretation. CCB members, regardless of educational background, should be able to understand the results of the assessment. This will call for "mixed translation methodologies" for presenting data and information taken from the survey. Thus, the analysts must first "do their homework" in understanding the CCB target audience, clearly understanding the goals of the CCB, and gaining a sense of the skill required to effectively translate the results.

Finally, the community assessment process represents a key step in the CEOD process. Its critical nature should be continuously highlighted to CCB members, some of whom may be interviewers themselves, as an important team accomplishment. Other than the 501(c) 3 incorporation phase of the CEOD process, the community assessment will serve as first official team activity of the CCB.

COLLABORATING WITH CCB FOR DEVELOPMENT AND IMPLEMENTATION OF HEALTH-PROMOTION INTERVENTIONS

Collaboration, Inclusion, and Engagement

Once the assessment phase is completed, and the results analyzed, and fully understood by all CCB members, the CCB can begin to discuss and decide to take action by designing a community health-promotion intervention. The public health practitioner should seek to further build the CEOD process by developing formal meetings that calls for "collaboration, inclusivity, and engagement" by all CCB members. The public health practitioner can facilitate this by inviting all CCB members to the table and establishing agendas where members have the opportunity to have input into planning and design of a community health promotion intervention program. This may take time, requiring several meetings, in order to give all members ample time to gain respect and share their viewpoints.

However, implementation of this inclusivity in a real-world environment has shown that such attempts do not always work out. Some people might, for one reason or another, opt out of the process. In some of these situations, a persistent attempt at inclusivity can cause its own problems. Be that as it may, this does not preclude giving all members the choice to express themselves in the intervention planning process.

In brief, here are a few examples of eventual benefits to CCB involvement in the community health-promotion intervention planning process:

1. *CCB Ownership:* Through involvement in planning of a community health-promotion intervention, CCB members begin to move to an even higher level of "ownership" and begin to feel that they will do whatever they can to see their work succeed.

   In the CEOD process, it has also been learned that in most low-income, high-disparity, or minority communities, individuals and groups feel that they are *talked down to and/or not listened to,* even when they are asked for their opinions. True involvement then calls for "dialogue" with and between members, discussing in a respectful manner methods and strategies to be used. Many times this means having respectful debates about what should or should not be done in the intervention. "Rubber stamping" ideas presented by CCB members just because they are community members or low-income and/or minorities can, in some instances, lead to reverse condescension, as if anything they say must be accepted as true and appropriate. Thus, a truly community-engaged intervention planning process means listening to everyone, but being prepared to disagree over ideas and goals, and to wrestle with new concepts.

2. *Credibility of the Intervention:* Because the intervention was planned by the CCB members and representatives of the community, other community residents will more easily respond to participating in the community health-promotion intervention activities.

3. *Reduces Possibility of Intervention Failures:* Involvement of CCB members in the community health-promotion intervention planning process can help bring forward the many values and norms specific to the community's culture. For instance, scheduling interventions on days when many community members are awaiting financial or food assistance checks to arrive in the mail, and so on will almost always guarantee high rates of "no shows" for recruitment and participation. Many CCB members will know what strategies have failed in the past and why, and can keep the intervention program developers from repeating past mistakes.

4. *Key CCB Members Buy-In:* Because of their involvement in the intervention planning process, CCB members identified to be "key players" many times make commitments to future cooperation, simply because they have been included in the planning from the beginning.

5. *Teaching Planning Skills:* The community health-promotion intervention planning process can help to improve the community over the long term. CCB members can learn to run meetings, to analyze data, to construct strategic plans—in short, to become community resources and leaders.
6. *Increases CCB Trust:* CCB member interaction in the intervention planning process, especially between community members and business leaders, can be not only be supportive of the intervention, but may help to create long-term relationships among members. This trust can serve as a foundation for future community development and community action.

In conclusion, collaboration, inclusiveness, and empowerment, embody the ideals that form the foundation of a true grassroots, community-based CEOD process. It respects everyone's intelligence, values everyone's ideas and experience, and affords everyone a measure of control. By empowering the community rather than imposing preexisting ideas of academics or public health professionals, one can assure an ethical approach to planning an evidence-based community intervention.

Designing the Community Intervention—Plan of Action

Asking Important Preliminary Questions

Before the actual designing of the community health intervention begins, the CO/health educator should assist the CCB in the developing an intervention *action plan*, which can be extensive. In short, the public health practitioner should assist the CCB to ask and answer the following questions:

- What *potential barriers* exist or can be anticipated in the community? How can they be minimized?
- What *resources* are available and needed (i.e., financially, politically, time-wise, and kind)?
- What *intervention components* should be implemented?
- Who should coordinate and implement *programs*?
- When should programs be scheduled (i.e., *mornings, evenings, noon*)?
- What *partnerships with individuals or organizations* need to be formalized?
- What *interventions programs have already worked* and could be replicated?

Identifying Core Intervention Program Components

Identifying appropriate *core program components* for the community health intervention will be the true nucleus of the intervention design. The public health practitioner should encourage the CCB to consider these core items closely when designing the intervention plan. This calls for the CCB to lay out appropriate, feasible, and culturally sensitive programs by its leadership. The CCB should identify, as closely as possible, appropriate, manageable timelines and activities that can be used in the implementation of the intervention. Examples include the following:

■ Identification of *where* to hold the intervention programs (i.e., community center, church, school, etc.)
■ Identification of *recruitment methods and strategies* for bringing in participants
■ Identification of *which days and hours* to conduct the intervention activities
■ Identification of *what culturally appropriate educational training materials* should be needed for each program
■ Identification of *who* (staff/personnel) should coordinate/conduct the intervention programs
■ Identification of *appropriate methods* for monitoring and evaluating program effectiveness (academic and private institutions can assist here)

Maintaining the Community Intervention

A successful community health intervention, with evidence-based and evaluable outcomes can and, in most cases, will take time to realize. Just as with intervening with an individual one-on-one, a community intervention can go through stages of development that require patience and ongoing monitoring.

For example, the *TTM of Behavior Change* assesses an individual's readiness to act on a new, healthier behavior, and provides strategies or processes of change to guide the individual through the stages of change to action and maintenance (see Figures 1.1 and 1.2). The public health practitioner will have to conduct ongoing periodic assessments of how the community as a whole responds to the new intervention program. Results from these assessments will help guide the public health practitioner to modify and revise the intervention to boost attendance and participation by the community. These "boosters" are vital to the ongoing maintenance, to the "upward spiral," and to the sustaining power of the intervention and can be the difference between success and failure (see Figure 1.2).

Let us take a look at the six Stages of Change involved in the TTM and imagine for a moment similar stages being a Community Intervention Method (CIM) process.

■ *Precontemplation:* "People are not intending to take action in the foreseeable future, and are most likely unaware that their behavior is problematic."
■ *Contemplation:* "People are beginning to recognize that their behavior is problematic, and start to look at the pros and cons of their continued actions."

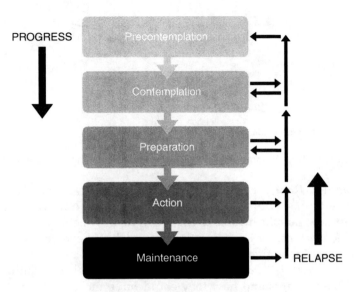

FIGURE 1.1 Transtheoretical Model (TTM) Stages of Change.

- *Preparation:* "People are intending to take action in the immediate future, and may begin taking small steps toward change."
- *Action:* "People have made specific overt modifications in their life style, and positive change has occurred."
- *Maintenance:* "People are working to prevent relapse, a stage which can last indefinitely."
- *Termination:* "Individuals have zero temptation and 100% self-efficacy...they are sure they will not return to their old unhealthy habit as a way of coping."

In general, as with the TTM, for community residents to take ownership and fully participate in a community health intervention, the public health practitioner will need to work with community participant to:

A. Develop a growing awareness that the advantages (the "pros") of the intervention change/outweigh the disadvantages (the "cons")—the TTM calls this decisional balance
B. Instill confidence that they can make and maintain changes in situations that lead to unhealthy behavior—the TTM calls this self-efficacy
C. Include the community in developing strategies that can help them make and maintain change—the TTM calls these processes of change.

The 10 processes are listed as follows:

1. *Consciousness Raising:* Increasing awareness via information, education, and personal feedback about the healthy behavior.

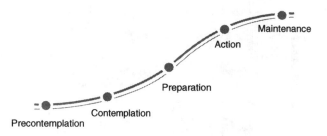

FIGURE 1.2   Transtheoretical Model (TTM) Stages of Change—Upward Spiral.

2. *Dramatic Relief:* Feeling fear, anxiety, or worry because of the unhealthy behavior, or feeling inspiration and hope when they hear about how people are able to change to healthy behaviors
3. *Self-Reevaluation:* Realizing that the healthy behavior is an important part of who they are and want to be
4. *Environmental Reevaluation:* Realizing how their unhealthy behavior affects others and how they could have more positive effects by changing
5. *Social Liberation:* Realizing that society is more supportive of the healthy behavior
6. *Self-Liberation:* Believing in one's ability to change and making commitments and recommitments to act on that belief
7. *Helping Relationships:* Finding people who are supportive of their change
8. *Counter-Conditioning:* Substituting healthy ways of acting and thinking for unhealthy ways
9. *Reinforcement Management:* Increasing the rewards that come from positive behavior and reducing those that come from negative behavior
10. *Stimulus Control:* Using reminders and cues that encourage healthy behavior as substitutes for those that encourage the unhealthy behavior

While the comparison of the processes of this model to that of the CEOD model may seem an oversimplication of the task at hand for the public health practitioner, it can serve as a valuable template in the planning, designing, implementation, and evaluation processes of the CIM.

CCB STRATEGIES FOR SUSTAINABILITY

Sustaining the CCB can be a challenging venture as ongoing changes and even burn-out will inevitably occur. The CCB will need to develop resilience to withstand these changes. For example, ongoing changes can occur in the number and composition of membership and partnerships, which are natural occurrences with any community-based organization for various reasons. Therefore, in order to maintain and sustain the CCB, its leadership must deploy ongoing strategies. This will keep members motivated and continue to build ownership and collective trust.

There are some key examples of strategies showing how this ownership and "stick-with-it-ness" spirit can be maintained and sustained:

1. 501 (c) 3—Institutionalization
Establishing and maintaining the nonprofit organization is essential to the CEOD process. This calls for ongoing identification and replacement of members, implementing new programs, ongoing development of new relationships, identifying new strategies and practices, and updating methodologies for approaching the community and the ongoing identification of resources. Thus, developing a plan for sustaining the 501 (c) 3 CEOD institution will increase its impact and perception in the community as an institution embedded there for the long run.

2. Subcommittee Development
The creation of subcommittees allows CCB members to engage and plan for community intervention activities. These committees are where members can agree and disagree, all the while working together for common goals.

3. CCB Education, Training, and Skills Development
Education, training, and skill building among CCB members are key components in the sustainability process. Such learning endeavors help to further motivate and build ownership among members.

Through ongoing participation in learning programs, members will themselves become high-achieving community health innovators and advocates. They will also begin to encourage each other, and their partner organization members, to bring on new learning initiatives that will assist the CCB to grow.

These learning efforts (i.e., education, training and skill building, etc.) can be achieved through various methods including: in-service courses, webinars, seminars, workshops, participation at conferences, and other learning experiences.

The overarching goal, in all cases, is to make sure that everyone on the CCB has the opportunity to constantly be engaged in ongoing learning. This will be a key factor in the building and sustaining of a truly empowered CCB.

4. Marketing, Partnering, and Resource Identification
Designing a CCB logo and developing an inventory of free giveaways can help in marketing the nonprofit groups. Partnering with other organizations is very important to the social capital network. This partnering can

occur in a variety of different ways, from writing grants together to the sharing of resources, such as:

- Time-share positions
- Office space and equipment
- Skilled staff persons
- Recommended volunteers
- Recommend student interns from academic institutions
- In-kind donations of time

Most of the items listed above can be categorized as *in-kind support*, which simply refers to resources *other than money* that comes available to the CCB.

5. Grant Funding

Seeking out grant funding is usually the primary method of acquiring financial sustainability for a CCB. These monetary grants may come from a variety of sources including local and federal government or private foundations. Each grant is usually awarded for the purpose of assisting in the implementation of a specific community intervention program or project.

6. Fundraising

Fundraising should be an ongoing part of the CCB agenda (i.e., quarterly, semi-annually, or yearly). Fundraisers usually require the CCB to provide a product, a service, or an event that will allow others to contribute money. Examples of fundraisers include bake sales, car washes, block parties, sporting events, and so on. In each case, the group charges money for a product to raise funds to support their cause.

SUMMARY

While the concepts shared in this chapter are by no means all that can be used to conduct CEOD activities, they are realistic and can be used as templates in the development of even better and more innovative CEOD approaches over time.

Public health practitioners will need to study and familiarize themselves with the basics before and after entering a grassroots community. Learning the do's and don'ts of working with community residents, while identifying the "how to" of fusing oneself into the community in a trustworthy and passionate way, is most paramount. Preparation and patience go hand-in-glove in the CEOD-building process. The old adage of hurry up and wait turns out to be a realistic concept. It means knowing when to be aggressive, so as not have missed opportunities, yet knowing when to be patient and prudent in the implementation of methods and strategies to avoid being disrespectful and presumptuous.

Knowing community is one thing, doing community is quite another! While this statement may seem an oversimplification of the matter, one only has to immerse oneself into community-based public health practice to realize the complexity that exists in successfully connecting the dots of the CEOD process. CEOD, in theory, may sound like a game of checkers, but, in practice, it is a high-stakes game of chess.

Case Study Exercises

Individually, or as a group, review the following case studies and follow the exercises suggested at the end of the study, as appropriate. Be sure to focus on the why, how, and what emphasized in each item. Your professor/instructor will provide you with specific guidance on how you are to report your findings for the class.

Case Study 1.1: Franklin County Health Department

In order to address the social conditions that lead to poor health, Franklin County is participating as one of the national Health for All Initiative grantees.

Franklin County public health officials recognize that the odds of being healthy can depend very much on which community you live in. Franklin County has been closely tracking inequities in health and using data on social determinants of health to inform community health improvement efforts. In-depth analysis of available census data has shown, in fact, that there is a 10-year difference in life expectancy between a child born in rural Franklin County and a child born in urban areas. The geographic area into which a child is born can also predict whether the child is likely to graduate from high school or the likelihood of developing medical conditions such as asthma.

Examining mortality and morbidity census data by urban or rural status shows gross, and growing, disparities. In fact, retroactive analysis has shown that the gap between life expectancy for urban and rural residents has increased since 1970.

Former Surgeon General, David Satcher, and his colleagues calculated that between 1991 and 2000 nearly 177,000 deaths were prevented because of advances in medical technology. The epidemiologist with the Franklin County Health Department calculated that if we were to eliminate the disparity between urban and rural residents, we would have avoided over 25,000 deaths.

Franklin County also examines the social gradient, which, in keeping with trends nationally, shows that the more income and wealth people have, the more likely they are to live longer, while people with less income and wealth can expect to live comparatively shorter lives.

Public health officials in Franklin County use these compelling data in reports and presentations to raise awareness about these inequities and the importance of addressing conditions for health at a fundamental level. They used these data to underscore the need for capacity-building and to address these systemic issues. These data point to the multiple and interrelated solutions that must be put in place to begin addressing these inequities, including social policies that affect education, housing, land-use decisions, and economic development. It also points to needed modifications to the physical environment that influence health, including reducing exposure to mining toxins; increasing the availability of open space and healthy foods; decreasing the prevalence of stores specializing in fast foods, alcohol, and tobacco; and encouraging residential patterns that promote interaction across boundaries of race and class.

Study Items

1. Identify a target community or county of your own (real or fictitious).
2. Identify and describe what data you would look for that might help see the broader conditions of disparity that lead to disparities just as in Franklin County.
3. List what sources you would contact and use to obtain such data.
4. Describe how you would use this information to select interventions.

Case Study 1.2: AbilityLinks Increases Employment for People With Disabilities

Background

AbilityLinks, established to increase employment opportunities for people with disabilities, works to increase awareness of the value of hiring people with disabilities. Founded in 2001 by Marianjoy Rehabilitation Hospital in Wheaton, Illinois, AbilityLinks's centerpiece is its award-winning website—www.AbilityLinks.org—which brings together businesses and job candidates with disabilities and is backed by AbilityLinks staff who provide ongoing support to website users.

AbilityLinks, a consortium of approximately 150 businesses, non-profits, and government agencies, holds periodic planning sessions to review its vision, mission, and objectives. These include advisory board meetings (three to four a year) and a more inclusive strategic planning session involving all the stakeholders held every year. One such planning session, "Charting Our Course for the Year Ahead," held in May 2004 was facilitated by an outside consulting firm. Participants looked carefully at past accomplishments, identified key focus areas for the consortium, clarified priorities, and defined committees needed to achieve these plans.

At this strategic planning meeting, the consortium considered many issues to ensure the project focus stayed on its mission to increase employment of people with disabilities. They determined that the vision, mission, and objectives are still relevant, but AbilityLinks had evolved beyond the start-up stage and was ready to progress to the next stage of self-sufficiency. Further and continuous planning was critical to continue to move the consortium forward. Such planning began at this meeting as the consortium reviewed previously established goals and strategies in more detail and recognized the need to restructure the committees to better fulfill the vision, mission, and objectives. Committee restructuring and developing work plans for the new committee became the focus of this planning meeting.

The consortium uses committees to carry out many of its actions set forth by the objectives, while AbilityLinks staff continue to carry out actions related to finance, administration, and website development. Because of the consortium's committee structure, membership becomes a critical element and likely stumbling block. Now, the AbilityLinks consortium has a strong, representative membership that it needs to use effectively, which requires continuous communication and meaningful involvement. Members may participate regularly or intermittently, depending on their organizational connection and time availability. The only foreseen concern that may hamper working relationships among consortium members and AbilityLinks relates to turf issues and competition for job placement and job leads.

Consortium members suggested ways to better manage the committees and membership in order to ensure active participation. They decided to form fewer committees with more membership represented on each committee in order to ensure that each committee has enough active participants to be successful.

Expanding and using the membership effectively involved tracking those who expressed interest in joining the consortium. In the past, businesses and service providers had signed up to be a part of the consortium, but were not contacted in a timely manner to become involved. Sophisticated record-keeping, tracking, and communication are necessary to ensure that contact information is kept current. These efforts should improve communication and encourage participation.

The AbilityLinks consortium is addressing the problem of unemployment among people with disabilities. Although many jobs exist in the community that people with disabilities are able to do, employers are just not aware of the untapped resource that exists. At the same time, people with disabilities need a central place to go to find these jobs, which AbilityLinks provides. The assumption guiding this work is that employment among people with disabilities will increase, if employers consider them good job candidates and they have a central place to look for employment.

Because the consortium is made up of those businesses that are hiring people with disabilities and promoting the hiring of people with disabilities, the larger the membership of the consortium is, the better for the employment of people with disabilities.

The goal of AbilityLinks is to have as many consortium members as possible. Each consortium member means that one more business or community organization has a better understanding of the value of hiring people with disabilities and may give someone with a disability a job in the future or promote employment of people with disabilities in some way. Member benefits include:

- Access to candidates who have equal job performance, low turnover, and low absenteeism, which reduces business costs for recruiting and training
- Access to education, training, and networking events for job seekers and consortium members
- Opportunity for businesses to demonstrate support for equal opportunity to employees, customers, and government agencies
- Free access to post jobs and search résumés on www.abilitylinks.org

Members are recruited through visual and written materials distributed to businesses and other community organizations. The Business Leadership Network in Chicago also specially developed an educational video to be shown at business gatherings. Other business events also have been used to educate businesses about AbilityLinks and recruit for the consortium.

In addition to businesses, the AbilityLinks consortium is made up of nonprofit groups, including those serving people with disabilities. These are essential members of the consortium who get the word out to people with disabilities who might be looking for jobs. The consortium targeted centers for independent living as a way to reach out to disability organizations in the community and expand to a more regional scope when recruiting.

Increase Level of Commitment

As with many coalitions, the AbilityLinks consortium has varying levels of involvement from the 150 entities that form the consortium. An annual strategic planning meeting will help increase the level of commitment from members. Members can be involved in a variety of ways, including education and training events, fundraising, and serving on committees.

Obstacles to participating in the consortium have related mostly to a lack of knowledge and understanding about the employment of people with disabilities. Many employers have incorrect ideas about employing people with disabilities such as thinking they have a high absenteeism rate or require a high cost for accommodation. One of the best ways to remove these myths is through education. AbilityLinks does this at its employer breakfasts, which it also uses to recruit new consortium members.

Over time, the consortium has become a more cooperative effort and has experienced less turf issues related to job placement. AbilityLinks also has gained name recognition and credibility among the business and disability communities, which has helped overcome resistance. Strategic planning meetings are used as a means to foster this cooperation and describe potential barriers or opposition to your partnership's success and strategies to overcome them.

Turf issues have surfaced as a barrier related to resistance by consortium members to join and become involved. Employment and job placement can be competitive with service providers competing for job placement credits and businesses competing for the best employees. AbilityLinks strives to serve as a neutral party to address turf issues and convince the parties that the cause is worthy.

Study Exercises

1. Describe the types of multiple organizations that have come together in common purpose.
2. The TTM of Stages of Change includes stages from precontemplation to maintenance. The consortium conducted activities to bring partners to the consortium. Identify what activities and what stages of TTM it may have influenced.
3. It is important to understand barriers to reaching goals. Identify and discuss some of largest possible stumbling blocks for this consortium.

BIBLIOGRAPHY

Blumenthal, D. B., & DiClemente, R. J. (2004). The view from the community. In N. Cruz, F. G. Murphy, N. Nyarko, & D. N. Yung Krall (Eds.), *Community-based health research* (pp. 63–81). New York, NY: Springer Publishing Company.

Braithwaite, R. L., Griffin, J. P., Stephens, T., Murphy, F., & Marrow, T. (1998). Perceived exercise barriers and participants in Tai Chi for elderly African Americans. *American Journal of Health Studies, 14,* 169.

Braithwaite, R. L., Murphy, F. G., Lythcott, N., & Blumenthal, D. S. (1989). Community organization and development for health promotion within and urban Black community: A conceptual model. *Health Education Journal, 20,* 56–60.

Elders, J. M., & Murphy, F. (1992/2001). Diabetes. In R. Braithwaite & S. Taylor (Eds.), *Health issues in the black community* (pp. 226–241). San Francisco, CA: Josey-Bass Health Series

Jack, L., Jr., Airhihenbuwa, C. O., Murphy, F., Thompson-Reid, P., Wheatley, B., & Dickson-Smith, J. (1993). Cancer among low-income African-Americans: Implications for culture and community-based health promotion. *Wellness Perspectives, 9*(4), 57–68.

KU Work Group for Community Health and Development. (2010). *Chapter 3, Section 10: Conducting Concerns Surveys.* Lawrence, KS: University of Kansas. Retrieved January 2, 2010, from the Community Tool Box http://ctb.ku.edu/en/tablecontents/section_1045.htm

Murphy, F. G., Bond, T. M., Warren, R. C., & Maclin, S. C. (2008). Globalization in the twenty-first century: Impact of gentrification on community health. *American Journal of Health Studies, 23,* 66.

Murphy, F. G., Jackson, P., Johnson, P., Ofili, E., Quarshie, A., & Nwigwe, C. (2004). Informing and consenting disadvantaged populations for clinical and community-based research studies. *American Journal of Health Studies, 19*(4), 246–248.

Murphy, F. G., Satterfield, D., Anderson, R. M., & Lyons, A. E. (1993). Diabetes educators as cultural translators. *The Diabetes Educator, 19*(2), 113–116.

Taylor, B., Murphy, F., Sheats, J. Q., Densler, M. W., & Crump, S. R. (Spring, 1998). Translating breast health information: The emerging role of community health workers. *American Journal of Health Studies.*

2

Defining Community Boundaries and Conducting Community Assessments: CEOD Methods and Practices

Karen E. Bouye, Ramal Moonesinghe, and Frederick G. Murphy

LEARNING OBJECTIVES

What you can learn by studying this chapter:

- What methods can be used for defining community boundaries
- How the World Health Organization (WHO) and the United Nations Children's Fund (UNICEF) define community
- How to identify community characteristics
- What methods and practices to use for analyzing community assessment data
- What data collection methods to use for community assessment
- How to design data collection methods
- How to choose an evaluation method
- How to identify data analysis methods for evaluation
- How to identify methods for reporting data and results

Identifying needs and assets can be helpful to any organization or community group at almost any point, but especially at the start of a new community health initiative dedicated to improving the health of disparate persons living in underserved communities. Identifying problems and assets can help to more clearly identify and prioritize what areas need to be addressed first, and also what and how resources need to be distributed to address these areas.

There are many ways to identify local needs and resources. You can focus on the needs or strengths in your community. You can interview key people, hold community meetings or focus groups, or follow one of the number of other methods. The most important part of identifying local needs and resources is *listening to the insights of group members, community members, leaders, and others, while incorporating community data and history into the analysis.*

Identifying needs can be defined as the gap between what is actually occurring in a given community and what could or should be occurring.

An individual, a group, or an entire community can feel a need. Examining needs helps us discover what is lacking, and helps in planning and guiding public health practitioners to the right direction as they seek to implement programs.

In this chapter, we briefly explore several concepts and models and methods to assess community needs and resources. These methods will assist the public health practitioner to plan and design community health-related programs.

DEFINING COMMUNITY BOUNDARIES

In defining community boundaries, the first step is considering the meaning of *community*. One person's definition of a community may be totally different from that of another's. The notion of community refers to a group of people united by at least one common characteristic (WHO, 2001). Such characteristics could include geography, shared interests, values, experiences, or traditions (WHO, 2001). Communities may be viewed as systems composed of individual members and sectors that have a variety of distinct characteristics and interrelationships (Thompson & Kinne, 1990). These sectors are populated by groups of individuals who represent specialized functions, activities, or interests within a community system. Each sector operates within specific boundaries to meet the needs of its members and those the sector is designed to benefit (WHO, 2001). In a study by Chappel, Funk, and Allan (2006), data revealed that the similarity of community boundaries was based on a sense of belonging with administrative boundaries. The communities differed significantly in income, community activities attended, and health measures. The typology indicated that the community rich in both income and sense of belonging had higher participation and health than did communities low in both or with mixed resources.

The WHO and UNICEF define community in three different ways:

1. An area or neighborhood: "a group of people living together within a fixed geographic location."
2. Social relationships: "a set of social relationships mostly taking place within a fixed geographic location."
3. Identity or common interest: "a shared sense of identity such as groups of substance users" (Howard, Rhodes, & Stimson, 1998).

In a systems view, healthy communities are those that have well-integrated, interdependent sectors that share responsibility to resolve problems and enhance the well-being of the community (Smith, 2001). Another definition of community was described as a group of people with diverse characteristics who are linked by social ties, share common perspectives, and engage in joint action in geographical locations or settings (MacQueen, 2001).

One useful way to describe a community and its sectors is through a technique known as mapping (Kretman & McKnight, 1993). Mapping allows an individual to describe the bounds of a community by identifying primary, secondary, and potential building blocks, or human and material resources. Each of these resources has assets that can be identified, mobilized, and used to address issues of concern and bring about change (Smith, 2001).

COMMUNITY CHARACTERISTICS

In preparing a needs assessment, it is important to find out about and mingle with the local population. The health status of the community, the health needs of the community, and local factors affecting the community's health are very important.

Characteristics of the Population

The total number of people within the community should include all people from birth to death. This will show the number of people the community assessment is designed to cover. The age distribution must be examined, which will have a major influence on the community's health needs. Most profiles divide the community into the following age groups: preschool children, school-age children and young people, adults, and elderly people (WHO, 2001).

Gender distribution is important when looking at specific health issues, such as family planning, maternity services, or diseases that are gender-specific, such as ovarian cancer. The ratio of males to females in a community obviously has a major bearing on the community's health needs. Gender distribution has some standard patterns on a large scale, such as more boys are born than girls and there are more women than men in the very old age group (Breen, 2002).

Minority ethnic and religious groups can be marginalized within a community; a lack of awareness can result in a community needs assessment that may not include the most vulnerable groups. Ethnic groups can be classified by racial origin, religion, color, or nationality. The national classification may be used in order to make comparisons with other areas. Different groups face different problems and require services that are sensitive to their cultural and linguistic background. Religious groupings are useful to know, as they can have a powerful influence over people's lives, are often a source of community support, and influence health behavior. Ethnicity and cultural background have a significant impact on health, and individuals, whatever their ethnic background, are entitled to equal access to health care (Shea et al., 1991).

Language and literacy play a large role in population profiling. There may be one or many languages in use within the community, together with local or regional dialects. Language and literacy are essential for communicating health information and for accessing services. Knowledge of local minority languages is vital to ensure equity and to enable the whole community to become involved in the community assessment process (Kosa, Molnar, McKee, & Adany, 2007). Data commonly used to identify the health of a population are mortality data, morbidity data, behavior measures, quality of life measures, use of service information, and health inequalities.

Mortality data: These data describe patterns of death in relation to age, gender, and cause of death. It is a basic measure of epidemiology—the study of disease in populations. Information is collected nationally, regionally, and sometimes at local levels, usually from death certificates. Mortality rates are most useful for large populations; in small communities, a little change can produce large statistical distortions. A problem in using mortality rates is that it depends on a shared understanding of the causes of death and do not describe the health of the living (LaVest, 2005).

Morbidity data: The data describe the types of illness and disability, their incidence, and prevalence. These data are derived from a wide variety of sources including hospital records, infectious disease notifications and disability registers, sickness records, general medical practice, child health records, census material, and other surveys. Information collected in this way should be treated with care, as it may be a measure of health service activity rather than true disease patterns. Morbidity data are a reflection of illness and not health (LaVest, 2005).

Behavior measures: These measures are often used as indicators of health. Smoking is one of the best examples. Smoking is an activity proven to cause ill health, so if a lot of people smoke, it is expected that there will be a large potential for illness in the population. Breastfeeding is considered the best of all infant feeding methods, so it is taken as an indicator of good health. These measures should be treated carefully as they are about behavior, yet are sometimes used as proxy measures for health (Oddy et al., 2010).

Quality-of-life measures: The quality-of-life measures are a means of assessing physical health, functional ability, and psychological well-being. The assessment scales are based primarily on an individual's own assessment (Hahn & Cella, 2003). These scales have been developed mostly in North America and the United Kingdom to measure health outcomes based on peoples' perception of their health. The reliability and validity of these tools vary, but they are still useful in providing people-based measures of health. Examples include the Barthel Index, the Nottingham Health Profile, and the Index of Activities of Daily Living (WHO, 2001).

Use of service information: The use of service information can help build a picture of morbidity, as it can describe the diseases that are being treated by the health services. It will cover both treatment, for example, hospital admissions, and uptake of preventive services, such as immunization and screening programs. In some cases, access to services may be limited through inadequate provision or because of an individual's inability to pay for treatment. Thus, this information will often be unreliable as an indicator of population health (WHO, 2001).

Health inequalities: It is essential to collect information about health inequalities. Most disease and illness patterns are related closely to economic circumstances, so that those in poverty suffer disproportionately high rates of poor health. Health statistics reveal that, even where death rates improve for a disease, this is less likely to be true for the poorer sections of the population (WHO, 2001). For this reason, it will be important to record patterns of health inequality in the targeted population.

Causal factors for poor health: There are a number of local factors that may affect health. However, in each community they will be different. Work and levels of employment and unemployment in a community are fundamental to health for the following reasons:

1. *Occupational Diseases:* All work affects health, both positively and negatively. However, some work is known to cause disease, such as silicosis in mine and quarry workers and machinery accidents among farm workers. New work-related illnesses are also being recognized, such as repetitive strain injury for keyboard operators.
2. *Income Levels:* The amount of income people earn has an important influence on their health, affecting their ability to choose a healthy lifestyle and to access health services. Levels of income also have an impact on the local economy within a community.
3. *Self-Worth:* The status of an occupation affects how people feel about themselves. People's level of satisfaction at work contributes to their well-being. Many define people by their work or lack of it. The unemployed may feel excluded, and lack of paid employment has been shown to contribute to poor health.
4. *Poverty and Income:* These can be absolute (inadequate to sustain health) or relative (how poor one person is compared to another). In health terms, it is not only the level of poverty that counts but also the gap between richest and poorest. A large gap results in a big difference in health and life expectancy between rich and poor. This is known as health inequality. It is one of the most significant factors affecting health across the world and therefore information on this issue will be essential (WHO, 2001).

5. *Environmental Factors:* Where we live, work, and play directly affect health. Some environmental factors that play a major role are as follows:

   a. Pollution of air and water causes disease and death, which is evident throughout the world. For instance, some pollution is caused by lead in gasoline or a chemical spill from a factory, or drinking water contaminated by sewage.
   b. Sanitation is an environmental factor that greatly affects health. Good sanitation eliminates diseases such as cholera and dysentery completely; in areas with poor sanitation, gastrointestinal illnesses are quickly evident.
   c. Housing affects all aspects of health. Shelter is needed to protect us from the weather and as an environment to sustain a family, a place to feel safe. The availability and type of housing will reflect local history, culture, economy, and political climate. Consideration should be given to such conditions as overcrowding, dampness, and poor heating, as these are significant factors affecting health. Also, consider how far homes are from work, pharmacies, schools, grocery markets, and shops.
   d. Social networks are essential for the well-being of a community. There are a number of elements that need to be considered when describing the extent of social cohesion in a community, such as social networks that are essential for the well-being of a community. There are other important elements that need to be considered when describing the extent of social cohesion in a community, such as networks that provide emotional support; migration which can cause disruption to a population; marginal groups that are outside the dominant community; and pleasure and leisure that provide nonwork social activities (WHO, 2001).

All communities have existing resources and assets with which they respond to the needs of individuals, families, or social groups. These resources may be formal services or informal networks. It is important to assess the extent of both types of resources as part of the profile information. It is too easy to focus on the problems and needs of a community; by ignoring the strengths, there is a danger that existing assets can be undermined. Research has shown that a sense of community, characterized by belonging, influence, fulfillment of needs, and shared connections, is related to self-reported general health, mental health, and well-being (Parker et al., 2001).

METHODS AND PRACTICES FOR ANALYZING COMMUNITY ASSESSMENT DATA

A *community needs assessment* identifies the strengths and resources available in the community to meet the needs of those who reside in the community. The assessment focuses on the capabilities of the community, including its citizens, agencies, and organizations. It provides a framework for developing and identifying services and solutions and building communities that support and nurture children and families (Cassell et al., 2005). A community assessment may be limited to a compilation of demographic data from census records, results of surveys conducted by others, and informal feedback from community partners. Or, assessments may be expanded to include focus group discussions, town hall meetings, interviews with stakeholders, and telephone or mailed surveys to partnership members and the community (Cassell et al., 2005). The assessment consists of (1) identifying the evaluation criteria, (2) establishing how to measure criteria, and (3) gathering data and conducting an analysis.

DATA-COLLECTION METHODS FOR COMMUNITY ASSESSMENT

Methods for conducting a community assessment are similar to conducting research using quantitative and qualitative methods. Often, these two methods are used together. *Quantitative methods* are those that establish specific questions and gather information to support or reject a specific hypothesis or theory. For example, a quantitative survey might discover that more than 50% of the people in a particular neighborhood don't use condoms. Quantitative methods produce information in the form of numbers that are then compared using statistics (Fink, 1993).

Qualitative methods, on the other hand, aim to study people in their natural social settings. Qualitative research involves field observations and talking to the target population to gather information in a less structured way than the methods dedicated to quantitative research. The advantage of qualitative methods is that this method can help in gaining more indepth knowledge than can quantitative research. Qualitative tools, like interviews and observations, are best used for exploring new topics, when little information is known about the target population, and in situations where word-based, interview-type data are preferred over numerical information (Patton, 1990). A further discussion of when to use quantitative versus qualitative methods will be provided later in this chapter.

Commonly utilized approaches for gathering new information on a community are primary data collection and secondary data collection (Burns, 2000). *Primary data-collection techniques* are data gathered directly from clients or the target population, or it is collected by researchers for a specific purpose. Primary data collection techniques include (1) surveys of the population, (2) survey of a subpopulation (purposeful or stratified survey), (3) survey of key informants (one form of a purposeful survey), (4) observations including situations where the researcher is known or unknown, as well as those where the researcher participates or doesn't participate,

(5) case studies that include a life history, an agency history, the history of an issue in a community, or a client focus, (6) social network analysis (focuses on relationships among social entities), (7) power actor techniques (techniques used to identify those in the community that are able to affect the outcome of most community issues) including reputational, decisional, and title or actual office holder, (8) group processes to generate data including focus groups, nominal group processes (participants assemble in groups, without interacting, and each person writes their views or opinions of an issue that is presented), Delphi technique (a method for consensus building by using a series of questionnaires delivered using multiple iterations to collect data from a panel of selected subjects), brain storming, formation of advisory or task forces, or the community forum concept, among many others, and (9) usual techniques for involving citizens in generating data or examining community information (Denzin & Lincoln, 1994).

Key informants can include respondents from client groups, service providers, community leaders, and so on. These informants can give information and/or point to other sources of information. It is useful to think of people in a community linked together and to focus on the modes of communication. Key informants can include town clerks, elected officials, fire persons, mail persons, historians, librarians, farmers, bartenders, general store keepers, factory workers, people associated with informal groups and clubs, town characters, secretaries, and so on (Patton, 1990).

Secondary data-collection techniques can come from general public sources. These might include (1) national data, such as the U.S. Census, the Behavioral Risk Factor Surveillance System (BRFSS), and the National Health Interview Survey (NHIS); (2) state data; (3) business data including the County Business Patterns and Standard Industrial Code information; (3) vital statistics; (4) service district statistics, including basic client counts, attributes, demographics, social conditions, and program information; (5) other social and economic indicators, such as the Consumer Price Index, unemployment figures, inflation indicators, and income tax information; (6) resource inventories and other needs assessments; (7) opinion polls taken by others; and (8) the Internet. Some unusual, but easily accessible, community data sources for gathering data are state tourist maps and other state road maps; topographic maps and aerial photos; the Yellow Pages; newspapers; bulletin boards; films, postcards, and old prints; high school yearbooks; and similar memorabilia (Patton, 1990).

The strengths of using secondary data are that it is less expensive, mostly consists of large sample sizes, and gives population estimates and trends that can be tested over time. Some weaknesses associated with using secondary data are the data are nonexperimental, its constructs are measured by fewer items (no scales), often the data requires special statistical techniques, and the data are mostly cross-sectional (Babbie, 1998).

DESIGNING DATA-COLLECTION METHODS

In designing a data-collection method, *statistical validity* and *reliability* are key criteria, meaning that the research instrument measures exactly what was intended (validity) and will generate similar results if repeated (reliability). *Random sampling* is also important, so that all people being researched have an equal chance of responding (Patton, 1990). The cultural perspectives of the targeted audience, as well as data-collection strategies, should be considered in the selection of the data-collection methods. Some racial–ethnic minority groups tend to be skeptical or mistrustful of the evaluation process. Their experiences have been that social scientists enter their communities and collect data, but frequently fail to share their findings or take viable and beneficial action. The challenge for the researcher is to build confidence in the purpose and benefits of the research results for the community. Try to involve respected community members and leaders in evaluation planning. Ask their cooperation in helping to recruit participants (Olney & Barnes, 2006).

Written questionnaires, telephone interviews, and face-to-face interviews are methods of collecting data from respondents. Respondents are the individuals who supply this information, so the measures are called *self-report*. Self-reported results are always influenced by the person's ability to recall accurately and report honestly (Olney & Barnes, 2006).

Surveys are instruments that present information to a respondent and require a written response—a check, circle, word, sentence, or several sentences. Surveys can be conducted by mail, in person, by telephone, or electronically. Survey research is one of the most common methods used in outreach evaluation (Olney & Barnes, 2006).

Interviews are structured dialogues conducted between two or more persons, in which a respondent answers questions posted by an interviewer. The questions may be predetermined, but the interviewer is free to pursue interesting responses. Focus group interviews take advantage of small group dynamics (usually 8–12 individuals). The open-ended nature of interviews or focus groups allows participants to provide answers in their own words and allows researchers to better understand issues from the perspective of the audience (Olney & Barnes, 2006).

Using small informal groups to discuss and reflect on issues surrounding their community is a way to start compiling a list of issues that will be included on the needs assessment survey. The focus group consists of people who share a common situation to some degree. For instance, you may want to organize a focus group in which participants are similar to each other since the primary goal of the discussion is to allow a free-flowing exchange of ideas and opinions. If there appears to be a great difference among members within a focus group discussion, the participants may become intimidated and limit their input. We suggest holding a few focus groups. One with community leaders; these include a person or group of people with influence in the community who are willing to guide others by defining common goals, listening, and understanding concerns. Another focus group would consist of the adult residents of the community. A third would consist of youth residents of the community (Patton, 1990).

Observations require that one or more observers devote attention to the behavior of an individual or group in a natural setting. Protocols about who or what to observe, when and how long, and the method of recording the information (e.g., a questionnaire or tally sheet) can guide observers. Or, an observer may simply record an account of events that occurred within the prescribed time period, without following a guide for what to observe, for how long, and so on (Smith, 2001).

Records are systematic account of regular occurrences consisting of such things as medical records in physicians' offices and hospitals, hospital discharge records, birth certificates, and death certificates. These records can be used to access barriers to medical care, health disparities, pregnancy outcomes, and health care performance (Li, Quan, Fong, & Lu, 2006).

Meetings are a good source of information for the formative planning stages of a program. For example, a meeting with contacts of the targeted audience and outreach staff will be helpful for effective planning of the implementation and evaluation. The meeting structure can be flexible to avoid limiting the scope of the information gained. Possible biases may occur if those involved feel they need to give "acceptable" responses rather than discussing their actual concerns (Olney & Barnes, 2006).

CHOOSING AN EVALUATION METHOD

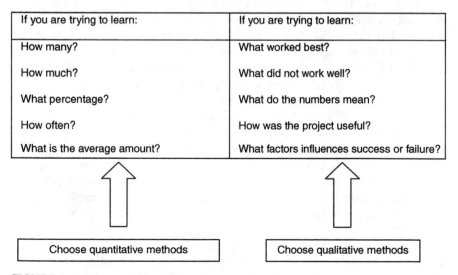

If you are trying to learn:	If you are trying to learn:
How many?	What worked best?
How much?	What did not work well?
What percentage?	What do the numbers mean?
How often?	How was the project useful?
What is the average amount?	What factors influences success or failure?
Choose quantitative methods	Choose qualitative methods

FIGURE 2.1   What are your evaluation questions?

Quantitative data are data that can be counted such as attendance at classes or events, participation or drop-out rates, test scores, and satisfaction ratings. Quantitative methods also show the degree to which certain characteristics are present, such as frequency of activities, opinions, beliefs, or behaviors within a group, as well as an average look at a group or population. Figure 2.1 shows examples of commonly used quantitative evaluation methods. The questions listed below are best answered using quantitative methods:

1. How long have you lived in the community?
   1–5 years_____   5–10 years_____   Over 10 years_____

2. Do you have access to grocery stores in your community?
   Yes_____   No_____

3. Are there any walking paths in your area?
   Yes_____   No_____

4. Are there any parks in your area?
   Yes_____   No_____

5. Do you walk regularly?
   Yes_____   No_____

6. Do you exercise regularly?
   Yes_____   No_____

7. In general, would you say that your health is:
   Excellent_____   Good_____
   Fair_____   Poor_____

8. In the last 12 months, have you seen a doctor?
   Yes_____   No_____

9. Do you have health care insurance?
   Yes_____   No_____
   Don't know_____

10. Have you been to the emergency room in the past 12 months?
    Yes_____   No_____
    Don't know_____

Case Study Exercises

Individually, or as a group, review the following case study and follow the exercises suggested at the end of the study, as appropriate. Be sure to focus on the why, how, and what emphasized in each exercise. Your professor/instructor will provide you with specific guidance on how you are to report your findings for the class.

Case Study 2.1: OYD Service Region Needs Assessment

Over the past decade, the state of Louisiana's Office of Youth Development (OYD) has demonstrated tremendous leadership on the national stage through its reform efforts—namely, by reducing the number of youth incarcerated in the state's juvenile secure and nonsecure care facilities and in reducing associated costs to taxpayers for these expensive and often ineffective services. In partnership with the MacArthur Foundation, however, OYD has set its sights on becoming not only an agency that successfully reduces its census of incarcerated youth, but also one that is truly a "model for change" for the rest of the nation.

The purpose of this needs assessment is to support OYD in assessing the status of community, family, and evidence-based treatment services available for youth in one OYD service region, identifying gaps in available services, including strategies for identification of appropriate youth, and recommending evidence-based assessment and treatment practices that would be appropriate to the development and service needs of youth in that region, as a model for the rest of the state.

Study Exercises

1. Design a data-collection instrument to capture practices and attitudes about services and collect the data.
2. Conduct focus group discussions with frontline probation staff.
3. Analyze data from the survey and focus group.
4. Develop a three- to five-page report based on data analysis from the survey and the focus group.

REFERENCES

Babbie, E. (1998). *The practice of social research* (8th ed.). Belmont, CA: Wadsworth Publishing.

Breen, N. (2002). Social discrimination and health: Gender, race, and class in the United States. In G. Seen, A. George, & P. Ostlin (Eds.), *Engendering international health* (pp. 223–255). Cambridge, MA: Massachusetts Institute of Technology Press.

Burns, R. B. (2000). *Introduction to research methods.* London, England: Sage Publications.

Cassell, C., Santelli, J., Gilbert, B. C., Dalmat, M., Mezoff, J., & Schauer, M. (2005). Mobilizing communities: An overview of the community coalition. *Journal of Adolescent Health, 37*(3), S3–10.

Chappel, N. L., Funk, L. M., & Allan, D. (2006). Defining community boundaries in health promotion research. *American Journal of Health Promotion, 21*(2), 119–126.

Denzin, N. K., & Lincoln, Y. S. (1994). *Handbook of qualitative research.* Thousand Oaks, CA: Sage Publications.

Fink, A. (1993). *Evaluation fundamentals: Guiding health programs, research, and policy.* Newbury Park, London: Sage Publication.

Hahn, E. A., & Cella, D. (2003). Health outcomes assessment in vulnerable populations: Measurement challenges and recommendations. *Archives of Physical Medicine and Rehabilitation, 84,* S35–S42.

Howard, J., Rhodes, T., & Stimson, G. V. (1998). *The rapid assessment and response guide on psychoactive substance use and especially vulnerable young people (EVYP-RAR).* World Health Organization. Unpublished manuscript.

Kosa, K., Molnar, A., McKee, M., & Adany, R. (2007). Rapid health impact appraisal of eviction versus a housing project in a colony-dwelling Roma community. *Journal of Epidemiology and Community Health, 61*(11), 960–965. Doi: 10.1136/jech.2006.057158

Kretman, J., & McKnight, J. L. (1993). *Building communities from the inside out: Centre for urban affairs and policy research.* Chicago, IL: ACTA Publications.

LaVest, T. A. (2005). *Minority populations and health: An introduction to health disparities in the United States.* San Francisco, CA: Jossey-Bass.

Li, B., Quan, H., Fong, A., & Lu, M. (2006). Assessing record linkage between health care and vital statistics databases using deterministic methods. *BMC Health Services Research, 6,* 48.

MacQueen, K. M. (2001). What is community? An evidence-based definition for participatory public health. *American Journal of Public Health, 91*(21), 1929–1938.

Oddy, W. H., Kendall, G. E., Li, J., Jacoby, P., Robinson, M., de Klerk, N., . . . Stanley, F. J. (2010). The long-term effects of breastfeeding on child and adolescent mental health: A pregnancy cohort study followed for 14 Years. *The Journal of Pediatrics, 156*(4), 568–574.

Olney, C. A., & Barnes, S. (2006). *Collecting and analyzing evaluation data.* Seattle, WA: National Library of Medicine.

Parker, E., Lichtenstein, R., Schulz, A., Israel, B., Schork, M., & Steinman, K. (2001). Disentangling measures of individual perceptions of community social dynamics: Results of a community survey. *Health Education & Behavior, 28*(4), 462–486.

Patton, M. Q. (1990). *Qualitative evaluation methods* (2nd ed). Newbury Park, CA: Sage Publications.

Shea, S., Stein, A. D., Basch, C. E., Lantigua, R., Maylahn, C., Strogatz, D. S., & Novick, L. (1991). Independent associations of educational attainment and ethnicity with behavioral risk factors for cardiovascular disease. *American Journal of Epidemiology, 134*(6), 567–562.

Smith, M. K. (2001). *Social capital.* The Encyclopedia of Informal Education. Retrieved from www.infed.org/biblio/social_capital.htm

Thompson, B., & Kinne, S. (1990). *Social change theory: Applications to community health.* Newbury Park, CA: Sage Publications.

World Health Organization. (2001). *Community health needs assessment: An introductory guide for the family health nurse in Europe.* Copenhagen, Denmark: WHO Regional Office for Europe.

3

Ethics and Servant Leadership in Public Health Practice

Frederick G. Murphy and Winifred Smith

LEARNING OBJECTIVES

What you can learn by studying this chapter:

- How to define ethics
- How to identify the principles of ethics
- How to identify and apply the basic ethical concepts of the Belmont Report
- What are the services and practices in community engagement, organization, and development (CEOD)
- How to define servanthood
- How to define servant leadership
- How to define trust
- Key components in CEOD servant leadership

Every person in a given community has the right to know what happens to information they disclose in the course of a community health-related activity. This "right to know" falls under the heading of ethics. A participant in a community health-related program—a health clinic, a community-based research project, a community health survey, or a community health intervention program—has a right to certain expectations relating to how they and the information they pass on are treated. They should also have expectations about the benefits, reliability, competence, and honesty of a program to and for their community.

In the CEOD process "service" is the key component. It involves the entrusting of oneself to the effort and care of another person's well-being. In this process, *"service,"* in and of itself, one takes on the responsibility for, and use of, everything entrusted to oneself by another. This responsibility extends itself to the commitment of one's time, skills, and knowledge to the well-being of the residents of the community targeted. In a nutshell, it involves the wise and unselfish work toward the benefit of others.

Trust is another key component to the community engagement, organization, and development process. It is the cornerstone upon which all other community ingredients are bolted. Public health practitioners (PHPs) of all stripes do well to establish and maintain this essential component as they venture out into the community to deliver public health services of all types.

In this chapter, we discuss each of those concepts, and the moral and professional obligations PHPs have to those they serve.

DEFINING ETHICS

One cannot begin to explore the relevance and importance of working in and with community groups and subpopulations today without first taking a look at what ethics really mean. To do so mandates that we look at important historical documents addressing the ethical and moral framework for community health-related work.

Ethics is a code of thinking and behavior governed by a combination of personal, moral, legal, and social standards of what is right. Although the definition of "right" varies with situations and cultures, its meaning in the context of a community intervention involves a number of guiding principles with which most community activists and public health service providers would probably agree.

Community health interventions can, in fact, sometimes harm participants by merely providing substitutes for what is really needed in the community. What they may really need, in most instances, is just simply to be viewed as a real community, or to be seriously regarded in terms of their capacities rather than their deficiencies, or to have access to a steady source of income. Thus, the PHP, medical practitioners, and research investigators should ask some basic ethical questions before embarking on any community health or medically related project. Examples of these questions include the following:

1. What are the positive and negative effects of the health service(s) proposed to assist this community?
2. What are the situations in which the proposed health service(s) may be integrated with other community services and what interactive negative effects will result?
3. Would a focus on building the capacity of the community be more effective than the health service programs slated to focus on health deficiencies and needs?
4. Will the resources allocated for the health service(s) to be provided be better expended differently that originally proposed?
5. Will incorporation of health practices into community life be even more beneficial than a one-time screening or medical service treatment program?

HISTORY OF ETHICS

The *Belmont Report* "Ethical Principles and Guidelines for the Protection of Human Subjects of Research" (The National Commission for the Protection of Human Subjects of Biomedical and Behavioral Research, 1979) is one of the most important historical documents in the field of public health practice and medical ethics. The report was created in 1979 and gets its name from the Belmont Conference Center where the document was drafted. The Belmont Report attempts to summarize the basic ethical principles identified by the Commission in the course of its deliberations. It is the outgrowth of an intensive 4-day period of discussions that was held in February 1976 at the Smithsonian Institute's Belmont Conference Center and supplemented by the monthly deliberations of the Commission held over a period of nearly 4 years. It is a statement of ethical problems that surround the conduct of research with human subjects This most important report was prompted primarily because of problems arising from the Tuskegee Syphilis Study conducted from 1932 to 1972.

The Belmont Report explains three unifying principles that form the basis for fundamental ethics when approaching communities for applying public health practice of any nature. These principles include the following:

1. Respect
2. Beneficence
3. Justice

In the 21st century, concepts espoused in the Belmont Report continue to be essential to public health and medical practitioners, in order to ensure that the interventions and research meets ethical foundations.

1. *Respect for Person* calls for protecting the autonomy of all people and treating them with courtesy and respect and allowing for education through such methods as "informed consent."

The principle of respect for persons divides into two separate, yet fundamental, moral requirements: first, to *acknowledge autonomy* and, second, to protect those with *diminished autonomy*.

An autonomous person is an individual capable of deliberating about personal goals and of acting under the direction of such deliberation. To respect autonomy is to give weight to an autonomous person's considered opinions and choices, while refraining from obstructing his or her actions unless they are clearly detrimental to others. To show lack of respect for an autonomous agent is to repudiate that person's considered judgments, to deny an individual the freedom to act on those considered judgments, or to withhold information necessary to make a considerate judgment, when there are no compelling reasons to do so. However, not every human being is capable of self-determination. Some persons are in need of extensive protection, even to the point of *excluding them from activities, which may harm them*; other persons require little protection beyond making sure they undertake activities freely and with awareness of possible adverse consequences. The extent of protection afforded should depend upon the *risk of harm and the likelihood of benefit*. The judgment that any individual lacks autonomy should be periodically reevaluated and will vary in different situations. Respecting persons, in most hard cases, is often a matter of balancing competing claims urged by the principle of respect itself.

In summary then, here are some important, yet basic, things to remember concerning respect prior to entering and while conducting health services in any community or culture:

- *Respect people as ends, not means:* Consider and treat everyone as a unique individual who matters, not as a number in a political or social or clinical calculation.
- *Respect participants' ability to play a role in determining what they need:* Do not assume that professional staff or program planners necessarily know what is best for a community or individual.
- *Respect everyone's human, civil, and legal rights:* This encompasses such issues as nondiscrimination and cultural sensitivity.
- *Do what is best for everyone under the circumstances:* You are not necessarily going to be able to help everyone all the time, but you can try to get as close as possible.
- *Don't abuse your position or exploit a participant to gain a personal advantage or to exercise power over another person:* This refers to taking advantage of participants or others for political, social, sexual, or financial gain.

2. **Beneficence:** *Beneficence means maximizing* benefits for the public health project, while minimizing risks to community participants. Persons are treated in an ethical manner not only by respecting their decisions and protecting them from harm, but also by making efforts to secure their well-being. Such treatment falls under the principle of beneficence.

The term beneficence is often understood to cover acts of kindness or charity that go beyond strict obligation. For purposes of this learning experience, beneficence is understood in a stronger sense as an obligation. Two general rules have been formulated as complementary expressions of beneficent actions in this sense:

1. Do not harm
2. Maximize possible benefits and minimize possible harms

The Hippocratic maxim "do no harm" has long been a fundamental principle of medical ethics. He put this in words over 2,000 years ago, and it's still Rule Number One. He spoke of *doing no harm* which, in its most fundamental terms, can mean not starting a community health/

medical intervention or research effort at all. The problem posed by this imperative is to decide when it is justifiable to seek certain benefits despite the risks involved, and when the benefits should be foregone because of the risks. The obligations of beneficence affect both individual investigators and society at large, because they extend both to particular research projects and to the entire enterprise of research. In the case of scientific research and health interventions in general, members of the larger society are obliged to recognize the longer-term benefits and risks that may result from the improvement of knowledge and from the development of novel medical, psychotherapeutic, and social procedures.

The principle of beneficence often occupies a well-defined justifying role in many areas of research involving human subjects. An example is found in research involving children. Effective ways of treating childhood diseases and fostering healthy development are benefits that serve to justify research involving children—even when individual research subjects are not direct beneficiaries. Research also makes it possible to avoid the harm that may result from the application of previously accepted routine practices that on closer investigation turn out to be dangerous. But the role of the principle of beneficence is not always so unambiguous. A difficult ethical problem remains, for example, about research that presents more than minimal risk without immediate prospect of direct benefit to the children involved. Some have argued that such research is inadmissible, while others have pointed out that this limit would rule out much research promising great benefit to children in the future. Here again, as with all hard cases, the different claims covered by the principle of beneficence may come into conflict and force difficult choices. Although, in practice, interventions designed solely to enhance the well-being of a particular individual are sometimes applied to one individual for the enhancement of the well-being of another. However, an intervention may have the dual purpose of enhancing the well-being of a particular individual and, at the same time, providing some benefit to others (e.g., vaccination, which protects both the person who is vaccinated and society generally). In summary, then, here are some basic things to remember concerning the beneficence recommendations, and questions to consider before entering a community or culture to provide or while conducting health services:

- *Evaluate fully just how the health/research effort you are seeking to provide will truly benefit this community:* If you are actively striving to do "good," how far does that obligation take you? If there are issues affecting the community that have nothing to do directly with the one you are concerned with, do you nonetheless have an obligation to become involved? What if you do not really understand the whole situation, and your involvement may *do as much harm as good*—do you still have an ethical obligation to support or become active on the right side? What if your support or activism endangers or compromises your community intervention?

- **Do not attempt an intervention in areas in which you are not trained and/or competent:** This goes along with "do no harm," but it's not always possible. Just as there are times when no intervention may be preferable to doing something counterproductive, there may be times when any intervention is better than none at all. In those circumstances, you may have to learn as you go, getting all the help you can and hoping you don't do anything harmful. It's important to distinguish between doing what you can and getting in over your head to the point where what you're doing becomes truly unethical and harmful.
- **Actively strive to improve or correct, to the extent possible, the situations of participants in your program and the community:** In other words, it is incumbent on you to try to create the best and most effective program possible to meet the needs of participants, and to address underlying conditions or situations in a way that will benefit the community as a whole.

While this guideline of beneficence is a valuable one, it is also difficult to follow. How do you determine what is best for anyone in a particular situation, let alone the best outcome for everyone? The best outcome for most parties may be dependent on a bad outcome for one; or the best outcome for everyone—one that leaves no one as a clear loser—may be relatively negative. It is not always easy to be fair and respectful, or to benefit and show justice for everyone's needs and values

3. *Justice:* Last but not least, there is justice, which focuses on ensuring that reasonable, nonexploitative, and well-considered methods and procedures are administered fairly (i.e., the fair distribution of costs and benefits).

Who ought to receive the benefits of research and bear its burdens? This a question of justice, in the sense of "fairness in distribution" or "what is deserved." An injustice occurs when some benefit to which a person is entitled is denied without good reason or when some burden is imposed unduly. Another way of conceiving the principle of justice is that equals ought to be treated equally. However, this statement requires explication. Who is equal and who is unequal? What considerations justify departure from equal distribution? Almost all commentators allow that distinctions based on experience, age, deprivation, competence, merit, and position do sometimes constitute criteria justifying differential treatment for certain purposes. It is necessary, then, to explain in what respects people should be treated equally. There are several widely accepted formulations of just ways to distribute burdens and benefits. Each formulation mentions some relevant property on the basis of which burdens and benefits should be distributed. These formulations are (1) to each person an equal share, (2) to each person according to individual need, (3) to each person according to individual effort, (4) to each person according to societal contribution, and (5) to each person according to merit. Questions of justice have long been associated with social practices such as punishment, taxation, and political representation. Until recently, these questions have not generally been associated with scientific research. However, they are foreshadowed even in the earliest reflections on the ethics of research involving human subjects. For example, during the 19th and early 20th centuries, the burdens of serving as research subjects fell largely upon poor ward patients, while the benefits of improved medical care flowed primarily to private patients. Subsequently, the exploitation of unwilling prisoners as research subjects in Nazi concentration camps was condemned as a particularly flagrant injustice. In this country, in the 1940s, the Tuskegee Syphilis Study used disadvantaged, rural black men to study the untreated course of a disease that is by no means confined to that population. These subjects were deprived of demonstrably effective treatment in order not to interrupt the project, long after such treatment became generally available. Against this historical background, it can be seen how conceptions of justice are relevant to research involving human subjects. For example, the selection of research subjects needs to be scrutinized in order to determine whether some classes (e.g., welfare patients, particular racial and ethnic minorities, or persons confined to institutions) are being systematically selected simply because of their easy availability, their compromised position, or their manipulability, rather than for reasons directly related to the problem being studied. Finally, whenever research supported by public funds leads to the development of therapeutic devices and procedures, justice demands both that these not provide advantages only to those who can afford them and that such research should not unduly involve persons from groups unlikely to be among the beneficiaries of subsequent applications of the research. These are not insignificant questions, and we will not pretend to answer them here. Many of history's great minds have struggled with them and have often come up with contradictory answers. But you need to be aware of them, and to make decisions about how you are going to address them if you are concerned about the ethics of your intervention and your organization.

THE 12 KEY PRINCIPLES OF ETHICAL PUBLIC HEALTH PRACTICE

The code, or principles, of ethics states the key ethical practices of public health. As stated in the section above, there are key *values and beliefs* inherent to a public health perspective upon which the ethical principles are based. Public health is understood within these 12 principles as what we, as a society, do collectively to ensure the conditions for people to be healthy. The World Health Organization defines health as *a state of complete physical, mental, and social well-being, and not merely the absence of disease or infirmity.* These principles are intended principally for the public and other institutions in the United States that have an explicit public health mission. Institutions and individuals that are outside of traditional public health, but recognize the effects of their work on the health of the community, may also find the code relevant and useful. The 12 Principles of Ethical Practice are as follows:

1. Public health should address principally the fundamental causes of disease and requirements for health, aiming to prevent adverse health outcomes.
2. Public health should achieve community health in a way that respects the rights of individuals in the community.
3. Public health policies, programs, and priorities should be developed and evaluated through processes that ensure an opportunity for input from community members.
4. Public health should advocate and work for the empowerment of disenfranchised community members, aiming to ensure that the basic resources and conditions necessary for health are accessible to all.
5. Public health should seek the information needed to implement effective policies and programs that protect and promote health.
6. Public health institutions should provide communities with the information they have that is needed for decisions on policies or programs and should obtain the community's consent for their implementation.
7. Public health institutions should act in a timely manner on the information they have within the resources and the mandate given to them by the public.
8. Public health programs and policies should incorporate a variety of approaches that anticipate and respect diverse values, beliefs, and cultures in the community.
9. Public health programs and policies should be implemented in a manner that most enhances the physical and social environment.
10. Public health institutions should protect the confidentiality of information that can bring harm to an individual or community if made public. Exceptions must be justified on the basis of the high likelihood of significant harm to the individual or others.
11. Public health institutions should ensure the professional competence of their employees.
12. Public health institutions and their employees should engage in collaborations and affiliations in ways that build the public's trust and the institution's effectiveness.

A *code of ethics* for public health clarifies the distinctive elements of public health and the ethical principles that follow from or respond to those distinct aspects. It makes clear to populations and communities the ideals of the public health institutions that serve them. A code of ethics thus serves as a goal to guide public health institutions and practitioners and as a standard to which they can be held accountable.

Codes of ethics are typically relatively brief; they are not designed to provide a means of untangling convoluted ethical issues. The process requires deliberation and debate over the multitude of factors relevant to a particular issue. Nor does a code typically provide a means of resolving a particular dispute. It does, however, provide those in a dispute over a public health concern with a list of issues and principles that should be considered in the dispute.

ETHICAL PRACTICE: PRINCIPLES, RATIONALE, AND VALUES

Another important document developed in the 21st century related to ethical practices is the *Principles of the Ethical Practice of Public Health, Version 2.2*. The Public Health Leadership Society (PHLS) developed this important document in 2002. Many public health professionals, most of them associated with the PHLS, came together to initiate the process of writing ethics code. Represented on the PHLS Public Health Code of Ethics Committee are public health professionals from local and state public health agencies, public health academia, the Centers for Disease Control and Prevention (CDC), and the American Public Health Association (APHA). They were formally encouraged in this effort during a town hall meeting attended by representatives from a wide variety of public health organizations at the 2000 APHA annual meeting. A draft code was reviewed and critiqued in May 2001 by 25 public health professionals and ethicists in a CDC-funded meeting held in Kansas City. A revised version of the code was presented for discussion at another town hall meeting at the 2001 APHA annual meeting. Prior to the meeting, the code was published on the APHA website and an e-mail address was provided for reactions and feedback. The present code reflects the input and discussion from all of these forums. It has been presented to various organizations for adoption or endorsement.

Until recently, the ethical nature of public health has been implicitly assumed rather than explicitly stated. Increasingly, however, society is demanding explicit attention to ethics. This demand arises from: technological advances that create new possibilities, and with them, new ethical dilemmas; new challenges to health such as the advent of human immunodeficiency virus; abuses of power, such as the Tuskegee Syphilis Study and an increasingly pluralistic society in which we can no longer simply adopt the values from a single culture or religion, but must work out our common values in the midst of diversity.

Historically, medical institutions have been more explicit about the ethical elements of their practice than have public health institutions. The concerns of public health are not fully consonant with those of medicine, however; we cannot simply translate the principles of medical ethics to public health. For example, in contrast to medicine, public health is concerned more with populations than with individuals, and more with prevention than with cure. Thus, the purview of public health includes those who are not presently ill, and for whom the risks and benefits of medical care are not immediately relevant.

Values and Beliefs

The following 11 *values and beliefs* are key assumptions inherent to a public health perspective. These are not to be confused with the 12 Principles of Ethical Public Health Practice, but are to be viewed as underlying foundational areas of human and civil rights that underpin the 12 Principles of Ethical Practice of Public Health to be listed subsequently.

1. *Humans have a right to the resources necessary for health.* The Public Health Code of Ethics affirms Article 25 of the Universal Declaration of Human Rights, which states in part "Everyone has the right to a standard of living adequate for the health and well-being of himself and his family...."
2. *Humans are inherently social and interdependent.* Humans look to each other for companionship in friendships, families, and communities and rely upon one another for safety and survival. Positive relationships among individuals and positive collaborations among institutions are signs of a healthy community. The rightful concern for the physical individuality of humans and one's right to make decisions for oneself must be balanced against the fact that each person's actions affect other people.
3. *The effectiveness of institutions depends heavily on the public's trust.* Factors that contribute to trust in an institution include the following actions on the part of the institution: communication, truth telling, transparency (i.e., not concealing information), accountability, reliability, and reciprocity. One critical form of reciprocity and communication is listening to, as well as speaking with the community.
4. *Collaboration is a key element to public health.* The public health infrastructure of a society is composed of a wide variety of agencies and professional disciplines. To be effective, they must work together well. Moreover, new collaborations will be needed to rise to new public health challenges.
5. *People and their physical environment are interdependent.* People depend upon the resources of their natural and constructed environments for life itself. A damaged or unbalanced natural environment,

and a constructed environment of poor design or in poor condition, will have an adverse effect on the health of people. Conversely, people can have a profound effect on their natural environment through consumption of resources and generation of waste.

6. *Each person in a community should have an opportunity to contribute to public discourse.* Contributions to discourse may occur through a direct or a representative system of government. In the process of developing and evaluating policy, it is important to discern whether all who would like to contribute to the discussion have an opportunity to do so, even though expressing a concern does not mean that it will necessarily be addressed in the final policy.

7. *Identifying and promoting the fundamental requirements for health in a community are of primary concern to public health.* The way in which a society is structured is reflected in the health of a community. The primary concern of public health is with these underlying structural aspects. While some important public health programs are curative in nature, the field as a whole must never lose sight of underlying causes and prevention. Because fundamental social structures affect many aspects of health, addressing the fundamental causes rather than more proximal causes is more truly preventive.

8. *Knowledge is important and powerful.* We are to seek to improve our understanding of health and the means of protecting it through research and the accumulation of knowledge. Once obtained, there is a moral obligation in some instances to share what is known. For example, active and informed participation in policy-making processes requires access to relevant information. In other instances, such as information provided in confidence, there is an obligation to protect information.

9. *Science is the basis for much of our public health knowledge.* The scientific method provides a relatively objective means of identifying the factors necessary for health in a population, and for evaluating policies and programs to protect and promote health. The full range of scientific tools, including both quantitative and qualitative methods, and collaboration among the sciences is needed.

10. *People are responsible to act on the basis of what they know.* Knowledge is not morally neutral and often demands action. Moreover, information is not to be gathered for idle interest. Public health should seek to translate available information into timely action. Often, the action required is research to fill in the gaps of what we do not know.

11. *Action is not based on information alone.* In many instances, action is required in the absence of all the information one would like. In other instances, policies are demanded by the fundamental value and dignity of each human being, even if implementing them is not calculated to be optimally efficient or cost beneficial. In both of these situations, values inform the application of information or the action in the absence of information.

Finally, every PHP must ask the question: Who is subject to the code of ethical behavior in any community? The short answer is that everyone—those who work in a community program of any kind or those who deal with other people in a professional or paraprofessional capacity—is subject to a code of ethics in community interventions. There are, however, a number of formal ethical codes—usually set down by professional organizations, but sometimes by law—that apply to people in particular professional or other positions.

Here are some examples of people expected to adhere to a formal code of ethics:

- Medical professionals (i.e., doctors, nurses, emergency medical technician [EMTs]). This category also includes such nontraditional medical workers as chiropractors and acupuncturists.
- Public health educators
- Mental health professionals (i.e., psychiatrists, psychologists, psychotherapists, and counselors)
- Community health workers
- Social workers
- Clergy
- Public officials
- Educators and youth workers
- People who work with young children or in child protective services
- Lawyers and paralegals
- Mediators
- Administrators of all types of community programs or their sponsoring organizations
- Nonprofessional line staff (home health aides, overnight staff at residential facilities and shelters)

In some states, many of these people—medical personnel, mental health workers, social workers, educators, and others who work with children and youth—are legally considered *mandated reporters*. A mandated reporter is required by law to report any suspected instance of child physical or sexual abuse or child neglect. (Most formal codes of professional ethics demand such reporting as well.) We will look at the implications of mandated reporter status later in this section.

In addition to its simply being the right thing to do, always acting ethically brings some particular advantages including the following:

1. *Program effectiveness.* Consistent ethical behavior in all aspects of a community intervention will lead you to finding the most effective and community-centered methods.
2. *Standing in the community.* An organization that has a reputation for ethical action is far more likely to be respected by both participants and

the community as a whole. A PHP or organization that is recognized as ethical is also apt to be seen as competent and trustworthy, making it easier to recruit staff, volunteers, board members, and participants, and to raise money and public support.

3. *Moral credibility and leadership.* Ethical action reflects why you started your community intervention in the first place. You have a moral obligation to yourself, the individuals you work with, and the community to be ethical in all you do.

4. *Professional and legal issues.* Many of the health and human service professions often involved in community interventions are held to specific codes of ethics by their professional certification or licensure organizations. If members of any profession violate these standards, they can be disciplined, or even lose their licenses to practice.

Key Ethical Practices in CEOD

Ethical behavior in community interventions relates to the treatment of people, information, and money, and to the general actions of the workers and the organization or initiative, even when they are not dealing directly with the community. Not all of the areas discussed below are covered by a specific legal or ethical code for every profession or community service, but are nonetheless related to ethical behavior for just about any program or organization. All should at least be considered as you define ethics for yourself and your program.

1. **Confidentiality.** Probably the most familiar of ethical issues—perhaps because it is the one most often violated—is the expectation that communications and information from participants in the course of a community intervention or program (including conversations, written or taped records, notes, test results, etc.) will be kept confidential. Programs' legal responsibilities in this area may vary, but as a general rule, confidentiality is the best policy. It protects both participants and the organization from invasion of privacy, and establishes a bond of trust between the participant and the program. Depending upon the program, the PHP's position, and the participant's needs, confidentiality may encompass a range of possibilities:

    ▪ *No one but the individual working with a particular participant will have access to information about or records of that participant without the participant's permission.* At this level of confidentiality, records and notes are usually kept under lock and key, and electronic coding or passwords should protect computer records.

    ▪ *Information is confidential within a program, but may be shared among staff members for purposes of consultation and delivering better health services to the participant.* The health teacher of a fitness class, for instance, may confer with other teachers about a student with a particular health condition or problem.

▪ *Information is confidential within a program or to a particular staff member, but may be shared with staff members of other programs in which the participant is involved, either to improve services for the participant, or to contribute to the other organization's reporting data.* This kind of arrangement usually requires that participants be told about it from the beginning, and that they sign release forms giving the program permission to share records and information under appropriate circumstances.

▪ *Information is confidential within a program, but is submitted to funding sources as documentation of services provided.* This situation can lead to problems if participants have been promised complete confidentiality. In that case, especially if threatened with withdrawal of funds, the program has to decide whether the money is more important than participants' anonymity, or what level of anonymity is sufficient. Some organizations simply provide the requested documentation without informing participants, on the assumption that funders are not likely to either have actual contact with participants or misuse an individual record; others feel they must honor their promise, and can't release anything without participants' permission.

▪ *Information is not confidential, or is only confidential under certain circumstances.* Participation in a program may be court-mandated or mandated by an agency as a condition of receiving benefits or services. Often, in those cases, participation implies an agreement to the sharing of records and information, and may even be a matter of public record.

In all circumstances, ethical treatment of participants demands that they be informed about the program's confidentiality policies. In most cases, they then have the choice of not participating if they are unhappy with those policies; in the case of court-mandated participation, at least they'll know what to expect. All of which brings us to the next two issues, which may intertwine with confidentiality and each other: consent and disclosure.

2. **Consent.** There are really three key types of consent. These include:

   a. Program participants giving program staff consent to share their records or information with others for purposes of service provision;
   b. Participants giving informed consent to submit to particular medical or other services, treatment, research, or program conditions; and,
   c. Community members consenting to the location or operation of an intervention in their neighborhood.

Let's discuss each of these consent types briefly.

Consent to sharing of information: As we found in the discussion of confidentiality above, most participant records and information collected by program staff can only be passed on with the consent of the participant. In general, this consent is embodied in a standard form signed by the participants, granting permission to a program in which they were formerly or are currently enrolled to share their information with another organization, in which they are also a former or current participant. In some programs, a participant might sign a blanket form on entrance, but a separate form is usually needed for each separate instance of information sharing outside the program itself. Informed consent means showing respect for persons, and requires that participants, to the degree that they are capable, be given the opportunity to choose what shall or shall not happen to them. This opportunity is provided when adequate standards for informed consent are satisfied. While the importance of informed consent is unquestioned, controversy prevails over the nature and possibility of an informed consent. Nonetheless, there is widespread agreement that the consent process can be analyzed as containing three elements: information, comprehension, and voluntariness.

Informed consent for services, treatment, research, or program condition: In some situations, services might be significantly different from participants' expectations (being asked to enter residential drug treatment as a result of psychotherapy, for example). In others—medical diagnoses, for instance—there are no "normal" expectations. A third possibility involves participants enrolling in a community intervention, which is also a study. In any of these instances, ethical practice demands that people be fully informed—and can ask and have answered any questions—about what they are about to take part in. An informed consent form is usually the vehicle by which participants give their permission to be involved in these interventions.

Community consent: It's difficult to draw lines here, or to find the absolute ethical standard. Is it ethically necessary to gain the consent of a neighborhood to place a community health clinic or dialysis center there, for instance? What if neighbors' attitudes stop at "not in my back yard"? Do you need the consent of a group—or its community leadership, council person, or president or director—to go forward?

Both confidentiality and consent bring up the issue of privacy, one that has been much discussed in the past 30 years or more. Technology has made information far more accessible to far more people, and individual privacy has consequently become far more threatened. Much of what is discussed above and below has been the subject of legal wrangling. While the question of the right to privacy, constitutional or otherwise, is much too broad to go into any detail here, it is always lurking behind any PHP's decision about releasing information.

3. **Disclosure.** Like consent, disclosure in this context has more than one meaning.

   ■ *Disclosure to participants of the conditions of the program.* These may include the disclosure of: program policies of confidentiality and when it might be breached, what kinds of services are available and what kinds are not, any time limits on the program, whether it will cost anything, and so on. Participants have a right to know if they will be part of a research study if they enter the program, and to understand the purpose of that study, as explained above. Some organizations or individuals put these disclosures in writing, and make sure that every participant has a copy and understands what's written on it. That participants know exactly what they're getting into and that they be treated as adults who can decide what makes sense for them are ethically important.

   ■ *Disclosure of participant information to other individuals, agencies, and so on.* The rules here are essentially those for confidentiality: Information, except in cases of mandated reporting, potential harm to self or others, or court testimony, can only be disclosed with the participant's permission. Exceptions to this rule have to be spelled out to participants as they enter the program, so that they can decide whether the services are worth any loss of privacy or anonymity.

4. **Competence.** By offering services of any kind, a PHP or organization is essentially making a contract with participants to do the job it says it will do. Implied in that contract is that those actually doing the work, and the organization as a whole, are competent to accomplish their goals under reasonable circumstances.

   Further, competence means more than simply having the appropriate training and experience. A competent organization hires competent staff members, provides supervision and staff development, and does everything it can to ensure that the services it offers are the best available. If service appears to be ineffective or harmful, it is the ethical responsibility of the program to seek out or develop and try more effective methods. If a staff member, even with help from supervisors and others, isn't able to do the job, that should be documented and the member should be dismissed.

   It is obvious that no program or individual will succeed 100% of the time. Some community interventions may succeed less than half the time and that may be the best anyone can do. But whatever the success rate, participants and the community have a right to expect that the program knows what it's doing and will make its best faith effort to provide effective services. This means that community services need to be offered by PHPs who are competent at what they do.

There are legal implications here as well. As explained earlier in this section, in some cases, service providers can lose their licenses or be sued for malpractice if they are found to be incompetent. It is up to a program to make sure that no one on its staff places himself in that position.

5. **Conflict of interest.** A conflict of interest is a situation in which someone's personal (financial, political, professional, social, sexual, family, etc.) interests could influence his judgment or actions in a financial or other decision, in carrying out his job or in his relationships with participants. In community interventions, conflicts of interest may change—to the community's disadvantage—how a program is run or how its money is spent.

Applications of the general principles to the conduct of research leads to consideration of the following requirements: informed consent, risk/benefit assessment, and the selection of subjects of research.

Information. Most codes of research establish specific items for disclosure intended to ensure that subjects are given sufficient information. These items generally include: the research procedure; their purposes, risks and anticipated benefits; alternative procedures (where therapy is involved); and a statement offering the subject the opportunity to ask questions and to withdraw at any time from the research. Additional items have been proposed, including how subjects are selected, the person responsible for the research, and so on. However, a simple listing of items does not answer the question of what the standard should be for judging how much and what sort of information should be provided. One standard frequently invoked in medical practice, namely the information commonly provided by practitioners in the field or in the locale, is inadequate since research takes place precisely when a common understanding does not exist. Another standard, currently popular in malpractice law, requires the practitioner to reveal the information that reasonable persons would wish to know in order to make a decision regarding their care. This, too, seems insufficient since the research subject, being in essence a volunteer, may wish to know considerably more about risks gratuitously undertaken than do patients who deliver themselves into the hand of a clinician for needed care. It may be that a standard of "the reasonable volunteer" should be proposed: The extent and nature of information should be such that persons, knowing that the procedure is neither necessary for their care nor perhaps fully understood, can decide whether they wish to participate in the furthering of knowledge. Even when some direct benefit to them is anticipated, the subjects should understand clearly the range of risk and the voluntary nature of participation. A special problem of consent arises where informing subjects of some pertinent aspect of the research is likely to impair the validity of the research. In many cases, it is sufficient to indicate to subjects that they are being invited to participate in research of which some features will not be revealed until the research is concluded. In all cases of research involving incomplete disclosure, such research is justified only if it is clear that (1) incomplete disclosure is truly necessary to accomplish the goals of the research, (2) there are no undisclosed risks to subjects that are more than minimal, and (3) there is an adequate plan for debriefing subjects, when appropriate, and for dissemination of research results to them. Information about risks should never be withheld for the purpose of eliciting the cooperation of subjects, and truthful answers should always be given to direct questions about the research. Care should be taken to distinguish cases in which disclosure would destroy or invalidate the research from cases in which disclosure would simply inconvenience the investigator.

Comprehension. The manner and context in which information is conveyed is as important as the information itself. For example, presenting information in a disorganized and rapid fashion, allowing too little time for consideration or curtailing opportunities for questioning, all may adversely affect a subject's ability to make an informed choice. Because the subject's ability to understand is a function of intelligence, rationality, maturity, and language, it is necessary to adapt the presentation of the information to the subject's capacities. Investigators are responsible for ascertaining that the subject has comprehended the information. While there is always an obligation to ascertain that the information about risk to subjects is complete and adequately comprehended, when the risks are more serious, that obligation increases. On occasion, it may be suitable to give some oral or written tests of comprehension. Special provision may need to be made when comprehension is severely limited—for example, by conditions of immaturity or mental disability. Each class of subjects that one might consider as incompetent (e.g., infants and young children, mentally disabled patients, the terminally ill, and the comatose) should be considered on its own terms. Even for these persons, however, respect requires giving them the opportunity to choose, to the extent they are able, whether or not to participate in research. The objections of these subjects to involvement should be honored, unless the research entails providing them a therapy unavailable elsewhere. Respect for persons also requires seeking the permission of other parties in order to protect the subjects from harm. Such persons are thus respected both by acknowledging their own wishes and by the use of third parties to protect them from harm. The third parties chosen should be those who are most likely to understand the incompetent subject's situation and to act in that person's best interest. The person authorized to act on behalf of the subject should be given an opportunity to observe the research as it proceeds in order to be able to withdraw the subject from the research, if such action appears in the subject's best interest.

Voluntariness. An agreement to participate in research constitutes a valid consent only if voluntarily given. This element of informed consent requires conditions free of coercion and undue influence. Coercion occurs when an overt threat of harm is intentionally presented by one person to another in order to obtain compliance. Undue influence, by contrast, occurs through an offer of an excessive, unwarranted, inappropriate, or improper reward or other overture in order to obtain compliance. Also, inducements that would ordinarily be acceptable may become undue influences if the subject is especially vulnerable. Unjustifiable pressures usually occur when persons in positions of authority or commanding influence— especially where possible sanctions are involved—urge a course of action for a subject. A continuum of such influencing factors exists, however, and it is impossible to state precisely where justifiable persuasion ends and undue influence begins. But undue influence would include actions such as manipulating a person's choice through the controlling influence of a close relative and threatening to withdraw health services to which an individual would otherwise be entitled.

Assessment of Risks and Benefits. The assessment of risks and benefits requires a careful array of relevant data, including, in some cases, alternative ways of obtaining the benefits sought in the research. Thus, the assessment presents both an opportunity and a responsibility to gather systematic and comprehensive information about proposed research. For the investigator, it is a means to examine whether the proposed research is properly designed. For a review committee, it is a method for determining whether the risks that will be presented to subjects are justified. For prospective subjects, the assessment will assist the determination whether or not to participate.

The Nature and Scope of Risks and Benefits. The requirement that research be justified on the basis of a favorable risk/benefit assessment bears a close relation to the principle of beneficence, just as the moral requirement that informed consent be obtained is derived primarily from the principle of respect for persons. The term "risk" refers to a possibility that harm may occur. However, when expressions such as "small risk" or "high risk" are used, they usually refer (often ambiguously) both to the chance (probability) of experiencing a harm and the severity (magnitude) of the envisioned harm. The term "benefit" is used in the research context to refer to something of positive value related to health or welfare. Unlike "risk," "benefit" is not a term that expresses probabilities. Risk is properly contrasted to probability of benefits, and benefits are properly contrasted with harms rather than risks of harm. Accordingly, so-called risk–benefit assessments are concerned with the probabilities and magnitudes of possible harms and anticipated benefits. Many kinds of possible harms and benefits need to be taken into account. There are, for example, risks of psychological harm, physical harm, legal harm, social harm, and economic harm and the corresponding benefits. While the most likely types of harms to research subjects are those of psychological or physical pain or injury, other possible kinds should not be overlooked. Risks and benefits of research may affect the individual subjects, the families of the individual subjects, and society at large (or special groups of subjects in society). Previous codes and federal regulations have required that risks to subjects be outweighed by the sum of both the anticipated benefit to the subject, if any, and the anticipated benefit to society in the form of knowledge to be gained from the research. In balancing these different elements, the risks and benefits affecting the immediate research subject will normally carry special weight. On the other hand, interests other than those of the subject may on some occasions be sufficient by themselves to justify the risks involved in the research, so long as the subject's rights have been protected. Beneficence thus requires that we protect against risk of harm to subjects and also that we be concerned about the loss of the substantial benefits that might be gained from research.

The Systematic Assessment of Risks and Benefits. It is commonly said that benefits and risks must be "balanced" and shown to be "in a favorable ratio." The metaphorical character of these terms draws attention to the difficulty of making precise judgments. Only on rare occasions will quantitative techniques be available for the scrutiny of research protocols. However, the idea of systematic, nonarbitrary analysis of risks and benefits should be emulated insofar as possible. This ideal requires those making decisions about the justifiability of research to be thorough in the accumulation and assessment of information about all aspects of the research, and to consider alternatives systematically. This procedure renders the assessment of research more rigorous and precise, while making communication between review board members and investigators less subject to misinterpretation, misinformation, and conflicting judgments. Thus, there should first be a determination of the validity of the presuppositions of the research; then the nature, probability, and magnitude of risk should be distinguished with as much clarity as possible. The method of ascertaining risks should be explicit, especially where there is no alternative to the use of such vague categories as small or slight risk. It should also be determined whether an investigator's estimates of the probability of harm or benefits are reasonable, as judged by known facts or other available studies. Finally, assessment of the justifiability of research should reflect at least the following considerations: (a) Brutal or inhumane treatment of human subjects is never morally justified. (b) Risks should be reduced to those necessary to achieve the research objective. It should be determined whether it is in fact necessary to use human subjects at all. Risk can perhaps never be entirely eliminated, but it can often be reduced by careful attention to alternative procedures. (c) When research involves significant risk of serious impairment, review committees should be extraordinarily insistent on the justification of the risk (looking usually to the likelihood of benefit to the subject or, in some rare cases, to the manifest voluntariness of the participation). (d) When vulnerable populations are involved in research, the appropriateness of involving them should itself be demonstrated. A number of variables go into such judgments, including the nature and degree of risk, the condition of the particular population involved, and the nature and level of the anticipated benefits. (e) Relevant risks and benefits must be thoroughly arrayed in documents and procedures used in the informed consent process.

Selection of Subjects. Just as the principle of respect for persons finds expression in the requirements for consent and the principle of beneficence in risk/benefit assessment, the principle of justice gives rise to moral requirements that there be fair procedures and outcomes in the selection of research subjects. Justice is relevant to the selection of subjects of research at two levels: the social and the individual. Individual justice in the selection of subjects would require that researchers exhibit fairness: thus, they should not offer potentially beneficial research only to some patients who are in their favor or select only "undesirable" persons for risky research. Social justice requires that distinction be drawn between classes of subjects that ought, and ought not, to participate in any particular kind of research, based on the ability of members of that class to bear burdens and on the appropriateness of placing further burdens on already burdened persons. Thus, it can be considered a matter of social justice that there is an order of preference in the selection of classes of subjects (e.g., adults before children) and that some classes of potential subjects (e.g., the institutionalized mentally infirm or prisoners) may be involved as research subjects, if at all, only on certain conditions. Injustice may appear in the selection of subjects, even if individual subjects are selected fairly by investigators and treated fairly in the course of research. Thus, injustice arises from social, racial, sexual, and cultural biases institutionalized in society. Thus, even if individual researchers are treating their research subjects fairly, and even if Institutional Review Boards (IRBs) are taking care to ensure that subjects are selected fairly within a particular institution, unjust social patterns may nevertheless appear in the overall distribution of the burdens and benefits of research. Although individual institutions or investigators may not be able to resolve a problem that is pervasive in their social setting, they can consider distributive justice in selecting research subjects. Some populations, especially institutionalized ones, are already burdened in many ways by their infirmities and environments. When research is proposed that involves risks and does not include a therapeutic component, other less burdened classes of persons should be called upon first to accept these risks of research, except where the research is directly related to the specific conditions of the class involved. Also, even though public funds for research may often flow in the same directions as public funds for health care, it seems unfair that populations dependent on public health care constitute a pool of preferred research subjects if more advantaged populations are likely to be the recipients of the benefits. One special instance of injustice results from the involvement of vulnerable subjects. Certain groups, such as racial minorities, the economically disadvantaged, the very sick, and the institutionalized may continually be sought as research subjects, owing to their ready availability in settings where research is conducted. Given their dependent status and their frequently compromised capacity for free consent, they should be protected against the danger of being involved in research solely for administrative convenience, or because they are easy to manipulate as a result of their illness or socioeconomic condition.

Conflicts can also affect an organization, especially where a Board of Directors is involved. If a staff member is also a Board member, that person should not take part in Board decisions about staff salaries, for instance, although it may in fact be helpful for that person to contribute to the discussion of that issue. It is usually considered a conflict of interest for programs to pay Board members for services (e.g., hiring a Board member to be the program's lawyer).

Conflicts of interest are virtually always unethical, to the point where the mere appearance of a conflict needs to be avoided. Even if decisions or actions are not actually influenced by personal interest, people in conflict of interest situations in their public or professional lives should do everything possible to resolve them.

If you find yourself in such a situation, the ethical remedy is two-pronged:

1. *Point it out to whoever needs to know:* Alert your employer, a funder, the community, the participant you're working with and discuss possible solutions.
2. *Eliminate the conflict situation:* Depending upon the situation, solutions might involve excusing yourself from taking part in a particular decision, refusing funding from a particular source, ceasing to work with a particular participant, or even changing jobs.

Some examples of conflict of interest (with possible solutions in parentheses):

- A decision by a program director to purchase office equipment for the program from a company his wife owns: The director has both a personal and a financial stake in the decision. (The director could remove himself and/or his wife's company from the purchasing process.)
- A staff member entering into a sexual relationship with an intern or someone he or she supervises. The supervisor has power over the other's employment and/or professional evaluation, which puts pressure on the subordinate to enter into and/or continue the relationship, even if the subordinate is reluctant, and may keep the supervisor from making objective decisions about the subordinate. (If the relationship is mutual and the attraction is strong on both sides, this can present a very difficult situation. If the supervisor simply transfers the supervi-

sory responsibility to someone else, there still remains the power in the program or organization itself. The best solution is probably for the supervisor to remove himself or herself *and* wait until the internship period ends before approaching an intimate relationship.)

6. **Grossly unethical behavior.** This is behavior far beyond the bounds of the normally accepted ethical standards of society. In some cases, grossly unethical behavior may stem from taking advantage of a conflict of interest situation. In others, it may be a simple case of dishonesty or lack of moral scruples. Both individuals and organizations can be guilty of some instances of it, and in both cases, it is often a result of someone managing to justify the unjustifiable. Community programs need to be clear about their own ethical standards and hold individuals to them and to any other standards their professions demand. In most cases, staff members guilty of grossly unethical behavior should be dismissed as quickly as possible, and prosecuted where that is appropriate. Some of the more familiar types of grossly unethical behavior include:

- Having sexual relationships—even consensual sexual relationships— with people with whom one has a professional relationship in which one holds the power. Doctor–patient, therapist–client, teacher–student, supervisor–intern, and youth worker–teen are all examples of such relationships. In some of these cases, a sexual relationship both violates the professional's code of ethics (and is therefore grounds for losing professional certification), and also may be the base for a sexual harassment or sexual assault lawsuit as well.
- Exploiting people for financial gain with whom one has a professional relationship. Moving someone to the head of a waiting list in return for free services from that person (car repair, for instance), or accepting gifts or money—essentially bribes—to do something out of the ordinary (e.g., accept someone who normally wouldn't qualify for your program).
- Defrauding funders: Billing for nonexistent services or inventing problems in order to deliver unnecessary services.
- Denying necessary medical services to those uninsured and unable to pay.
- Discriminating in service delivery by race, gender, ethnicity, and so on.
- Outright criminal behavior: redirecting program funds for personal use, for instance, or sexually abusing children in a day care center. This can also include criminal behavior that a staff member engages in on his or her own time—for example, selling drugs or robbing a warehouse.

7. **General ethical responsibilities.** Ethical behavior for a community intervention is more than simply following particular professional codes and keeping your nose clean. It means actively striving to do

what is right for participants and for the community, and treating everyone—participants, staff members, funders, and the community at large—in an ethical way. By doing what you do in the community, you take on a number of responsibilities:

Responsibility to funders: You are responsible for being fiscally account-able, for using funds properly, and for trying to do what you promised to do when you took the money.

Responsibility to staff members: You are responsible for making sure everyone is treated fairly in all dealings with the program; that everyone is paid for the work he or she do; that everyone has a reasonable amount of control over his or her job; and that everyone has the opportunity to con-tinue to develop skills and effectiveness through staff development and/ or supervision. You are also responsible for protecting staff from harm to the extent possible, and for warning and training staff if some physical or other danger is part of their jobs.

Responsibility to participants: You are responsible for trying, throughout the life of the program, to provide the best and most effective services possible. This means constantly searching for better methods and ideas; paying attention to participant feedback; building on program successes; and acknowledging, learning from, and correcting program weaknesses. You are also responsible for respecting participants' rights, and for treat-ing all with the respect due to them, not only as program participants, but also as human beings.

Responsibility to the community: You are responsible for trying to under-stand and meet the needs of the community; for being responsive to com-munity attitudes and opinions (without compromising your own mission or philosophy); and for trying, through your intervention, to improve the quality of life in some way for both program participants and the com-munity as a whole.

The participatory nature of community interventions that these obliga-tions imply can also raise ethical questions. It usually makes both ethical and practical sense to involve the target population and/or the community at large in planning a community program. There are many good reasons for this involvement—fostering community ownership of the program, having the input of people with a sense of community history, respecting people enough to pay attention to what they say they need, and so on— but there can be drawbacks as well. What if you think the community's ideas are completely wrongheaded or they want more control over the program than you'd feel comfortable with? What are the ethical solutions to these situations?

The reality is that there aren't specific answers to most ethical ques-tions. It's important to consider the questions, but to understand that tak-ing what you see as the ethical path can sometimes land you in a briar patch. It helps to have clear sense of what you believe is right, and to also consider carefully what will actually benefit the situation and the people involved.

In the case of community participants giving wrongheaded advice, for instance, is the principle of respecting the community's wishes more or less important than that of creating the most effective way to meet community needs? And which will be more likely to actually get the job done in the community? The answers will probably vary in different places and times.

DEFINING SERVANTHOOD AND SERVANT LEADERSHIP

The world is crying out for ethical and effective leadership that serves others, invests in their development and fulfills a shared vision. The world has been shown how to lead by people who gave examples of serving throughout many different generations and in many ways. On the one hand, the concept of *servant leadership* appears to be so complex as to defy simple definition—it is multidimensional, rich in hues, and wideranging in its meanings. Further, *servanthood* has been shown through numerous examples of both women and men (Gandhi, Martin Luther King Jr., Mother Teresa, etc.), especially in the church history. There are examples of persons who have given their entire lives in service. Many of these showed what it meant to do good deeds of kindness, sacrificing personal time and resources for others without ever expecting to be repaid. In the Christian world, for example, Jesus Christ gave the premier example of how one is to be a true servant, choosing to serve rather than be served. This is the embodiment of true servanthood. One writer sums it up this way: "The only greatness is the greatness of humility. The only distinction is found in devotion to the service of others...there is in man a disposition to esteem himself more highly than his brother, to work for self, to seek the highest place, and often this results in evil surmising and bitterness of spirit" (White, 1970). Another term for servanthood is "stewardship." Stewardship, as with servanthood, involves service to others and being willing to share anything that might benefit another including skills, time, and talents. It elevates service above one's education, position, wealth, or fame.

Service, especially in community service, manifests itself in daily life only if a person chooses to lead by serving. So then, serving others fully is one of the most effective ways to "lead" them. Leading others moves the person serving into that of servant leadership. The CEOD model fully embraces this concept for use by PHPs.

Basically, service covers two areas: *servanthood* and *servant leadership*. With respect to servanthood aspects: The leader develops and empowers the community residents, who then, in turn, assist the leader to edify the community. The focus here is on the leader's *character* and *desire* to serve. Being just a service-oriented person, in the traditional notion of servanthood, does not qualify one as a servant leader. However, servanthood can be viewed as the first phase to servant leadership. Therefore, in servant leadership, the leader builds the community by effectively using people as resources; the emphasis here is on leadership skills, such as *vision-casting* and *team-building*. Effective PHPs should find themselves rotating back and forth in these two definitions.

For the purpose of this chapter will use the three terms of servanthood, servant leader, and PHP interchangeably. Thus, we will define servant leadership as: A leader whose primary purpose for leading is to serve communities by investing in their development and well-being for the benefit of accomplishing health-related tasks and goals for the improvement of the communities' overall quality of life (Wong & Page, 2003).

Scholars have observed that at the very heart of servant leadership is the genuine desire to serve others for the common good. In servant leadership, self-interest gives way to collective human development. In addition, servant leadership must not be seen as a model for weak leaders. As is inevitable in all leadership situations, the servant leader must be just as tough-minded and resilient as any other kind of leaders. What distinguishes servant leaders from other hierarchical styles of leadership is not only the quality of the decisions they make, but how they exercise their responsibility and whom they consult in reaching these decisions. Therefore, servant leadership is an "attitude" toward the responsibilities of leadership as much as it is a style of leadership (Hall, 1991) Hall, A. S. 1991. "Why a Great Leader." In K. Hall Living Leadership: Biblical Leadership Speaks to Our Day. Anderson, IN: Warner Press (14). Several authorities on servant leadership have suggested that to learn servant leadership, individuals need to undergo a journey of self-discovery and personal transformation. The secrets of servant leadership are gradually revealed to them through listening to their inner voices, as well as the voices of those who have discovered the truth. In spite of these caveats about understanding the true nature of servant leadership, we must nevertheless provide a clear and comprehensive view of servant leadership in order to properly measure its value.

Doing menial chores does not necessarily indicate a servant leader. Instead a servant leader is one who invests self in enabling others, in "helping them be and do their best." In addition, servant leadership should not be equated with self-serving motives to please community persons or to satisfy one's need for acceptance and approval. At the very heart of servant leadership is the genuine desire to serve others for the common good. In servant leadership, self-interest gives way to collective human development. Servant leadership must not be seen as a model for weak leaders or "losers." When the going gets tough or when difficult decisions have to be made, as is inevitable in all leadership situations, the servant leader must be just as tough-minded, passionate, and resilient as other kinds of leaders.

Servant leadership takes into account the fact that traditional forms of leadership are inadequate for motivating today's community residents.

For our purposes of the CEOD process, there are three basic elements that can assist the professionally trained PHP to be an effective servant leader. These include:

1. Character development
2. Engagement and involvement
3. Impacting community and culture

Let's briefly review each one of these elements.

Character Development

Leadership begins from within. Thus, *character development* is central to servant leadership. Character is what kind of people we are inside and out. In servant leadership, this means a fundamental commitment to serving others with integrity and humility. It is placed at the core of the circle because everything else a leader does flows from this inner reality. Followers demand it and leaders must live it. It is this fundamental attitude of servanthood that influences how leaders work with followers and how they carry out the task of leadership. Too often, leaders have been task- or process-oriented without the heart and passion for serving others.

True character breeds true commitment as an internal attribute. Commitment is a by-product of character, and it too comes from within. It is born of an "inner burn" to learn and to serve others. It, like character, is a "mustard seed" of *servanthood* and is a originator of the burning desire to help others, to engage and share with others, and to partner with them to improve their health status. Proof of commitment means that one pledges or vows to carry out the task to the fullest of his or her ability, and then demonstrates intent to carry out the task through subsequent behavior and action (Bender, 1997).

Engagement and Involvement

Akin to commitment is the "action" manifested by ongoing engagement, community involvement, and relationship building. Simply stated, these are commitment in action. It is taking the theoretical textbook definition of the terms and putting them to work. It is the putting of one's knowledge, attitudes, and skills into motion. Both call for the constant study and immersion of oneself into the day-to-day activities of the community targeted for public health service. It matters not whether one is planning to conduct a community health fair, design and implement a community-based research investigation, provide primary care services, or initiate an ongoing community-based health intervention program.

Genuine engagement and involvement can only be realized if there is ongoing evidence-based action. Just talking engagement and involvement is a far cry from the dynamic implementation called for by these terms.

Impacting Community and Culture

Students and practitioners of public health many times find themselves in uncharted terrain when they enter a new community or culture to pursue a health-related initiative. They are immediately faced with new symbols, values, languages, and ecological environments. The context of public health practice changes in an instant, right before their eyes. Servant leadership suggests that to truly be a leader, the PHP will need to undergo a journey of self-discovery and personal transformation. The components of servant leadership unfold to the student/ practitioner only through listening and learning, trial and error, and committed and consistent community involvement. Servant leadership incorporates the ideals of empowerment, total quality, team building, participatory management, and the service ethic into a leadership philosophy.

The concern that effective servant leadership means giving up power stems from the seeming oxymoron that one can be a humble servant and at the same time wield a big stick. This apparent contradiction in terms can be easily resolved by recognizing that effective servant leaders use a variety of social skills techniques and they will resort to only coercive power in dealing with immature and irresponsible individuals or institutions. Leaders who are opposed to the sharing power and/ or empowering others fear that these others may use this new-found freedom and power against their leadership. In order to feel secure in their position, they resort to subversive, unethical, and coercive tactics to keep control.

TRUST AND LEADERSHIP

In the CEOD process, the concept and practice of "trust" is an imperative component to the leadership credibility and community service. It is the bedrock upon which all other community ingredients are laid. PHPs do well to understand that this component takes time and effort to establish, but it is an essential ingredient in the success or failure to deliver evidence-based community health services of all types.

As a servant leader, one's word is one's bond. Thus, in the whole trust-building rubric, one can and must deliver on promises made, both in the short and long run. Community residents expect, and deserve, delivery on promises made. In many instances, health professionals are determined to get what they want out of communities no matter what they have to say or do to get it. In the long run, they promise to come back into the community to assist with environmental clean up efforts, or to mentor young people, or provide health lectures at the community church. However, many times and more often than not they leave and never return. Trust plays a central role in building all public health and medical relationships with communities, and is an important contributor to positive therapeutic outcomes. In medical practice and research protocols, lack of patient trust is associated with less doctor–patient interaction, poor clinical relationships that exhibit less continuity, reduced adherence to recommendations, worse self-reported health, and reduced utilization of health care services. African Americans' relatively lower trust in the health care system puts them at greater risk of all these negative outcomes. Distrust of research and researchers is commonly believed to be a major, ongoing impediment to minority participation. African Americans, in particular, have many reasons to distrust the medical research enterprise. These reasons include the persistence of racially segregated medical facilities in the 1960s and the infamous Tuskegee Syphilis Study. In that 40-year study, federally funded investigators, in the name of understanding how syphilis behaved in African Americans, purposefully withheld effective treatment from infected African American men. The study was finally stopped in 1972 after a whistleblower divulged the story to the press (Gamble, 1997).

Some might wonder whether these decades-old events still affect attitudes today. In the current era of the Belmont Report, the federal Office for Human Research Protections, and vigilant institutional review boards, does minority distrust in research still persist? In a recent issue of *Archives*, the study by Rajakumar and colleagues reminds us that it does. In a survey of parents visiting an academic pediatric clinic, African American parents expressed greater distrust in research than White parents did. Parental distrust was in turn associated with less positive attitudes toward research and less willingness to enroll children in a clinical study (Rajakumar, Thomas, Musa, Almario, & Garza, 2009). PHPs, as servant leaders, must fully understand what all this really means. Part of what it means is that they cannot just be presumptuous and "vanish into the hills" never to be seen or heard from again, once they have collected valuable data and gained valuable community experiences for themselves and/or their students. They must stay or return to follow-up and deliver on the promises made in the deal they struck with community residents during the days and weeks when they first engaged them. They must exit in a proper and respectful manner.

SUMMARY

PHPs and community leaders must have the courage to try new ideas and to encourage robust dialogue among politicians, administrators, companies, associations, and individuals. It is people that make the difference. So, it follows that the communities of the future need leaders of the future. The number-one task for today's and tomorrow's public health leaders is to "put people first." They must develop an ethical, trustworthy leadership style that addresses the needs of both the institutions they represent and the community residents they need to serve. This can make both groups happy by fulfilling their dreams and visions. PHPs as leaders, therefore, have one of the future's most important roles. They have the opportunity to create growth and development for the broadest number of individuals with a stake in the future. The interesting paradox with leadership is the relationship between leading and following: If no one is leading, no one can follow; and if no one is following, no one is leading. These two statements underline that leadership is relationship based. Therefore, the PHP must be a creative leader with a passion for the public health task at hand. The successful PHP will seek to integrate both strategic management (direction) and leadership (relationship) to provide the framework for success and the means to achieving it. They must learn to do this while also seeking to inspire and empower the culture they are serving.

Many PHPs tend to focus on the importance of translating the ideas and research findings of the institutions they represent, rather than defining the culture of the community and translating its intelligences and resources back to the institution. PHPs as leaders will need to find a balance between maintaining the existing culture of the community they seek to serve, while simultaneously translating new ideas and research methodologies designed and espoused by their respective institutions. They must create "opportunity space" where community residents and institutions compromise for the good of the community's health. Further, PHPs will need to set a clear vision for the future, and help steer the community, and their institution, toward realistic public health evidence-based outcomes. As servant leaders, they must forecast and interpret trends and create opportunities for growth and development. Similarly, they must respond to the global, national, and local challenges to help sustain a high quality of life for community residents. They have a key servant leadership role to play in developing the strong brand and rich cultural scene, which can elevate communities into the future.

Successful servant leaders do not place themselves at the center; they place others there. They do not seek the attention of people; they give it to others. They do not focus on satisfying their own aims and desires; they look for ways to respond to the needs and interests of their constituents. They seek to serve a purpose and the people who have made it possible for them to lead. In serving a purpose, leaders strengthen credibility by demonstrating that they are not in it for themselves; instead, they have the interests of the institution, department, or team and its constituents at heart. Being a servant may not be what many PHP leaders had in mind when they chose to take responsibility for the community public health vision and/or the direction of their organization or team, but ethical, trustworthy, and passionate service to others is the most glorious and rewarding of all leadership tasks.

Case Study Exercises

Individually, or as a group, review the following case study and follow the exercises suggested at the end of the study, as appropriate. Be sure to focus on the why, how, and what emphasized in each exercise. Your professor/instructor will provide you with specific guidance on how you are to report your findings for the class.

Case Study 3.1: Situational Ethics and Leadership

One difficulty in practicing ethics and servant leadership in America is that we are in a culture of individualism and competitiveness, which foster egotistic pride. The Founding Fathers were correct in creating a system of checks and balances, because they were fully aware of the dangers of egotism and corruption of power. Individualism coupled with authoritarian hierarchy has proven to be a fertile ground for egotistical, arrogant leaders.

When there is no trust, ethics, and checks and balances, self-serving leaders are free to elevate themselves and expand their territory of influence. Such egotistical leaders can be found mostly in many research institutes and other organizations. The celebrity syndrome, the pedestal syndrome, and rankism are just some of the symptoms of egotism running rampant in hierarchical organizations. The leaders exude power and success and carry themselves as the "king of the hill." They demand to be the center of attention and claim credits, which are due to others. They will use whatever means necessary to achieve numerical and material success, just as they will do anything to perpetuate their grip on power. Egotism is contradiction to servanthood, which is based on self-giving rather than self-serving.

Study Exercises

1. Describe how you and your team would go about serving communities in an ethical and trustworthy manner.
2. List the steps you would take to establish and engage yourself with this community.
3. Describe how you would convince your health institution that "servant leadership" is a key means in implementing community-based public health practice.
4. Describe how you would go about exiting a community in an ethical way after completing your public health work there.

REFERENCES

Bender, P. U. (1997). *Leadership from within.* Toronto, ON: Stoddart.

Bok, S. (1999). *Lying: Moral choice in public and private life.* New York, NY: Vintage.

Dass, R., & Gorman, P. (1985). *How can I help: Stories and reflections on service.* New York, NY: Knopf.

Fried, C. (1978). *Right and wrong.* Cambridge, MA: Harvard University Press.

Greenleaf, R. K. (1991). *The servant as leader.* Indianapolis, IN: The Greenleaf Center, p.30.

Greenleaf, R. K. (1977). *Servant leadership: A journey into the nature of legitimate power and greatness.* New York, NY: Paulist Press.

Hall, A. S. (1991). Why a great leader. In K. Hall (Ed.), *Living leadership: Biblical leadership speaks to our day* (p. 14). Anderson, IN: Warner Press.

Hall, M. A., Dugan, E., Zheng, B., & Mishra, A. K. (2001). Trust in physicians and medical institutions: What is it, can it be measured, and does it matter? *Milbank Quarterly, 79,* 613–639.

Kouzes, J., & Posner, B. (1993). *Credibility: How leaders gain and lose it, why people demand it.* San Francisco, CA: Jossey-Bass, p. 185.

McKnight, J. (1995). *The careless society: Community and its counterfeits.* New York, NY: Basic Books.

Mechanic, D., & Schlesinger, M. (1996). The impact of managed care on patients' trust in medical care and their physicians. *JAMA, 275,* 1693–1697.

Musa, D., Schulz, R., Harris, R., Silverman, M., & Thomas, S. B. (2008, October 15). *Trust in the health care system and the use of preventive health services by older Black and White adults.* Retrieved from http://dx.doi.org/10.2105/AJPH.2007.123927.

Pearson, S. D., & Raeke, L. H. (2000). *Patients' trust in physicians: Many theories, few measures, and little data. Journal of General Internal Medicine, 15,* 509–513.

Public Health Leadership Society. (2002). *Principles of the ethical practice of public health.* Version 2.2. Atlanta, GA: Centers for Disease Control and Prevention.

Singer, P. (1993). *Practical ethics.* Cambridge, England: Cambridge University Press.

The National Commission for the Protection of Human Subjects of Biomedical and Behavioral Research. (1979, April 18). *Belmont Report. Ethical principles and guidelines for the protection of human subjects of research.* The Superintendent of Documents, U.S. Government Printing Office, Washington, D.C

Thom, D. H., Hall, M. A., & Pawlson, G. (2004). Measuring patients' trust in physicians when assessing quality of care. *Health Affairs, 23,* 124–132.

BIBLIOGRAPHY

Gamble, V. N. (1997). Under the shadow of Tuskegee: African Americans and health care. *American Journal of Public Health, 87*(11), 1773–1778.

Rajakumar, K., Thomas, S. B., Musa, D., Almario, D., & Garza, M. A. (2009). Racial differences in parents' distrust of medicine and research. *Archives of Pediatrics & Adolescent Medicine, 163*(2), 108–114.

White, E. (1970). Servant of servants. In *Desire of ages* (p. 380). Boise, ID: Pacific Press Publishing.

Wong, P. T., & Page, D. (2003, October). *Servant leadership: An opponent process model.* Langley, BC: 1 Servant Leadership Roundtable Trinity Western University.

4

Culture Competency and CEOD Process: Immigrant Populations, Health Care, Public Health, and Community

Emanuel Joseph and Frederick G. Murphy

LEARNING OBJECTIVES

What you can learn by studying this chapter:

- How to define culture
- What culture is in real life
- The importance of establishing relationships between different cultures
- The impact of 21st-century immigration trends in cultural change
- How to create organizations in which diverse groups can work together for better community health status
- To identify current demographic challenges and trends in the United States
- What the historical basis is behind trends
- To understand the role and impact of nativity, language, culture, and personal characteristics among immigrant populations
- To understand the role of assimilation in absorption of immigrants into the American "mainstream" and the limitations of that process
- To identify the difference between cultural competence and cultural humility in working with immigrant populations and different cultures

Relationships are powerful. Our one-to-one connections with each other are the foundation for change. And building relationships with people from different cultures, often many different cultures, is key in building diverse communities that are powerful enough to achieve significant goals.

Whether you want to make sure your children receive a good education, or you want bring quality health care into your communities or promote economic development, there is a good chance you will need to work with people from several different racial, language, ethnic, or economic groups. And in order to work with people from different cultural groups effectively, you will need to build sturdy and caring relationships based on trust, understanding, and shared goals (see also Chapter 3 on ethics and service).

Why? Simple; trustworthiness in relationships is the glue that holds people together as they work on common problems. As people work on challenging problems, they will have to hang in there together when things get hard. They will have to support each other to stay with an effort, even when it feels discouraging. People will have to resist the efforts of those who use divide-and-conquer techniques—pitting one cultural group against another.

Whether your origin is Latino, Caribbean, Chinese, Korean, Vietnamese, African, Caucasian Protestant, Irish Catholic, Jewish, or any other racial, ethnic, religious, or socioeconomic group, many times the community engagement, organization and development process calls for establishing relationships with people whose group you may know very little about.

Each cultural group is unique, just as each individual is unique. Each one of us can build relationships and friendships around ourselves that provide us with the necessary strength to achieve community goals. If each person builds a network of diverse and strong relationships, they can come together and solve problems that we have in common. One must ask themselves: Why is culture important?

Culture is a strong part of people's lives. It influences their views, their values, their humor, their hopes, their loyalties, and their worries and fears. If you are from New Mexico or Montana; if your parents are Cambodian, French Canadian, or Native American; if you are German Catholic or African American; if you are Jewish or Mormon; if you are straight or gay; if you are a mixture of cultures, your culture has affected you. So when you are working with people and building relationships with them, it helps to have some perspective and understanding of their cultures.

At the same time, we can't pretend that our cultures and differences don't matter. We can't gloss over differences and pretend they don't exist, wishing that we could be alike. And we can't pretend that discrimination doesn't exist.

There are many benefits to diversity, such as the rich resource of alternative ideas for how to do things, the opportunity for contact with people from all cultures and nationalities that are living in your community, the aid in strategizing a quick response to environmental change, and a source for hope and success in managing our work and survival.

This chapter will discuss and provide practical information for practicing health professionals to better define what culture is, understand culture in real life, understand the importance of establishing relationships between persons from different cultures, explore the impact of 21st-century immigration trends in cultural change, and recognize the importance of creating organizations in which diverse groups can work together for better community health status.

DEFINING AND EXPLORING CULTURE

Culture is a complex concept, with many different definitions. But, simply stated, "culture" can be defined as a group or community with whom one shares common experiences that shape the way they understand the world. It includes groups that they are born into, such as gender, race, national origin, class, or religion. It can also include groups they become part of as they move through life. For example, one can take on a new culture by entering or moving to a new community or district, or by a change in economic status, or by a change in one's health status. How might this apply to you as a public health practitioner (PHP)?

In the 19th century, the term *culture* was commonly used as a synonym for Western *civilization*. The British anthropologist Sir Edward B. Taylor (1871) popularized the idea that all societies pass through developmental stages, beginning with "savagery," progressing to "barbarism," and culminating in Western "civilization." It's easy to see that such a definition assumes that Western cultures were considered superior. Both Western cultures, beginning with ancient Greece, and Eastern cultures, most notably imperial China, believed that their own way of life was superior. The study of multiple cultures without imposing the belief that Western culture was the ultimate goal was slow to develop.

Cultures are not synonymous with countries. Cultures do not respect political boundaries. For example, border cities such as Juarez, El Paso, Tijuana, and San Diego can develop cultures that in some ways are not like Mexico or the United States. In this context, other definitions of culture can include the following: a community or population sufficiently large enough to be self-sustaining, that is, large enough to produce new generations of members without relying on outside people; or a group or community that shares common experiences that shape the way its members understand the world. When one thinks of culture this broadly one realizes one can belong to many cultures at once (Jandt, 2007).

The totality of a group's thought, experiences, and patterns of life evolves through contact with other cultures. Hofstede (1994) classified these elements of culture into four categories: symbols, rituals, values, and heroes.

Symbols refer to verbal and nonverbal language.
Ritual is the socially essential collective activities within a culture.
Values are the feelings not open for discussion within a culture about what is good or bad, beautiful or ugly, normal or abnormal, which are present in a majority of the members of a culture or at least in those who occupy pivotal positions.
Heroes are the real or imaginary people who serve as behavior models within a culture. A culture's heroes are expressed in the culture's myths, which can be the subject of novels and other forms of literature (Rushing & Frentz, 1978). Rushing (1983) has argued, for example, that an enduring myth in U.S. culture, as seen in films, is the rugged individualist cowboy of the American West.

Collier and Thomas (1988) describe cultural identity, as the identification with and perceived acceptance into a group that has a shared system of symbols and meanings as well as norms for conduct. What does knowing an individual's cultural identity tell you about that individual? If you assume that that individual is like everyone else in that culture, you have stereotyped all the many, various people in that culture into one mold. Each individual knows that they are different from others in their culture. The diversity within cultures probably exceeds the differences between cultures. So just knowing one person's cultural identity doesn't provide complete or reliable information about that person. Knowing another's cultural identity does, however, help you understand the opportunities and challenges that each individual in that culture had to deal with.

One can have no direct knowledge of a culture other than their own. Experience with and knowledge of other cultures many times can be limited by the perceptual bias of one's own culture. An adult Venezuelan will never fully understand the experience of growing up a Japanese. To begin to understand a culture, one needs to understand all the experiences that guide its individual members through life: such things as language and gestures; personal appearance, environment, and so on.

Some define *subculture* or *co-cultures* as meaning "a part of the whole," in the same sense that a subdivision is part of—but no less important than—the whole community. Other scholars reject the use of the prefix *sub* as applied to the term *culture* because it seems to imply being under or beneath and being inferior or secondary. As an alternative, the word coculture is suggested to convey the idea that no one culture is inherently superior to any other coexisting culture (Orbe, 1998).

However, mutuality may not be easily established. Assume the case of homogeneous culture. One of the many elements of a culture is its system of laws. The system of laws in a hypothetical homogeneous culture, then, was derived from and reflects the values of that culture. Now assume immigration of another cultural group into the hypothetical culture. New immigrants may have different understandings of legal theory and the rights and responsibilities that individuals should have in a legal system.

Let's briefly define four concepts associated with culture.

Cultural knowledge means that you know about some cultural characteristics, history, values, beliefs, and behaviors of another ethnic or cultural group.

Cultural awareness is the next stage of understanding other groups—being open to the idea of changing cultural attitudes.

Cultural sensitivity is knowing that differences exist between cultures, but not assigning values to the differences (better or worse, right or wrong). Clashes on this point can easily occur, especially if a custom or belief in question goes against the idea of multiculturalism. Internal conflict (intrapersonal, interpersonal, and organizational) is likely to occur at times over this issue. Conflict won't always be easy to manage, but it can be made easier if everyone is mindful of the organizational goals.

Cultural competence brings together the previous stages—and adds operational effectiveness. A culturally competent organization has the capacity to bring into its system many different behaviors, attitudes, and policies and work effectively in cross-cultural settings to produce better outcomes. Cultural competence is nonthreatening because it acknowledges and validates who people are. By focusing on the organization's culture, it removes the need to place blame and assume guilt. Since becoming culturally competent focuses on the "how-to" of aligning policies and practices with goals, everyone is involved in the process. This "inside-out" model relieves the outsiders (or excluded groups) from the responsibility of doing all the adapting.

Building culturally competence means changing how people think about other cultures, how they communicate, and how they operate. It means that the structure, leadership, and activities of an organization must reflect many values, perspectives, styles, and priorities. Changing how an organization looks is only the first step. A culturally competent organization also emphasizes the advantages of cultural diversity, celebrates the contributions of each culture, encourages the positive outcomes of interacting with many cultures, and supports the sharing of power among people from different cultures. To really change, an organization has to commit to continuing programming, evaluation, and the creation of a place that is inclusive of all cultures and celebrates diversity. Benefits of building an organization's cultural competence include the following:

- Increases respect and mutual understanding among those involved
- Increases creativity in problem solving through new perspectives, ideas, and strategies
- Decreases unwanted surprises that might slow progress
- Increases participation and involvement of other cultural groups
- Increases trust and cooperation
- Helps overcome fear of mistakes, competition, or conflict. For instance, by understanding and accepting many cultures, everyone is more likely to feel more comfortable in general and less likely to feel the urge to look over their shoulders to be sure they are being "appropriate" in majority terms
- Promotes inclusion and equality

LEARNING CULTURES

It may seem odd that in order to learn about people in other cultures, one first needs to begin to become more aware of one's own culture. If a person hasn't had a chance to understand how his or her own culture has affected that person's life, it will likely be more difficult to understand how it could affect anyone else or why it might even be important to others. If one is comfortable talking about one's own culture, then one is more likely to become better at listening to others talk about theirs. Or, if one understands how discrimination has affected oneself personally, then one may be more aware of how it has affected others.

To begin to learn about one's own culture, or another culture, there are fundamental questions that should be explored. For example, these questions should include the following:

- Does one have a culture?
- Does one have more than one culture?
- What exactly is one's cultural background?

Even if one doesn't know who their ancestors are, they still have a culture. This stands true even if a person is a mix of many cultures. Culture evolves and changes all the time. It comes from ancestry from many generations before, and it comes from one's family and community today. For example, one's parents or grandparents almost certainly handed down values, customs, humor, and worldviews that played a role in shaping one's growing-up environment and life as it is today. Views toward family, work, health and disease, celebrations, and social issues are all influenced by heritage or by the experiences of family and community.

In addition to the cultural groups one belongs to, one also has some group with which one identifies, such as being a parent, an athlete, an immigrant, a small business owner, or a wageworker. These kinds of groups, although not exactly the same as a culture, have similarities to cultural groups. For example, being a parent and an immigrant may be an identity that influences how you view the world and how the world views you. Becoming aware of different identities can help one understand what it might be like to belong to a cultural group.

There are many ways that people can learn about other people's cultures and build relationships at the same time. Here are some examples/ steps one can take to do so:

1. Make a conscious decision to establish friendships with people from other cultures.
2. Put yourself in situations where you will meet people of other cultures.
3. Examine your biases about people from other cultures.

4. Ask questions about the cultures, customs, and views.
5. Read about other people's cultures and histories.
6. Listen and show caring.
7. Observe differences in communication styles and values; don't assume that the majority's way is the right way.
8. Risk making mistakes.
9. Learn to be an ally.

Let's now take a look at each of these in more detail.

Make a Conscious Decision to Establish Friendships With People From Other Cultures

Making a decision is the first step. In order to build relationships with people different from oneself, make a concerted effort to do so. There are societal forces that serve to separate individuals from each other. People from different economic groups, religions, ethnic groups, and races are often isolated from each other in schools, jobs, and neighborhoods. So, if one wants things to be different, one would need to take active steps to make them different.

You can join a sports team or club, ride the same rapid transit systems, become active in an community organization, volunteer, or even move into neighborhoods that puts one in direct and constant contact with people of cultures different from your own. Also, one may want to take a few minutes to notice the diversity that is presently nearby. If one begins to think about the people one sees and interact with everyday, one may become more aware of the cultural differences that exist.

Once the decision is made to make friends with people different from yourself, you can go forward and make friends with them in much the same way as with anyone else. It may take more time, and you may need to be more persistent, and reach out and take the initiative more than you are used to. People who have been mistreated by society may take more time to establish "trust" than those who haven't. There may be good reasons why people have built up defenses, but it is not impossible to overcome them and make a connection. This engagement effort is totally worth it.

Put Yourself in Situations Where You Will Meet People of Other Cultures

One of the first and most important steps is to show up in places where you will meet people of cultures other than your own. Go to meetings and celebrations of groups whose members you want to get to know. Or hang out in restaurants and other gathering places where different cultural groups go. You may feel embarrassed or shy at first, but your efforts will pay off. People of a cultural group will notice if you take the risk of coming to one of their events. If it is difficult for you to be the only person like yourself attending, you can bring a buddy with you and support each other in making friends.

Examine Your Biases About Other Cultures

We all carry misinformation and stereotypes about people in different cultures. Especially when we are young, we acquire this information in bits and pieces from TV, from listening to people talk, and from the culture at large. We are not bad people because we acquired this; no one requested to be misinformed. But in order to build relationships with people of different cultures, we have to become aware of the misinformation we acquired.

An excellent way to become aware of your own stereotypes is to pick groups that you generalize about and write down your opinions. Once you have, examine the thoughts that came to your mind and where you acquired them.

Another way to become aware of stereotypes is to talk about them with people who have similar cultures to your own. In such settings, you can talk about the misinformation you acquired without being offensive to people from a particular group. You can get together with a friend or two and talk about how you acquired stereotypes or fears of other different people. You can answer these kinds of questions:

- How did your parents feel about different ethnic, racial, or religious groups?
- What did your parents communicate to you with their actions and words?
- Were your parents friends with people from many different groups?
- What did you learn in school about a particular group?
- Was there a lack of information about some people?
- Are there some people you shy away from? Why?

Ask Questions About Cultures, Customs, and Views

People, for the most part, want to be asked questions about their lives and their cultures. Many of us were told that asking questions was nosy; but if we are thoughtful, asking questions can help you learn about people of different cultures and help build relationships. People are usually pleasantly surprised when others show interest in *their* cultures. If you are sincere and you can listen, people will tell you a lot.

For example, you might ask a person of African heritage if they want to be called Black or African American. Or you can ask a Jewish person what it is like for them at Christmas time when practically every store, TV commercial, and radio station focuses almost entirely on Christmas.

Read About Other Cultures and Histories

It helps to read about and learn about people's cultures and histories. If you know something about the reality of someone's life and history, it shows that you care enough to take the time to find out about it. It also gives you background information that will make it easier to ask questions that make sense.

However, you don't have to be an expert on someone's culture to get to know them or to ask questions. People who are, themselves, from a culture are usually the best experts anyway.

Listen and Care

It is easy to forget that the basis of any relationship is caring. Everyone wants to care and be cared about. Caring about people is what makes a relationship real. Don't let your awkwardness around cultural differences get in the way of caring about people. If one gets an opportunity to hear someone tell his or her life story first hand, much can be learned and a strong relationship built at the same time. Every person has an important story to tell. Each person's story tells something about his or her culture.

Listening to people's stories, we can get a fuller picture of what people's lives are like, their feelings, their nuances, and the richness of their lives. Listening to people also helps us get through our numbness—there is a real person before us, not someone who is reduced to stereotypes in the media.

Additionally, listening to members of groups that have been discriminated against can give us a better understanding of what that experience is like. Listening gives us a picture of discrimination that is more real than what we can get from reading an article or listening to the radio.

Observe Closely Differences in Communication Styles and Values

We all have a tendency to assume that the way that most people do things is the acceptable, normal, or right way. As community workers, we need to learn about cultural differences in values and communication styles, and not assume that the majority way is the right way to think or behave.

Risk Making Mistakes

As you are building relationships with people who have different cultural backgrounds than your own, you will probably make mistakes at some point. That happens. Don't let making mistakes keep you from going ahead and building relationships.

If you say or do something that is insensitive, you can learn something from it. Ask the affected person what you did that or offended them, apologize, and then go on in building the relationship. Don't let guilt bog you down.

Learn to Be an Ally

One of the best ways to help build relationships with people of different cultures is to demonstrate that you are willing to take a stand against discrimination when it occurs. People will be much more motivated to get to know you if they see that you are willing to take risks on their behalf.

We also have to educate ourselves and keep informed so that we understand the issues that each group faces and we become involved in their struggles instead of sitting on the sidelines and watching from a distance.

Trust is powerful. Servicing and caring for others is often what motivates one to make change(s). And establishing connections with people from diverse backgrounds can be key in making significant changes in any community.

The CEOD process is an essential approach to bring about change in communities for better health. It sets up neighborhoods and institutions in which people commit themselves to working to form strong relationships and alliances with people of diverse cultures and backgrounds. Also, it can help to establish networks and coalitions in which people are knowledgeable about each other's disparities and health concerns.

UNDERSTANDING CULTURE FOR CEOD

Communities throughout the United States are becoming increasingly diverse. The gentrification of the inner cities is rapidly integrating persons from all social and economic, ethnic, religious and racial strata. At the turn of the next century one out of every three Americans will be a person of color. Therefore, concepts such as racial profiling and stereotyping will become key discussion points when engaging and developing communities around public health practice. Profiling can be defined as a law enforcement practice of scrutinizing certain individuals based on characteristics thought to indicate a likelihood of criminal behavior. For example, it is believed that a person traveling alone is more likely to engage in terrorist activity. Profiling also refers to, for example, conducting traffic stops or airline screenings based on a person's perceived race, ethnicity, gender, or economic status. The September 11, 2001 attacks on the United States created an accelerated climate that gave law enforcement agencies wider latitude to engage in more intensive airport security checks of people who appear to be of Middle Eastern descent. The question then becomes: Is profiling a useful and necessary law enforcement tool, or is it a form of stereotyping that unfairly targets minorities?

Although one may consider stereotypes as being negative judgments, they can also be positive. Some people hold positive stereotypes of other individuals based on their professional group membership. For example, some people assume that all doctors are intelligent and wise.

Stereotypes can be harmful because they impede communication, engagement, and development in several ways:

1. They create assumptions that a widely held belief is true when it may not be.
2. Continued use of the stereotype reinforces the belief about certain groups. For example, stereotypes of women as ornaments, or people of color as being less intellectual or more licentious, or gay men as promiscuous.
3. Stereotypes also impede communication when they cause one to assume that a widely held belief is true of any one individual.

It is becoming clear that in order to successfully engage, organize, and develop communities for improving public health conditions, and resolving high-risk health problems, health professionals will need to build strong alliances with different cultural groups. Additionally, nonmainstream groups must be brought into the center of all CEOD activities.

CEOD AND CULTURES OF THE FUTURE

People have very different views of what a multicultural society or community should be like or could be like. In the past few decades there has been a lot of discussion about what it means to live and work together in a society that is as diverse as ours. People struggle with different visions of a fair, equitable, moral, and harmonious society. They struggle with these kinds of questions: What do you think about these questions? Which issues do you struggle with? What other issues are important to you or your cultural group?

As you envision this kind of diverse community, you and your neighbors may want to consider these kinds of questions. These are some of the real and tough questions that people grapple with on a daily basis. These questions point to some of the tensions that arise as we try to build harmonious, active, and diverse communities in a country as a complex as ours.

There are no easy answers; we all must learn as we go. So, when attempting to determine what kind of community one envisions developing or even living in there are many questions that must be considered, or even answered before moving forward. For example, here are some questions that may help one to engage, organize, and develop a healthy community of the future:

- If you could have your ideal community right now what would it look like?
- If you can't have your ideal community right now, what will be the next steps in building the kind of cultural community you desire?

- Who lives in your community right now?
- What kinds of diversity already exist?
- How will diversity be approached in your community?
- What kinds of relationships are established between cultural groups?
- Are the different cultural groups well organized?
- What kind of struggles between cultures exists?
- What kind of struggles within cultural groups exists?
- Are these struggles openly recognized and talked about?
- Are there efforts to build alliances and coalitions between groups?
- What issues do different cultural groups have in common?

These are just a few of the questions that can get one thinking about how to build a healthy community.

CULTURE BUILDING AND CONTEXT

Contextualization is communicating or providing a service in such a way that it addresses the needs of the people it seeks to serve. While the PHP is free to reach out in different ways to different groups, this freedom to contextualize does not mean that respect, beneficence, and justice should in any way be compromised. While contextualization is not always easy, for the PHP to contextualize public health approaches, methods, and strategies without compromising content will take preparation, patience, and perseverance.

In the book *Healing into Action*, authors Cherie Brown and George Mazza list principles that, when put into practice, help create a favorable environment for building diverse communities.

In order for people to commit to working on diversity, every person needs to feel that they will be included and important. Whether the person is a Japanese American woman, a White man, a Jew, a gay person, an African American, an Arab American, a fundamentalist Christian, or speaks with an accent, has a disability, is poor, or is wealthy—each person needs to feel welcomed in the effort to create a diverse community. And each person needs to know that his or her culture is important to others.

Guilt doesn't work in fostering diversity. Blaming people as a way of motivating them is not effective. Shaming people for being in a privileged position only causes people to feel bad; it doesn't empower them to take action to change. People are more likely to change when they are appreciated and liked, not condemned or guilt-tripped.

Treating everyone the same may be unintentionally oppressive. Although every person is unique, some of us have been mistreated or oppressed because we are a member of a particular group. If we ignore these present-day or historical differences, we may fail to understand the needs of those individuals. Often people are afraid that recognizing differences will divide people from each other. However, learning about cultural differences can actually bring people closer together, because it can reveal important parts of each other's lives. It can show us how much we have in common as human beings.

People can take on tough issues more readily when the issues are presented with a spirit of hope. We are bombarded daily with newspapers and TV reports of doom and gloom. People have a difficult time functioning at all when they feel there is no hope for change. When you present diversity issues you can say things like, "This is an excellent opportunity to build on the strengths that this organization has," or "There is no reason why we can't solve this problem together."

Building a team around us is the most effective way of creating institutional and community change around diversity issues. You will be more effective if you have a group of people around you that works together closely. People often try to go it alone, but we can lose sight of our goals and then become discouraged when operating solo. It is important to take the time to develop strong relationships with a core of people, and then work together as a group.

Recognize and work with the diversity already present in what appear to be homogenous groups. In working to combat racism and other forms of oppression many people become discouraged when they are unable to create a diverse group. Start by recognizing differences in religion, sexual orientation, socioeconomics, parenting, and class backgrounds, which will help create a climate that welcomes differences. It will also lay the groundwork for becoming more inclusive.

To sum up this section, sometimes "speaking the truth" can have negative connotations, especially in these days and times. Speaking the truth nowadays can be very unpleasant and can even be viewed as an insulting, hard-hitting tactic of conveying the facts. But in many instances, it is not the "what" of the content as much it is the "how" the content is delivered. In public health, PHPs may be called upon to deliver important, yet stinging, health messages because they know the community needs to hear them. The challenge in the 21st century is to establish methods for addressing communities within the proper context and, therefore, the need for proper "contexualization" of all methods. This does not mean that respect, trust, justice, and all other fundamental truths required for working in disparate communities, or any others for that matter, should be compromised.

In working toward engaging, organizing, and developing diverse cultures or communities, there is much more to consider that cannot be covered here. Each PHP can help build healthy communities by engaging families, organizations, institutions, and neighborhoods. To this end, everyone can make a commitment not to remain isolated from those who are different.

THE DEMOGRAPHIC CHALLENGE: BIRTH DEARTH
OR POPULATION BOMB

Although the problem itself may be complex, the essence of the demographic challenge is rather simple: The United States will be a truly multicultural country in the 21st century whether we like it or not. The only
question unanswered is whether the country will embrace the future (and
the social and economic challenges thereof) or fight tooth and nail to preserve the status quo.

In 1987 conservative author and scholar Wattenberg released a book
called *The Birth Dearth* whose subtitle asks *What Happens When People
in Free Countries Don't Have Enough Babies?* The unstated but obvious
implication was that America and the Western world were on the verge
of being overrun, not simply by people from "nonfree" countries but
by (mostly) brown people who had no such problems "having enough
babies."[1]

In *The Birth Dearth*, Wattenberg cites the projection of demographers
Bouvier and Gardiner (1986) that the White European share of the U.S.
population will be no greater than 60% of the population by 2080. He was
off by about 30 years. Here are a few brief statistics.

Thirty-seven million Americans alive today were foreign born, and one
in five Americans is a first- or second-generation immigrant (U.S. Census
Bureau, 2010). Among the foreign born, nearly half were born in Latin
America, and almost one-third were born in Mexico. First generation
immigrants (or as designated in census terminology "foreign born") in
2009 comprised 12.5% of the U.S. population.

In the 2010 census, Hispanics (both immigrant and native born) made
up 16.3% of the U.S. population, compared to 12.5% in the 2000 census, the
largest increase of any ethnic group (see Table 4.1).

For the period from 2005 to 2050, new immigrants and their descen-
dants will account for 82% of the population increase. Births in the United
States (in contrast to immigration of the foreign born) will play a growing
role in Hispanic and Asian population growth. As a result, a smaller proportion of both groups will be foreign born in 2050 than is the case now.
The non-Hispanic White population will increase more slowly than other
racial and ethnic groups; Whites will become a minority (47%) by 2050.
Programs and social interventions will increasingly have to acknowledge
not only the increased "browning" of America, but the younger age of
these first- and second-generation immigrants.[2]

As of 2007, children of immigrants accounted for 22% of all American
children. Of these, eight out of 10 children are racial or ethnic minorities,
and 55% are Hispanic. Contrary to stereotype, 81% of children in immigrant families speak English very well; however only 37% of parents
report satisfactory English proficiency (Mather, 2009).

TABLE 4.1   Overview of Race and Hispanic Origin 2010

	2000 CENSUS	2010 CENSUS	CHANGE (%)
U.S. Population	281.4 million	308.7 million	+27.3 million (9%)
Non-Hispanic White	194.6 (69%)	196.8 (64%)	+2.3 (1.2%)
Hispanic	35.3 (12.5%)	50.5 (16.3%)	+15.2 (43%)
Black	34.7 (12.3%)	38.9 (12.6%)	+4.3 (12.3%)
Asian	10.2 (3.6%)	14.7 (4.8%)	+4.4 (43%)

Source: U.S. Census Bureau (2011).

Of those children under six years of age in immigrant families, 93% are U.S. citizens. For 29% of these children, however, at least one parent is an undocumented immigrant, often affecting the child's likelihood of receiving social benefits or medical coverage for which they are eligible (Capps, Fix, Ost, Reardon-Anderson, & Passel, 2005).

Many of these children are at risk for poverty, and four principal factors account for much of their risk of living in poverty: (1) parents' education, (2) parents' citizenship status, (3) length of time in the country, and (4) language proficiency. Poverty rates for immigrants range from 9% for children with none of these risk factors, to 48% for those children with all four (Mather, 2009).

Most immigrants in the United States are not here illegally. Although numerical estimates of undocumented immigrants are often controversial, most undocumented immigrants are recent arrivals, while most long-term residents have normalized their status. The Pew Hispanic Center estimated that there were about 11.2 million undocumented immigrants in the United States in 2010 (3.7% of the population), with 8 million of these in the workforce (5.2% of the workforce) (Passel & Cohn, 2011).

PEW HISPANIC CENTER DATA, 2003[3]: RECENT IMMIGRANTS RESIDENT IN THE UNITED STATES FEWER THAN 10 YEARS

Undocumented[4]	46%
Legal noncitizens	42%
Temporary residents	6%
Naturalized citizens	5%

RESIDENT IN THE UNITED STATES MORE THAN 10 YEARS

Undocumented	17%
Legal noncitizens	31%
Temporary residents	0%
Naturalized citizens	52%

IMMIGRATION POLICY AND PRACTICE IN THE
UNITED STATES: A HISTORICAL PERSPECTIVE

An understanding of the place of immigrants in American society and their human potential requires a brief review of American policy toward immigration and the role it has historically played in shaping the nature of U.S. immigration, both legal and illegal.

A timeline of contemporary U.S. immigration policy would have to consider at least four major events:

The McCarran Walter Act of 1952, conceived during the cold war, closed the door on many immigrants, and created the first comprehensive barrier to immigration since the 19th century Asian Exclusion Act. Related to this was the subsequent 1953 Refugee Relief Act creating a special category of immigration favoring refugees from Communist countries, affecting Cuban immigrants in particular.

The Hart-Cellar Act of 1965, signed by Lyndon Johnson during an era of increasing race and civil rights consciousness, repealed 1952 nationality quotas and set up a radically new immigration policy. This policy gave preferential treatment for family members, set hemispheric quotas, and liberalized employment preferences. It heralded a wave of legal immigration of working class migrants from the Caribbean, Asia, and Latin America. Ironically it had the reverse effect with respect to Mexican immigration, which no longer had favored status relative to other Latin American and Caribbean countries. Combined with the ending of the Bracero program[5] in 1964, the Mariel boatlift in 1980, and civil wars in El Salvador and Nicaragua, these actions had a direct and immediate effect of increasing illegal migration from Mexico, and from Central America through Mexico.

The 1990s legislative backlash occurred in response to increasing numbers (and visibility) of undocumented immigrants throughout the 1980s and 1990s. This anti-immigrant sentiment was focused primarily at Spanish-speaking immigrants—and more pointedly, at those from Mexico. Much of this reaction was notably focused on three key factors with life-altering impact on immigrants' health status: (1) jobs, (2) education, and (3) utilization of health care resources. A significant weapon in this war on illegal immigration was the Illegal Immigration Reform and Immigrant Responsibility Act of 1996. This federal law allowed for mandatory detention and periods of exclusion, and generally placed more severe sanctions on undocumented immigrants than had heretofore been the case. Along with the 1996 Personal Responsibility and Work Opportunity Reconciliation Act (more commonly called the 1996 Welfare Reform Act), these measures made undocumented immigrants ineligible for Medicaid, food stamps and welfare services, placed a 5-year bar on legal immigrants receiving Medicaid and other federal services (with the exception of emergency medical services covered by Medicaid), and required that sponsors of legal migrants commit to pay for Medicaid or other federal assistance received by legal immigrants. These measures, as far as health and social services access was concerned, appeared to deprive both legal and undocumented immigrants of needed health services (Fragomen, 1996; Okie, 2007; Pati & Dasnagoulian, 2008).[6]

After 13 years of this national policy, during which the ranks of uninsured swelled from 36.5 million in 1994 to 46.5 million in 2006, and uninsured immigrants increased from 8.8% to 12.8% of the total, Congress partially reversed itself. The 2009 CHIP Reauthorization Act (CHIPRA) dispensed with the prohibition banning newly arriving legal immigrants from receiving Medicaid for 5 years, but only as it relates to pregnant women and children, and only "allowed" but did not require states to offer services.

The events of September 11, 2001, closed the door on both legal and illegal immigration, and heralded a new wave of anti-immigrant sentiment. Although the process had started years before, the 9/11 crisis allowed anti-immigration activists to couch their arguments in terms of national security. Illegal immigration from Mexico became "the next great threat" to the country, and whatever national sentiment existed for immigration reform (including amnesty for those already residing in the U.S.) rapidly disintegrated. Among the new legislative proposals is one that would abolish the 14th Amendment of the Constitution guaranteeing citizenship to all persons born in the United States. This move targets the U.S.-born children of undocumented immigrants. The residual impact of the events of 9/11 on national attitudes and sentiment is still evolving.

THE RESPONSE OF NATIVE BORN TO IMMIGRANT: MELTING POT OR CAULDRON

America is coming to be, not a nationality, but a transnationality, a weaving back and forth of many threads of all sizes and colors. Any movement which attempts to thwart this weaving, or to dye the fabric any one color, or disentangle the threads of the strands, is false to this cosmopolitan vision.

—Randolph Bourne, "Trans-National America" (1916)

Nativist sentiment in the United States is neither a new idea nor novel in its actions. Nativism, defined as intense opposition to an internal minority on the grounds of its foreign connections (Higham, 1955), is understandably linked to racism and ethnocentrism, and has emerged variously over the years as pledges to "take our country back" and "exert control over our borders." Unfortunately, in this argument, sentiments are often divorced from reality (see, for example, Dittgen, 1997).

Connected to the concept of nativism is the principle of assimilation. However, where nativism has distinctly negative connotations, assimilation has (traditionally) not only been an acceptable sentiment, but one overtly championed as a necessary part of becoming American—the much vaunted American "melting pot." Under this rubric, America is a melting pot where different elements can "melt together" into a harmonious whole with a common culture. The metaphor (and its earlier incarnations) are centuries old.

While the American melting pot has remained a persistent feature of American folklore (as well as the manifesto of some serious-minded intellectuals), arguments questioning this vision of America have existed for almost as long. Bourne, as early as 1916 (long before any influx of Mexicans, Asians, or Africans), questioned the concept of an Anglo-Saxon America in a now classical essay called "Trans-National America." In it, he decries "hard-hearted old Brahmins virtuously indignant at the spectacle of the immigrant refusing to be melted," and calls for a trans-national America, able to accept a variety of immigrants without requiring they strip themselves of "the literature and cultural traditions of their homeland." Neither nativism nor ethnocentrism are new concepts in American thought or politics. In the 21st century they have simply taken on the added baggage of language and skin color.

Curiously, one aspect of the 21st-century world that Bourne could scarcely have imagined is the truly trans-national impact of America on the world. It seems oddly out of step for America to fear being overwhelmed by foreign influences when the United States is currently the source of a global cultural tsunami—American movies, sports, television personalities, fast-food, and on and on. The list is endless. Ironically, English is now so well established as the Lingua Franca of the business world (and popular culture) that French politicians are caught campaigning against American language hegemony.

A second aspect of transnationalism not envisioned in 1916 is that which is enabled and encouraged by modern transportation and communication. The immigrant in that era was separated from the native country by distance and time. Travel to the "homeland" and maintenance of a "foreign" culture were both equally difficult. There was, therefore, a rationale in adopting an American White Anglo-Saxon Protestant way of life. For today's immigrant, isolation from their country of nativity is not only unnecessary but illogical.

In this context, assimilation is not a process that starts when immigrants land in this country; it is an ongoing evolution that permeates globally.

HEALTH STATUS OF IMMIGRANT POPULATIONS

For be it remembered, these children, with the training they receive—or do not receive—with the instincts they inherit and absorb in their growing up, are to be our future rulers, if our theory of government is worth anything.

—Jacob Riis, *How the Other Half Lives* (1997)

A summary assessment of immigrant health status (if such is possible) would state that the health of immigrants is generally better than that of native-born Americans of the same race and ethnicity, often declines after migration, improves with the second-generation, and declines thereafter—the so-called "immigrant paradox." Because the immigrant population is quite heterogeneous, however, that summary statement requires some qualification.

Immigrants have been found to do better than native-born Americans over a wide range of specific health indicators—adult perinatal, and infant mortality; self-assessed health status; disability days; work-loss days and physician visits; and hospitalization rates[7] (Cunningham, Reuben, & Narayan, 2008; Lucas, Barr-Anderson, & Kington, 2003). Some cause-specific mortality rates are higher for immigrants—for example, stomach cancer and homicide—whereas other cause-specific rates are appreciably lower: cardiovascular disease, overall adjusted cancer mortality, prostate cancer, COPD, unintentional injuries, suicide and firearm injuries (Singh & Siahpush, 2001).

Considerable differences also exist between immigrant populations of different nativity—for example, Vietnamese women have a rate of cervical cancer that is higher than that of both Black and White women, and is about 6 times that of Japanese and Chinese women (Williams, 2002). Correspondingly, while immigrant women *as a group* have lower infant mortality rates than native-born, rates vary considerably by race, ethnicity and country of origin. For example, Liu and Laraque (2006) in New York City found that the immigrant's advantage over native-born was almost entirely due to Asian, European, and South American immigrants, whereas immigrants from Africa, Central America, and the Caribbean had infant mortality rates higher than the U.S. average, but lower than the average for U.S.-born Blacks. Mexican immigrants report lower self-assessed health status than other Hispanic immigrant groups, a difference that is moderated but not abolished by controlling for socioeconomic status (Akresh & Frank, 2008).

Compared to the U.S.-born population, immigrants tend to have more positive health behaviors and fewer negative health behaviors (Lucas et al., 2003; Singh & Siahpush, 2001). However, over successive generations (and in some cases, over time within a single generation), immigrants tend to become more American in likes, dislikes, culture, and practices. Thus, their socioeconomic status, health status, health behaviors, and health care utilization might be expected to also become more "American." This is true in some cases (Broman, Neighbors, Delva, Torres, & Jackson, 2008; Jackson et al., 2007; Williams et al., 2007) but in others is not quite so straightforward (Kalmijn, 1996; Singh, Kogan, & Yu, 2009). In particular, a drift toward the negative health characteristics of the host population is often found—adoption of poor diet, sedentary lifestyle, increased prevalence of drug use, and so on—a scenario some have attributed to negative effects of acculturation, and termed "unhealthy assimilation" (Antecol & Bedard, 2006).

What, then, is one to make of these disparities in health status? As a group, one could assume that the immigrant population is doing well. However, hidden in those reassuring statistics are some consistent patterns—language barriers play a large role in adverse heath outcomes, and immigrants from non-English-speaking countries tend to do less well when compared to English speaking immigrants (although there are exceptions, for example, among South American and European immigrants). Poverty appears to play an even greater role than language, and education likewise. Moreover, while socioeconomic status (SES) is often controlled for in evaluations of immigrant health, racial/ethnic differences often exist not only in socioeconomic status, but in its subcategories—"quality" of education, purchasing power of income, stability of employment, and health risks of working in a particular occupation (Williams & Collins, 1995).

In reality, the health status of current immigrants is very much tied to their progress in a number of overlapping dimensions, health care being only one, and in many respects not the most important one when compared to socioeconomic well-being. Working with these communities must therefore take a much broader view of "health" than might be necessary in dealing with more stable, more affluent individuals and communities.

THE IRONY OF HEALTH CARE FOR IMMIGRANTS: THE INEQUITY SURPRISE

As interns and residents, young doctors get their training by practicing on the hospital ward and clinic patients—generally non-white. Later they make their money by practicing for a paying clientele—generally white. White patients are "customers;" black patients are "teaching material." White patients pay for care with their money; black patients pay with their dignity and their comfort.

—Ehrenreich and Ehrenreich, *The American Health Empire* (1971)

Any evaluation of the health status of immigrants and children of immigrants in America necessarily requires attention to health care quality and health care access. These in turn raise the inevitable question of health insurance (public or private), which in America is unavoidably linked to an individual's chances of accessing any but the most basic services. A few statistics follow.

Recent census figures for 2009 place the total uninsured population at 50.7 million, including an estimated 676,000 elderly uninsured (65+ years of age), and 7.5 million uninsured children (Kaiser Commission on Medicaid and the Uninsured, 2010). While native-born Americans account for three-quarters of all uninsured, immigrants account for an estimated 12.3 million uninsured, or 26.6% of the total uninsured (Current Population Survey data, 2004–2006, cited in Fronstin, 2008). On average the uninsured incur less than half the annual health care costs of the insured ($1,668 in 2008 versus $4,463 per person for insured individuals); about one-third of that cost is paid for out of pocket by the uninsured (Kaiser Commission on Medicaid and the Uninsured, 2010).

Immigrants as a group spend only one-half to two-thirds the medical expenditure of native-born Americans, even when fully insured. When controlled for other factors, they averaged 14% to 20% less than the native born. Recent immigrants are responsible for a little more than 1% of public (governmental) expenditure on health care although they constitute 5% of the adult population (Ku, 2009). Contrary to stereotype, immigrants as a group are sparing users of health services.

With respect to the burden of the uninsured immigrant population, a mere four states—California, Texas, Florida, and New York—account for over half (58.8%) of the total of uninsured immigrants in the United States. These states also account for a significant proportion of uninsured in general—41% of the nonelderly uninsured (immigrant and native born) reside in these four states (Fronstin, 2008). In California, not only is the burden of the uninsured high (6.6 million), but 48% of their uninsured populace is accounted for by immigrants. California, as a whole, accounts for a 27.1% share of the nation's total uninsured immigrants.

Despite the common belief that immigrants drive up the cost of health care, the uninsured (immigrant and native born) are responsible for only 2% overall of the cost of health care in the United States ($57 billion in 2008, a not insignificant amount, but by no means a major contributor to the $2.4 trillion cost of U.S. health care in 2008 [Kaiser Commission on Medicaid and the Uninsured, 2010]).[8] Using the estimate of 26.6% of the uninsured being immigrants (Fronstin, 2008) means immigrants would account for approximately $15.2 billion of uncompensated care or 0.53% of total U.S. health care cost.[9] This total is slightly misleading since cost is not born equally, but falls disproportionately on the states with the highest proportions of immigrants. Moreover, 60% of uninsured costs are born by hospitals, and among hospitals the burden is similarly not shared equally, but invariably borne by a handful of "charity hospitals" and inner city hospitals serving the poor and near poor.

Concern for the health of immigrants cannot be divorced from concern for the children of immigrants. An almost universal article of faith held by immigrants (legal and illegal) is belief in a better life for their children. From a public health perspective, the objective of keeping children healthy is both altruistic and one of self-interest. There can be only limited improvement in the health status of the nation at large without success in addressing health disparities.[10] And there can be no success in addressing disparities without including the immigrant populations in this "nation of immigrants" (Hernandez & Charney, 1998; Mahoney, 2004; Portes & Rumbaut, 2001; Telles & Ortiz, 2008).

Most private health insurance in the United States is employer-provided. However, only 39% of noncitizen immigrants have employer-provided health care, whereas 64% of native-born and 64% of foreign-born U.S. citizens do, largely because new immigrants are disproportionately employed in low-income occupations that do not provide health insurance[11] (Carrasquillo, Carrasquillo, & Shea, 2000).

Ironically, immigrants who lack insurance are faced with a contradictory costing mechanism that few are familiar with from their native countries. Because insurance companies negotiate rates with providers and hospitals, patents *with* insurance are charged significantly less than those *without* insurance. This results in the somewhat incongruous (and definitely illogical) situation where those least able to pay are charged the most. For example, Anderson (2007) found rates charged to uninsured and self-pay patients were often 2.5 times rates charged to insured patients, and more than three times Medicare allowable charges.[12] Because "nobody actually pays billed charges" this inequity is justified (or so the argument goes). Unfortunately, the argument fails to ask what happens to the self-paying patient who, for reasons of conscience or culture, feels obligated to pay what was charged.

The 2010 Health Reform Law (Patient Protection and Affordable Care Act of 2010) is expected to expand health care coverage to significant numbers of poor uninsured, mainly through expansion of Medicaid and CHIP programs and subsidies for insurance premiums, but will not provide any provision for medical care to undocumented immigrants and maintains most of the existing prohibitions from the 1996 Illegal Immigration Reform and Immigrant Responsibility Act, and the Welfare Reform Act of 1996. Barring any unexpected change in legislation, the health care status of immigrants is expected to remain in limbo for the foreseeable future.

GENERATIONAL DIFFERENCES AND GENERATIONAL CHANGE: ASSIMILATION—YES OR NO?

Traditional thinking with respect to immigrant assimilation has historically proposed that over successive generations, immigrants become more closely approximated to the host population, progressively erasing deficits in educational attainment, economic achievement and health status along seven dimensions—cultural, structural, marital, identity, prejudice, discrimination, and civic assimilation (Gordon, 1964). Unfortunately, while this model might hold true for successive generations of European immigrants, its validity has been questioned with respect to major Segments of today's immigrant populations, as documented in exhaustive detail by Portes and Rumbaut (2001) and Telles and Ortiz (2008). Asian and White

Europeans consistently appear to fare better than other immigrants of color, both in health and socioeconomic spheres. This disparity exists even when factors such as schooling and parental education are controlled.

Among generations of Hispanic immigrants there is a ready explanation for their inability to do well. Whether one accepts the view or not, one can easily identify language, parent's education, and immigration status—so-called "social capital"—as factors that probably are responsible for their failure to do well.[13] This hypothesis, applied to the Cuban American experience, however, presents a mixed picture: Cuban Americans in Miami are an ethnic enclave of immigrants who are not native English speakers. Cuban Americans have had a number of advantages, however. As professionals fleeing communist Cuba, the first Cuban immigrants were highly educated and highly entrepreneurial, two significant contributors to social capital. Additionally, Miami's post-1960 Cuban immigrants were granted refugee status, making them eligible for federal assistance, training, and resettlement programs not available to other immigrant groups—more social capital. So, as described by Portes and Rumbaut (2006): "Instead of complaining about discrimination or arguing about minority rights, Cubans laid claim to the city."

As a result, Cuban Americans are the most successful Hispanic group, both politically and economically. Although doing better than other Hispanics, however, they still rank lower in income, occupation, and education levels than the American average (Boswell, 2002). Moreover, assimilation does not seem to have included overcoming the ethnic enclave.

Among Asian immigrants, East Indian, Chinese, and Korean immigrants likewise do significantly better than Vietnamese, Laotians, and Cambodians, again largely attributable to differences in social capital—education level, employability in high-wage jobs, and language competency. These allow the former group upward mobility and the latter a legacy of social and economic marginalization (Uba, 1994).

Telles and Ortiz's 35-year follow-up of the 1965 Mexican American Study Project is a particularly important signpost because it follows an immigrant cohort through four individual generations, assessing the U.S.-born children of U.S.-born parents and grandparents. Most analyses aggregate these "children of immigrants" as part of the native-born comparison group. Telles and Ortiz's analyses, however, confirm a failure of traditional assimilation among later generations, with most improvement shown in the second generation and deterioration or stagnation in subsequent generations. Contrary to assimilation theory, they found generation since immigration did not improve socioeconomic status (Telles & Ortiz, 2008).

For immigrant Blacks, assimilation often means absorption into the African American mainstream. For many West Indian Blacks, with an awareness of American prejudices and the limited social standing of American Blacks, that is not an option. Hence, the tendency of first and second generation West Indians is to cling to their ethnic self-identity (Foner, 2001; Kasinitz, 1992; Waters, 1999); hence, also, the appeal of conservative (and some radical) intellectuals who identify West Indians as a separate subcategory from African Americans, possessed of greater ambition, education, initiative, and drive (Sowell, 1984; Williams, 1982; Wilson, 1978). While this may have been true for early West Indian immigrants (and there is some doubt in that respect), it is probably less characteristic of the later immigrant wave (see also Farley & Allen, 1989).

In contrast to Gordon's linear model of assimilation, others have outlined a model of "segmented assimilation," most prominently, Alba and Nee (1997, 2003; Portes & Rumbaut, 2001). This theorizes that rigid boundaries—most significantly racism and ethnicity—place a limit on some groups' ability to fully integrate into the American mainstream, while other factors, such as human capital, urbanization, and the extent of spatial segregation, also affect the likelihood of assimilation. Thus, not all immigrants can be expected to assimilate into American society at the same rate, or to the same extent (Telles & Ortiz, 2008).

Finally, there is "downward assimilation." This option is available when other options are not. Thus, the adoption of a counterculture life-style—dropping out of school, drug use, gang membership, an adversarial social outlook, teen pregnancy, and crime. This is most likely an outlook to be found in second or third generations who do not share their parents' willingness to work long hours in low-paying jobs, but who lack the social capital for upward mobility. This is the least desirable outcome of assimilation.

The American dream beckons us. In the words of James Banks, "Our nation's motto is e pluribus unum—out of many, one." The changing ethnic texture of the United States intensifies the challenge of educating citizens and creating an authentic unum that has moral authority. An authentic unum reflects the experiences, hopes, and dreams of all the nation's citizens. An imposed unum, the kind that has existed throughout most of the nation's history, reflects one dominant cultural group. Our challenge, in this 21 century, is to establish an authentic unum that has moral authority and yet create moral, civic, and just communities in which citizens from diverse racial, ethnic, and cultural communities will participate and to which they will have allegiance.

EFFECTING CHANGE AND ESTABLISHING DIALOGUE: ORGANIZATION AS EDUCATION

...Dialogue cannot exist without humility. The naming of the world, through which men constantly re-create the world, cannot be an act of arrogance.

Dialogue, as the encounter of men addressed to the common task of learning and acting, is broken if the parties (or one of them) lack humility. How can I dialogue if I always project ignorance onto others and never perceive my own?

Paulo Friere, *Pedagogy of the Oppressed* (1986)

Previous chapters have already outlined both the theoretical and practical framework for successful community organization and development. The specific needs of immigrant populations (first generation and subsequent generations) in many ways mirror the approaches necessary for working with U.S.-born minorities. Central to this is "cultural competency," a well-intentioned concept that unfortunately has now achieved the status of a buzz-word.

Much independent research has been published during recent years addressing health inequities, both with respect to native-born minorities and immigrants. Predictably, this abundance of research and reports, documenting glaring disparities that "are with few exceptions, remarkably consistent across a range of illnesses and health care services," has evoked some criticism, deriding it as "... a data deluge that has led many observers to suggest that it is time to stop documenting disparities and turn our efforts to doing something about them" (Lurie, 2005).

While the 2003 Institute of Medicine report—*Unequal Treatment: Confronting Racial and Ethnic Disparities in Health Care*—does address "cross-cultural communication," it does so mainly within the context of the clinical encounter, and largely within the setting of formal medical education. It offers three possible alternatives: the conventional approaches of enhancing knowledge (the multicultural/categorical approach) or attitudes (the sensitivity/awareness approach), and a more current approach, focusing on "tools and skills" (the cross-cultural approach). While it acknowledges that very little has been published on the impact of these training approaches, it does stress that the attitudes necessary for cross-cultural care "are those central to professionalism—humility, empathy, curiosity, respect, sensitivity, and awareness of all outside influences *on the patient.*" [emphasis added] This emphasis on humility and empathy has since become a recurring theme.

Without overtly acknowledging it, many of today's efforts to enhance "cultural competence" owe a practical, if not ideological, debt to Paulo Friere. His approach to working with rural peasants in Brazil four decades ago (minus its Marxist rhetoric) is often mirrored in current paradigms of cultural competency (see also Casale & Clancy, 2009).

Friere terms the traditional approach to education (and here one can insert "traditional health education" or "traditional doctor-patient relationship") the banking concept of education, wherein the student (community member/patient) is a "receptacle" to be "filled" by the teacher (health educator/doctor). In this paradigm, he notes: "The teacher teaches and the students are taught; the teacher knows everything and the students know nothing; the teacher thinks and the students are thought about; the teacher talks and the students listen—meekly" (1986, p. 59).

The alternative—*authentic education*—is characterized by humility, and "...is not carried about by 'A' *for* 'B' or by 'A' *about* 'B,' but rather by 'A' *with* 'B,'..." (Friere, 1986, p. 82). This is a concept that is easy to enunciate, harder to implement. One attempt to do so is the process of practicing cultural competency by embracing *cultural humility*.

Cultural humility has been described as a process of cultural competence "...defined not by a discrete endpoint but as a commitment and active engagement in a lifelong process that individuals enter into on an ongoing basis with patients, communities, colleagues, and with themselves" (Brown, quoted in Tervalon & Murray-Garcia, 1998). It is a process that, by definition, cannot be limited to the individual but needs to include social context and a community approach that considers, and works toward, a concept of community health and well-being, rather than mere diagnosis and treatment of disease.

A necessary component to this lifelong learning process or "dialogue" is the question of humility—not to negate the knowledge base of the physician/health educator or community organizer but to allow for the merest possibility of relevant knowledge in the patient/community/individual. Integral to this approach is a deliberate and conscious attitude of self-reflection and humility. Indeed, as Tervalon notes, "...an isolated increase in knowledge without a consequent change in attitude and behavior is of questionable value." At the community level, this calls for "mutually beneficial, nonpaternalistic and respectful working relationships with community members and organizations" (Tervalon & Murray-Garcia, 1998). In this setting, stereotypes can be avoided, and interactions between the health care provider and patient or community can take place not merely in a single dimension (teacher/student) but in a multidimensional context. Ridley (1995) gives a useful example of how such a multidimensional picture can be painted. Consider (for example) a Mexican American who is not simply an ethnic cutout, but holds "conjoint membership in eight cultural roles...as a Mexican American, male, father, husband, Catholic, mechanic, night-school student, and resident of East Los Angeles" (Ridley, 1995, quoted in Tervalon & Murray-Garcia, 1998).

Culture (and thus cultural competency) is *never* one-dimensional. Like the Mexican American/Catholic/student/mechanic above, personal culture is shaped "not only by our ethnicity and skin color, but also by our class, age, experiences, physical abilities, gender, language(s), religion, politics, education, sexual orientation, socioeconomic status, and residential status" (California Health Advocates, 2007). Understandably this approach is especially germane in any attempt to deal constructively with immigrant groups, just as it is with individuals.

The process of listening, if it is to be genuine, may need to delay or divert goals and objectives that health professionals or planners may have. It may require fluidity not only in methods to achieve an objective, but perhaps reexamination of the objectives themselves, not an easy task in grant-funded or time-limited projects.

There is also an alternative approach. That is an approach to cultural competency that consists of "a veritable laundry list of traditional beliefs and practices ostensibly characteristic of particular ethnic groups" (Hunt, 2001). Such pigeonholing by race or ethnicity does nothing to promote dialogue, and ironically, often promotes community passivity and reinforces stereotypes. The negative impact becomes magnified when information is not only stereotypical, but wrong.

What, therefore, can be done in concrete terms? A number of tested alternatives have been suggested: The formation of ethnic mutual assistance associations (MAAs) is one of several possible community strategies, as is a role for ethnically based service providers (EBSPs). Moreover, since these approaches are not mutually exclusive, there are also complementary roles for more traditional organizational structures—such as traditional community organizations, immigrant rights organizations, and crossover organizations (Applied Research Center, 2002). Where numbers and status allow, organized political advocacy and direct political representation are a possible step toward formal participation in the political system. In the current political landscape, this could be a potent addition to a community's toolkit (see, for example, Rogers, 2006).

Mutual assistance associations are, in essence, ethnically based organizations that may be structured around religion, families or clans, common politics, or cultural organizations. They are not a new idea, but have existed for decades as mutual benefit and relief societies among both immigrant and African American communities, and have roots in late 19th-century migrations from the South and the Caribbean (Watkins-Owens, 1996). They address self-identified needs of the ethnic community. They may also be eligible for grants or public funding and may choose to incorporate as non-profits to better avail themselves of such funding, but may need to draw a delicate balance between being an authentic community organization or a grant-driven "corporation" divorced from the community by its very sustenance.

WEST INDIAN IN AMERICA: IDEAL MINORITY OR DUST IN THE WIND

According to 2009 census estimates, there are an estimated 2.54 million Americans of West Indian ancestry and 2.85 million of African ancestry

(U.S. Census Bureau, 2009). West Indians comprise roughly 6% of the Black population, and a miniscule portion of the overall U.S. population, but fully one-third of New York's Black population (Rogers, 2006).

The number of West Indian immigrants is modest in comparison to other immigrant groups. However, their influence on America has always been disproportionate to their numbers. The roster of Caribbean immigrants who have played critical roles in American history has also served to boost the profile of the Caribbean immigrant as a class (James, 1998; Watkins-Owens, 1996).

The West Indian population (in some ways like the Indian subcontinent) is distinct in that its immigrants are from former colonies of Great Britain, are native English speakers, and have traditionally benefitted from a standardized English school system. In this respect there are, in some ways, closer cultural connections between Southeast Asian immigrants and West Indians than there are between West Indians and African Americans, more so when considering that 40% of Trinidadians and 51% of Guyanese are, in fact, East Indian in origin, and retain many of the characteristics of that culture—Hindu or Muslim religion, language competency, and food preferences. Moreover, much of the Afro-West Indian population also has absorbed the cross-cultural character of their Indo-Caribbean compatriots. This colonial inheritance has both positive and adverse consequences.

Among commonly held assumptions is one often repeated regarding Caribbean immigrants—the characterization of Black immigrants from the Caribbean as more successful, more educated, and higher in educational status and earnings than African Americans. Over decades, the argument has been used to support the thesis that African Americans were not so much disadvantaged by racism but rather by a lack of social capital relative to other "successful" minorities—Jews, West Indians, and Asians (Glazer & Moynihan, 1963; Sowell, 1978). Although repeated often, this hypothesis has proven vulnerable to empirical evidence (Model, 1991; Woodbury, 1993). As noted by Hintzen (2001): "These claims about West Indians' success are much more important for the part they play in the ideology of race relations than for what they say about the reality of the West Indian immigrant presence." In fact, while several recent studies have confirmed some advantage of first and second generation Caribbean Blacks over native-born African Americans, the differences have generally proven smaller than commonly believed, were often limited to English-speakers, and by no means approximated the SES of Whites. In fact, part of the discrepancy may simply be due to the fact that West Indians, as a whole, have settled almost exclusively in the Northeast (where salaries and SES are higher) and native-born Blacks in substantial numbers in the South (Kalmijn, 1996).

As noted by Farley and Allen: "If we had found that West Indian migrants consistently earned more than native Blacks, the evidence would have supported Sowell's hypothesis that immigrants have a culture differentiating them from native Blacks. If we additionally had found that foreign-born Blacks earned as much as comparable Whites, the evidence would have challenged the hypothesis that racial discrimination accounts for the current economic status of Blacks" (Farley & Allen, 1989).

The status of West Indians as an ideal minority seems pretty well discredited. Likewise the idea that a seamless integration of migrants of every color, creed, and race can (or should) be the goal of American assimilation. Still, there is sufficient history of successful organization within enclaves of West Indian residents, as well as a considerable record of successful social cooperation and political alliance with African Americans (Rogers, 2006; Watkins-Owens, 1996), to make the possibility of future alliances both feasible and desirable.

Case Study Exercises

Individually, or as a group, review the following case studies and respond to the questions posed at the end of the study, as appropriate. Be sure to focus on the why, how, and what emphasized in each question or exercise. Your professor/ instructor will provide you with specific guidance on how you are to report your findings for the class.

Case Study 4.1: U.S. Immigration and the West Indian Phenom

Perhaps 50% of all West Indians in America live in or around the five boroughs of the City of New York, spatially segregated in ethnic enclaves that they share to a limited extent with native-born African Americans, Asian immigrants, and Hispanics (mainly Puerto Ricans), but largely separate from the non-Hispanic White population. Immigration figures suggest that over half of the Jamaicans and Trinidadians, and three-quarters of the Guyanese legally entering the United States have settled in the New York region (Immigration and Naturalization Service, cited in Foner, 2001)

About two-fifths of the "Black" population of New York City is of West Indian ancestry. Jamaicans are the most numerous, followed by Trinidadians and Guyanese. Both the latter countries (and their New York communities) contain large population segments of East Indian ancestry, who do not normally self-identify as Black West Indian, but do strongly identify by nationality (as Trinidadian, Guyanese, or West Indian).

The borough of Brooklyn is home to the largest number of West Indians. Central Brooklyn has the largest concentration and has more diverse West Indian nationalities than any other borough. The area is also home to a large segment of Haitian immigrants, who share many cultural characteristics with English-speaking West Indians.

The central Brooklyn enclave is 30% West Indian, 52% African American, 10% Hispanic, and 8.8% non-Hispanic White. The largest West Indian segments are Jamaicans (8.6% of the total), Haitians (6.8%), "other" West Indians (4.4%), Trinidadians (3.8%), and Guyanese (3.2%). Many of these West Indians are recent first-generation immigrants.

In the middle of this West Indian enclave is an enclave-within-an-enclave of Orthodox Hassidic Jews, with whom the Black community has little social interaction. In fact, whatever interaction has occurred has often been confrontational.

Jamaicans come from a country of 2.8 million; Trinidadians, a country of 1.3 million; Haitians from a country of 9 million, which because of its poverty, is often not given as much standing within the West Indian community as its population might suggest. Because Haitians are native French and French-Creole speakers, they may also not be as easily assimilated into the English-speaking West Indian community. This is important because a hierarchy sometimes exists in West Indian immigrant neighborhoods—Jamaicans often referring to the other West Indian countries (including the South American nation of Guyana) as "small islands" and their inhabitants as "small-islanders"—a source of some resentment among small-islanders (particularly Trinidadians, whose home country, because of oil and natural gas reserves is doing considerably better economically than Jamaica). Because Jamaicans are also better known internationally, their community leaders often feel a "natural leadership" of West Indian immigrant communities—again a traditional source of conflict between "Trinidadian leaders" and "Jamaican leaders" in the diaspora.

Most West Indians in this enclave are working class, and often employed in a number of niche industries—private and public hospitals, trucking and private transport (primarily taxi services), public transport (bus and subway), service industries (hotels, restaurants, and department stores), and the public sector (schools, administration, human resources). A relatively small number are self-employed or are business owners (Foner, 2001).

New York health officials have identified a significant public health problem among West Indians in Central Brooklyn to be infant mortality rates consistently higher than city averages among all West Indian nationalities, with the exception of women from Guyana and Trinidad and Tobago (Bayne-Smith et al, in Mahoney, 2004). Interviews with focus groups have found reluctance to use prenatal services based primarily on physical accessibility, perceived need, and cost. Other authors have found similar results (Pallotto, Collins, & David, 2000).

Study Questions

1. How would you describe/assess the assimilation experience of the West Indian population in New York City?
2. What would you do to address the problem of high infant mortality?

3. What additional information would help you design and outline a long-term community intervention to address health problems in this enclave?
4. How would you go about improving relations between the Hassidic Jewish community and the West Indian community? Would you attempt to?
5. What of the African American majority in this community?
6. What sort of community organization(s) do you think might be feasible in a community such as this?
7. What would be the potential strengths of such an approach? Weaknesses? Obstacles? Threats?

Case Study 4.2: CEOD, Public Health Practitioners, and Cultural Sensitivity

In some cultures, people feel uncomfortable with silence, so they speak to fill the silences. In other cultures, it is customary to wait for a period of silence before speaking. If there aren't any silences, people from those cultures may not ever speak. Also, members of some groups (women, people of low income, some racial and ethnic minorities, and others) don't speak up because they have received messages from society at large that their contribution is not as important as others; they have gotten into the habit of deferring their thinking to the thinking of others. When some people don't share their thinking, we all lose out. We all need the opinions and voices of those people who have traditionally been discouraged from contributing.

The PHP must work to support and respect minority and immigrant families and their values. It may already be a huge concession on the part of a family to allow a teenager to participate in extracurricular activities at all. We need to make allowances for the cultural differences and try to help young people feel that they can have both worlds—instead of having to reject one set of values for another.

For example, as a community builder, it can help for the PHP to develop relationships with parents. If a young person sees her parents having relationships with people from the mainstream culture, it can help her feel that their family is accepted. It supports the teen in being more connected to her family and her community—and also, both relationships are critical protective factors for drug and alcohol abuse and other dangerous behaviors. In addition, in building relationships with parents, we develop lines of communication, so when conflicts arise, they can be more easily resolved.

Study Exercises

1. Describe how becoming impatient with people for not speaking is usually counter-productive.
2. Describe what steps can be taken to structure a meeting to encourage the quieter people to speak.

3. Discuss how people from different cultures can go about better understanding of persons not from their own culture.
4. Discuss how immigrant families who grow up in the United States often feel torn between the majority culture and the culture of their families.
5. Discuss how they can feel pressure from each culture to live according to its values, and feel they have to choose between the two.

NOTES

1. Wattenberg (2006) has repeatedly refuted the idea that the book is anti-immigrant, but in it he has conceded that racial imbalance caused by the birth dearth could cause social turbulence among "those who feel that America must absolutely remain a nation with a majority of citizens with a White European heritage."
2. In the 1990s, some in the gay community, faced with the challenge of organizing in response to the AIDS epidemic, came up with a novel slogan "We're here. We're queer. Get used to it." The immigrant community could well adopt a similar mantra: "We're here. We ain't going nowhere. Get used to it."
3. Passel and Pew Hispanic Center (2008), personal communication, quoted in Ku (2009).
4. The terms "illegal immigrant" or "illegal alien," though technically and etymologically correct, are often considered politically charged or "loaded" terms. Some authors prefer the less judgmental term "undocumented immigrants" (or in the case of the Pew Center, "unauthorized immigrants"). The use here of undocumented immigrant, which is the most commonly used term in public health literature, is not meant to be a judgment on the morality of cross border migration, legal or illegal.
5. The Bracero (or strong arm) program refers to a set of immigration policies initiated by the U.S. and Mexican governments during and after World War II, initially aimed at providing substitute labor for Americans fighting abroad, and subsequently to provide mostly cheap unskilled labor for the agricultural industry—an idea recently resurrected as a "guest worker" component in contemporary immigration reform proposals. At its height, in the 1950s, the Bracero program was responsible for the legal employment of as many as 444,000 Mexican guest workers annually, and almost 4.5 million over the life of the program (Garcia & Griego, 1996).
6. The Pew Center and others report that legal U.S. citizen children of undocumented immigrants are often deprived of services they may be legally entitled to because of the reluctance of parents to access government services through fear of arrest or deportation (Ku, 2006). It should also be noted that although non citizens are about three times more likely to be uninsured than citizens, they are not the primary burden of the uninsured population—81% of the uninsured are native born or naturalized U.S. citizens (Kaiser Commission on Medicaid and the Uninsured, 2010).
7. Acculturation and assimilation effects are often defined by age at arrival. Various authors have highlighted "critical periods" for behaviors such as

smoking, use of health care services, and obesity-related dietary habits. Bates and Teitler (2008), for example, note that immigrant women arriving in the United States after a threshold age of 12 years had three-quarters the odds of having a low birthweight infant compared to the native born, whereas the odds for those arriving after age 12 were indistinguishable from the native born.

8. Approximately 75% of health care for the uninsured is paid for by state or federal funds.

9. RAND Corporation researchers, using the estimate of undocumented immigrants comprising 3.2% of the U.S. population, estimated undocumented immigrants account for about 1.5% of U.S. medical costs (Goldman, Smith, & Sood, 2006).

10. The 2010 AHRQ National Healthcare Disparities Report, which measures 250 measures across six dimensions (AHRQ, 2011), found that although quality of care was increasing overall, fewer than 20% of disparities faced by Blacks, American Indians and Alaskan Natives, Hispanics, and poor people showed evidence of improvement, and of core access measures, only one showed reduction in disparity (see also Clancy, 2006).

11. While immigrants were 11% of the U.S. population in 2002, they comprised 14% of all workers and 20% of low-wage workers (Capps, Fix, Passel, Ost, & Perez-Lopez, 2003).

12. Using payments actually received rather than hospital charges, Melnick and Fonkych (2008) found the uninsured paid 18% to 20% more than was paid for Medicare patients.

13. Waldinger and Reichl (2006) note both the tendency for Mexican American immigrants to leave school earlier, and have lower levels of high school graduation and subsequent schooling compared to other immigrants. On the other hand, they note that Mexican immigrant men who are early school leavers are the most likely out-of-school youth to be working (89% vs. 87% for White native-born males and 67% for African American males). In the second generation, the percentage of Mexican immigrants in school at age 16 to 20 years increases from 40% to 60%, and for those age 21 to 25 years, from 7% to 24%. (Neither of these is anywhere near what one might consider acceptable levels of education for a 21st-century society.) The confluence of early school leaving, low high school graduation rates, and employment in low-paying jobs at the bottom tier of the job market combine to give first generation Mexican immigrants earnings that average half as much as that of White. While the second generation improved, it was only to 76% of native-born Whites.

REFERENCES

AHRQ. (2011, March). *Highlights from the 2010 agency for health care quality national healthcare disparities report*. AHRQ Publication No. 11–0004-1. Rockville, MD: Author.

Akresh, I. R., & Frank, R. (2008). Health selection among new immigrants. *American Journal of Public Health, 98*, 2058–2064.

Alba, R., & Nee, V. (1997). Rethinking assimilation theory in a new era of immigration. *International Migration Review, 31*(4), 826–874.

Alba, R., & Nee, V. (2003). *Remaking the American mainstream: Assimilation and contemporary immigration.* Cambridge, MA: Harvard University Press.

Anderson, G. F. (2007). From "soak the rich" to "soak the poor": Recent trends in hospital pricing. *Health Affairs, 26*(4), 780–789.

Antecol, H., & Bedard, K. (2006). Unhealthy assimilation: Why do immigrants converge to American health status levels? *Demography, 43*(2), 337–360.

Applied Research Center. (2002). *Mapping the immigrant infrastructure—Executive summary.* Report prepared for the Annie E. Casey Foundation, Spring 2002. Oakland, CA: Author. Retrieved May 26, 2011, from www.aecf.org/upload/PublicationFiles/01–013.pdf

Boswell, T. D. (2002). *A demographic profile of Cuban Americans.* Miami, FL: Cuban American National Council. Retrieved June 30, 2011, from www.eric.ed.gov/PDFS/ED480201.pdf

Bourne, R. (1916, July). Trans-National America. *Atlantic Monthly, 118,* 86–97. Retrieved June 26, 2011, from www.theatlantic.com/magazine/print/1916/07/trans-national-america/4838

Bouvier, L. F., & Gardiner, R. W. (1986). Immigration to the US: The unfinished story. *Population Bulletin, 41*(4), 1–50.

Broman, C. L., Neighbors, H. W., Delva, J., Torres, M., & Jackson, JS. (2008). Prevalence of substance use disorders among African Americans and Caribbean Blacks in the national survey of American life. *American Journal of Public Health, 98,* 1107–1114.

California Health Advocates. (2007, April). *Are you practicing cultural humility? The key to success in cultural competence.* Retrieved June 16, 2011, from http://cahealthadvocates.org/news/disparities/2007/are-you.html

Capps, R., Fix, M., Ost, J., Reardon-Anderson, J., & Passel, J. (2005, February). *The health and well being of young children of immigrants.* The Urban Institute Immigration Studies Program. Immigrant Families and Workers Brief No. 5. Retrieved May 26, 2011, from http://fcd-us.org/sites/default/files/HealthandWellbeingofYoungChildrenbrief.pdf

Capps, R., Fix, M., Passel, J., Ost, J., & Perez-Lopez, D. (2003). *A profile of the low-wage immigrant workforce.* Immigrant Families and Workers Brief No. 4. Washington, DC: The Urban Institute.

Carrasquillo, O., Carrasquillo, A. I., & Shea, S. (2000). Health insurance coverage of immigrants living in the United States: Differences by citizenship status and country of origin. *American Journal of Public Health, 90,* 917–923.

Casale, C. R., & Clancy, C. M. (2009). Commentary: Not about us without us. *Academic Medicine, 84*(10), 1333–1335.

Clancy, C. M. (2006). Closing the health care disparities gap: Turning evidence into action. *Journal of Health Care Law & Policy, 9*(1), 121–135.

Collier, M. J., & Thomas, M. (1988). Cultural identity: An interpretive perspective. *International and Intercultural Communications Annual, 2,* 99–120.

Cunningham, S. A., Reuben, J. D., & Narayan, K. M. (2008). Health of foreign-born people in the United States: A review. *Health & Place, 14*(4), 623–635.

Dittgen, H. (1997). The American debate about immigration in the 1990s: A new nationalism after the end of the Cold War? *Stanford Electronic Humanities Review, 5*(2). Retrieved June 20, 2011, from www.stanford.edu/group/SHR/5-2/dittgen.html

Ehrenreich, J., & Ehrenreich, B. (1971). *The American health empire: Power, profits, and politics*. A Report from the Health Policy Advisory Center (Health-Pac). New York, NY: Vintage Books, p. 14.

Farley, R., & Allen, W. R. (1989). *The color line and the quality of life in America*. New York, NY: Oxford University Press.

Foner, N. (2001). *Islands in the city. West Indian migration to New York City*. Berkley, CA: University of California Press.

Fragomen, A. T. (1996). Welfare Bill severely curtails assistance to noncitizens. *International Migration Review, 30*(4), 1087–1095.

Friere, P. (1986). *The pedagogy of the oppressed*. New York, NY: Continuum Publishing.

Fronstin, P. (2008). The impact of immigration on health insurance coverage in the United States, 1994–2006. Employee Benefit Research Institute. *EBRI Notes, 29*(8), 2–8.

Garcia y Griego, M. (1996). The importation of Mexican contract laborers to the United States, 1942–1964. In D. G. Guitierrez (Ed.), *Between two worlds: Mexican immigrants in the United States*. Jaguar Books on Latin America. No. 15. Wilmington, DE: Scholarly Resources Books.

Glazer, N., & Moynihan, D. P. (1963). *Beyond the melting pot*. Cambridge, MA: MIT Press.

Goldman, D. P., Smith, J. P., & Sood, N. (2006). Immigrants and the cost of medical care. *Health Affairs (Millwood), 25*(6), 1700–1711.

Gordon, M. (1964). *Assimilation in American life: The role of race, religion and national origins*. New York, NY: Oxford University Press.

Hernandez, D. J., & Charney, E. (Eds). (1998). *From generation to generation: The health and well-being of children in immigrant families*. National Research Council, Institute of Medicine. Washington, DC: National Academy Press.

Higham, J. (1955). *Strangers in the land: Patterns of American nativism, 1860–1925*. Piscataway, NJ: Rutgers University Press. Paperback Edition 2002.

Hintzen, P. (2001). *West Indian in the West: Self-representations in an immigrant community*. New York, NY: New York University Press.

Hofstede, G. (1994). Business cultures. *UNESCO Courier, 47*(4), 12–16.

Hunt, L. M. (2001). *Beyond cultural competence: Applying humility to clinical settings*. Park Ridge Center Bulletin. Issue 24, Nov/Dec 2001. Retrieved June 16, 2011, from www.parkridgecenter.org/Page1882.html

Jackson, J., Neighbors, H. W., Torres, M., Martin, L. A., Williams, D. R., & Baser, R. (2007). Use of mental health services and subjective satisfaction with treatment among Black Caribbean immigrants: Results from the National Survey of American life. *American Journal of Public Health, 97*(1), 60–67.

James, W. (1998). *Holding aloft the banner of Ethiopia: Caribbean radicalism in early twentieth century America*. New York, NY: Verso.

Jandt, F. E. (2007). *An introduction to intercultural communication: Identities in a global community* (5th ed.). Thousand Oaks, CA: Sage Publications.

Kaiser Commission on Medicaid and the Uninsured. (2010, December). *The uninsured: A primer—Key facts about Americans without health insurance*. Retrieved May 2, 2011, from www.kff.org/uninsured/upload/7451–06.pdf

Kalmijn, M. (1996). The socioeconomic assimilation of Caribbean American Blacks. *Social Forces, 74*(3), 911–930.

Kasinitz, P. (1992). *Caribbean New York*. New York, NY: Cornell University Press.

Ku, L. (2006). *Hardship among children of immigrants: Findings from the 1999 National Survey of America's Families*. Washington, DC: The Urban Institute.

Ku, L. (2009). Health insurance coverage and medical expenditures of immigrants and native-born citizens in the United States. *American Journal of Public Health, 99*, 1322–1328.

Liu, K., & Laraque, F. (2006). Higher mortality rate among infants of US-born mothers compared to foreign-born mothers in New York City. *Journal of Immigrant and Minority Health, 8*(3), 281–289.

Lucas, J. W., Barr-Anderson, D. J., & Kington, R. S. (2003). Health status, health insurance, and health care utilization patterns of immigrant Black men. *American Journal of Public Health, 93*(10), 1740–1747.

Lurie, N. (2005). Health disparities—Less talk, more action. *The New England Journal of Medicine, 353*, 727–729.

Mahoney, A. M. (Ed.). (2004). *The health and well-being of Caribbean immigrants in the United States*. Binghamton, NY: The Haworth Social Work Practice Press.

Mather, M. (2009, February). *Children in immigrant families chart a new path*. Washington DC: Population Reference Bureau Reports on America.

Melnick, G. A., & Fonkych, K. (2008). Hospital pricing and the uninsured: Do the uninsured pay higher prices? *Health Affairs, 27*(2), 116–122.

Model, S. (1991). Caribbean immigrants: A black success story? *International Migration Review, 25*(2), 248–276.

Okie, S. (2007). Immigrants and health care—At the intersection of two broken systems. *The New England Journal of Medicine, 357*(6), 525–529.

Orbe, M. P. (1998). *Constructing co-culture theory: An explication of culture, power and communication*. Thousand Oaks, CA: Sage.

Pallotto, E. K., Collins, J. W., & David, R. J. (2000). Enigma of maternal race and infant birth weight: A population-based study of U.S.-born black and Caribbean-born black women. *American Journal of Epidemiology, 151*(11), 1080–1085.

Passel, J., & Pew Hispanic Center. (2008). Personal communication, quoted in Ku, L.: Health insurance coverage and medical expenditure of immigrants and native-born citizens in the United States. *American Journal of Public Health, 99*, 1322–1328.

Passel, J. S., & Cohn, D. (2011, February 1). Unauthorized immigrant population: national and state trends, 2010. Pew Hispanic Center; Pew Research Center. Accessed on 6/1/2011 at http://pewresearch.org/pubs/1876/unauthorized-immigrant-population-united-states-national-state-trends-2010

Pati, S., & Dasnagoulian, S. (2008). Immigrant children's reliance on public health Insurance in the wake of immigration reform. *American Journal of Public Health, 98*(11), 2004–2010.

Portes, A., & Rumbaut, R. G. (2001). *Legacies: the story of the immigrant second generation*. Berkeley and Los Angeles, CA: University of California Press.

Portes, A., & Rumbaut, R. G. (2006). *Immigrant America: A portrait* (3rd ed). Berkeley, CA: University of California Press.

Ridley, C. (1995). *Overcoming unintentional racism in counselling therapy*. Thousand Oaks, CA: Sage. Quoted in Tervalon (1998).

Riis, J. (1997). *How the other half lives*. New York, NY: Penguin Books. Originally published by Charles Scribner's Son, New York, 1890.

Rogers, R. R. (2006). *Afro-Caribbean immigrants and the politics of incorporation*. New York, NY: Cambridge University Press.

Rushing, J. H. (1983). The rhetoric of the American Western myth. *Communication Monographs, 50*, 15–32.

Rushing, J. H., & Frentz, T. S. (1978). The rhetoric of Rocky: A social value model of criticism. *Western Journal of Speech Communication, 42*, 63–72.

Singh, G. K., Kogan, M., & Yu, S. M. (2009). Disparities in obesity and overweight prevalence among US immigrant children and adolescents by generational status. *Journal of Community Health, 34*(4), 271–281.

Singh, G. K., & Siahpush, M. (2001). All-cause and cause-specific mortality of immigrants and native born in the United States. *American Journal of Public Health, 91*(3), 392–399.

Sowell, T. (Ed.). (1978). *Essays and data on American ethnic groups*. Washington, DC: Urban Institute.

Sowell, T. (1984). *Civil rights: Rhetoric or reality?* New York, NY: Morrow.

Taylor, E. B. (1889). *Primitive culture: Researches into the development of mythology, philosophy, religion, language, art, and custom* (Vol. 1). New York: Holt.

Telles, E. E., & Ortiz, V. (2008). *Generations of exclusion: Mexican Americans, assimilation, and race*. New York, NY: Russell Sage Foundation.

Tervalon, M., & Murray-Garcia, J. (1998). Cultural humility versus cultural competence: A critical distinction in defining physician training outcomes in multicultural education. *Journal of Health Care for the Poor and Underserved, 9*(2), 117–125.

Uba, L. (1994). *Asian Americans: Personality patterns, identity, and mental health*. New York, NY: The Guilford Press.

U. S. Census Bureau. (2009). *Fact finder*. Table B04003. Total Ancestry Reported, 2009 American Community Survey 1-Year Estimates. Retrieved June 25, 2011, from http://factfinder.census.gov/servlet/DTTable?_bm=y&-geo_id=D&-ds_name=D&-_lang=en&-state=dt&-mt_name=ACS_2009_1YR_G2000_B04003

U. S. Census Bureau. (2010, October 9). *Nation's foreign-born population nears 37 million*. US Census Bureau. Press Release. Retrieved June 16, 2011, from www.census.gov/newsroom/releases/archives/foreignborn_population/cb10-159.html

U. S. Census Bureau. (2011). *Overview of race and Hispanic origin: 2010*. Census Brief—Issued March 2011. Retrieved June 12, 2011, from www.census.gov/prod/cen2010/briefs/c2010br-02.pdf

Waldinger, R., & Reichl, R. (2006). *Second-generation Mexicans: Getting ahead or falling behind*. Migration Information Source. Retrieved June 7, 2011, from www.migrationinformation.org/Feature/display.cfm?id=382

Waters, M. (1999). *Black identities: West Indian immigrant dreams and American realities*. New York, NY: Russell Sage Foundation.

Watkins-Owens, I. (1996). Blood relations; Caribbean immigrants and the Harlem community, 1900–1930. Bloomington and Indianapolis, IN: Indiana University Press.

Wattenberg, B. (2006, April 18). *Open to greatness: We need immigrants*. National Review Online. Retrieved June 11, 2011, from http://old.nationalreview.com/comment/wattenberg200604180659.asp

Wattenberg, B. J. (1987). *The birth dearth: What happens when people in free countries don't have enough babies?* New York, NY: Pharos Books.

Williams, D. R. (2002). Racial/ethnic variations in Women's health: The social embeddedness of health. *American Journal of Public Health, 92*(4), 588–597.

Williams, R. A. (2007). *Eliminating healthcare disparities in America: Beyond the IOM report*. Totowa, NJ: Humana Press.

Williams, W. E. (1982). *The state against Blacks*. New York, NY: McGraw-Hill.

Williams, D. R., & Collins, C. (1995). U.S. socioeconomic and racial differences in health: Patterns and explanations. *Annual Review of Sociology, 21,* 349–386.

Wilson, W. J. (1978). *The declining significance of race: Blacks and changing American institutions*. Chicago, IL: University of Chicago Press.

Woodbury, S. A. (1993). *Culture, human capital, and the earnings of West Indian Blacks*. Upjohn Institute Working Paper. No. 93–20. Kalamazoo, MI: WE Upjohn Institute for Employment Research. Retrieved May 22, 2011, from http://research.upjohn.org/cgi/viewcontent.cgi?article=1032&context=up_workingpapers

BIBLIOGRAPHY

AHRQ. (2011, March). *Agency for health care quality national healthcare disparities report 2010*. AHRQ Publication No. 11–0005. Rockville, MD: Author.

Buff, R. (2001). *Immigration and the political economy of home: West Indian Brooklyn and American Indian Minneapolis, 1945–1992*. Berkeley, CA: University of California Press.

Capps, R., Fix, M., Henderson, E., & Reardon-Anderson, J. (2005). *A profile of low-income working immigrant families*. New Federalism National Survey of America's Families. Series B, No. B-67. Washington, DC: The Urban Institute.

Centers for Disease Control and Prevention. (2011). CDC health disparities and inequalities report—United States, 2011. *Morbidity and Mortality Weekly Report, 60,* 1–116.

Crawford, J. (1992). *Language loyalties: A source book on the official English controversy*. Chicago, IL: University of Chicago Press.

Crawford, J. (2008). *Frequently asked questions about official English*. James Crawford— President, Institute for Language and Education Policy. Retrieved June 12, 2011, from www.diversitylearningk12.com/articles/Crawford_Official_ English_FAQ.pdf

Cruse, H. (1987). *Plural but equal: A critical study of Blacks and minorities and America's plural society*. New York, NY: William Morrow, pp. 286–342.

Ehrlich, P. (1968). *The population bomb* (Rev. ed.). New York, NY: Ballantyne Books.

Fruchter, R. G., Nayeri, K., Remey, J. C., Wright, C., Feldman, J. G., Boyce, J. G., & Burnett, W. S. (1990). Cervix and breast cancer incidence in immigrant Caribbean women. *American Journal of Public Health, 80,* 722–724.

Fruchter, R. G., Remy, J. C., Burnett, W. S., & Boyce, J. G. (1986). Cervical cancer in immigrant Caribbean women. *American Journal of Public Health, 76,* 797–799.

Galindo, R., & Vigil, J. (2004). Language restrictionism revisited: The case against Colorado's 2000 anti-bilingual education initiative. *The Harvard Latino Law Review, 7,* 27–61.

Guitierrez, D. G. (1996). *Between two worlds: Mexican immigrants in the United States.* Jaguar Books on Latin America. No. 15. Wilmington, DE: Scholarly Resources Books.

Kasinitz, P., Mollenkopf, J. H., Waters, M. C., & Holdaway, J. (2008). *Inheriting the city: The children of immigrants come of age.* New York, NY: Russell Sage Foundation.

Purcell, T. W. (1993). *Banana fallout: Class, color and culture among West Indians in Costa Rica.* Los Angeles, CA: Center for Afro-American Studies Publications, UCLA.

Smedley, B. D., Stith, A. Y., & Nelson, A. R. (Eds.). (2003). *Unequal treatment. confronting racial and ethnic disparities in health care.* Institute of Medicine Report. Washington, DC: National Academies Press.

Trivendi, A. N., Zaslavsky, A. M., Schneider, E. C., & Ayanian, J. Z. (2005). Trends in the quality of care and racial disparities in Medicare managed care. *The New England Journal of Medicine, 353,* 692–700.

Williams, D. R., Haile, R., Gonzalez, H. W., Neighbors, H., Baser, R., & Jackson, J. S. (2007). The mental health of Black Caribbean immigrants: Results from the national survey of American life. *American Journal of Public Health, 97,* 52–59.

5

Academic–Community Partnerships for CEOD

Daniel S. Blumenthal

LEARNING OBJECTIVES

What you can learn by studying this chapter:

- How to identify the characteristics of an equitable academic–community partnership
- How to define and describe community-based participatory research (CBPR)
- To identify and list at least three challenges faced by persons conducting CBPR
- To identify the challenges to sustainability of an academic–community partnership
- To identify what service-learning is and is not
- To identify the types of academic–community partnerships that are developed for the purpose of providing community service

George Will, the conservative newspaper columnist, supposedly originated the joke, now a cliché:

> *The American condition can be summed up in three sentences we're hearing*
> *these days: "Your check is in the mail."*
> *"I will still respect you in the morning."*
> *"I am from the government and I am here to help you."*
>
> (Shapiro, 2006)

This joke is not likely to create much mirth in low-income minority communities, where most of the little help that is available does, in fact, come from the government. The line that is more likely to produce a bitter chuckle is: *"I'm from the university and I'm here to help you."* The reason for the cynical response is clear: university professors and their students have exploited poor communities for years, especially for research but often for teaching as well. Many faculty conduct studies in these communities, administering questionnaires, taking samples, or conducting physical examinations. The faculty then return to campus, publish papers, win grants, and get promoted, while the community enjoys no benefit. Alternatively, as a teaching exercise, the faculty may take their students on "poverty tours" or send them to gather data on behalf of the professor. This has come to be known as "mosquito research": "They show up in the summer, they suck your blood, and then they disappear."

But times and ethics are changing. Universities, their faculty, and their students have begun to appreciate that communities and the people who live in them deserve to be treated with respect regardless of their economic or educational status. The model that is being discarded as a relic of the 20th century spoke of the "community laboratory" and the "community classroom." And at Thanksgiving and Christmas, students conducted clothing drives or collected canned goods for the poor. A more contemporary approach calls for this perspective:

- The community is not a laboratory: To regard it as a laboratory relegates the people who live there to the status of guinea pigs.
- The community is not a classroom: To regard it as a classroom relegates the people who live there to the status of props for a teaching exercise.
- The community is not a charity case: To regard it as a charity case denies the people who live there their dignity.

Rather, in research, education, and service, the community is a *partner*, engaging with university faculty and students in activities that benefit both.

In this chapter, we discuss academic–community partnerships that are created for the purpose of research, teaching, or service, or any combination of them. We recognize that communities may partner with entities other than academic institutions—for instance, businesses, nonprofit organizations, churches, foundations, or government agencies. In fact, it has become fashionable for almost any type of relationship with a community, no matter how tenuous, transient, or one sided, to label itself a "partnership." However, this chapter will focus primarily on partnerships in which one party is a university, college, or professional school, and we will draw some fairly definite boundaries around what can legitimately be called a partnership.

GENERAL PRINCIPLES OF ACADEMIC–COMMUNITY PARTNERSHIPS

Whether the purpose of the partnership is to conduct research, offer students an educational experience, or provide services to needy (or not-so-needy) people, it is the partnership itself that requires the most attention and effort. The organization Community–Campus Partnerships for Health has developed a widely accepted set of principles for such partnerships (2000), and this is as good a place to start as any. These supersede a very similar set of principles about which the organization published a book-length discussion (Blumenthal, 2009).

1. Partnerships form to serve a specific purpose and may take on new goals over time.
2. Partners have agreed upon mission, values, goals, measurable outcomes and accountability for the partnership.
3. The relationship between partners is characterized by mutual trust, respect, genuineness, and commitment.
4. The partnership builds upon identified strengths and assets, but also works to address needs and increase capacity of all partners.
5. The partnership balances power among partners and enables resources among partners to be shared.
6. Partners make clear and open communication an ongoing priority by striving to understand each other's needs and self-interests, and by developing a common language.
7. Principles and processes for the partnership are established with the input and agreement of all partners, especially for decision making and conflict resolution.
8. There is feedback among all stakeholders in the partnership, with the goal of continuously improving the partnership and its outcomes.
9. Partners share the benefits of the partnership's accomplishments.
10. Partnerships can dissolve and need to plan a process for closure.

One might view an academic–community partnership as a marriage, and couples will recognize that an ideal marriage is built on these same principles. However, not all marriages, and not all academic–community partnerships, are ideal. A less-than-ideal marriage or partnership can continue to exist for a time even if some principles are not adhered to. Eventually, however, repair must take place or principle number 10 will take effect: The partnership or the marriage will end.

Probably the most important principle is number #3. The other principles can be "put on hold" for a time. It may be, for instance, that communication (#6) or feedback (#8) about a particular project will fail to take place, or that one partner will benefit more than the other from a particular accomplishment (#9). These shortcomings can be repaired as long as there is trust and commitment. Without trust and commitment, however, the partnership will surely dissolve.

What is the relationship between these principles and the process of community organization and development (COD)? They both promote the same mission: permanent change in the community that leads to greater empowerment, prosperity, and good health. For many entities (health departments and other public agencies, community organizations, etc.), pursuing this mission is a "given," and COD merely constitutes a recipe for achieving it. The same is not true of academic institutions; community improvement is not part of their traditional mission, at least not in any direct sense. Universities focus on education of their students and on the generation of new knowledge through research. Academicians are also charged with providing service, but "service" usually means service to the institution (for instance, by serving on committees) or to the profession (for instance, by reviewing grant proposals or serving as an officer of a professional organization). At a medical school, service includes providing patient care.

The academic argument is that colleges and universities provide community benefit by creating a more well-educated populace and by discovering (for instance) new treatments and cures that will improve overall health. There is some truth to this argument but the isolationist attitude of many academic institutions has created their "ivory tower" reputation and the widespread view that they benefit only the elite. To add to this reputation, many large universities are surrounded by poverty-stricken neighborhoods in which residents understandably feel like poor medieval serfs living resentfully within easy view of the castle of the wealthy lord.

THE COMMUNITY AS PATIENT

The relationship between academic health centers and communities has changed in recent years, just as the relationship between individual physicians and individual patients has changed. It is instructive to consider these parallels (Gamble, 1997).

Individuals previously known as "research subjects" are now "research participants," and are to be treated as partners with doctors or scientists in conducting research. The informed consent process is to provide the participant with a full understanding of the purpose, risks, and potential benefits of the research.

In education, patients are no longer described as "teaching material." Again, the patient is ideally part of a triad with the attending physician and the medical student—a full partner in the teaching exercise. And in clinical care, patients are no longer expected to follow "doctor's orders;" instead they participate in "shared decision making" with their treating physician in selecting the best tests or treatments in accord with their personal values and preferences.

There are also differences, of course. The "community as patient" model teaches us to treat communities with respect, but it does not tell us how to organize a community, or how to create a partnership with a community. Some guidelines on the partnership development process follow.

RESEARCH PARTNERSHIPS

In many low-income minority communities, the term "research" has acquired a negative connotation. This is often attributed to the notorious Tuskegee Study of Untreated Syphilis in the Negro Male (see case study; Viswanathan, et al., 2004). But there are numerous other examples of exploitative research and even among people who cannot cite specific examples, there is often a great deal of suspicion of research and researchers.

As a result, faculty proposing to do community-based research may find themselves shunned by those of whom they wished to be their research subjects (or participants). Alternatively, they may be able to circumvent established community structures to recruit subjects, a strategy that can enable the completion of the research but is ultimately harmful to the community, violates the goals of community organization and development, and certainly does not represent a partnership.

COMMUNITY-BASED PARTICIPATORY RESEARCH

The unfortunate history of community-based research has led contemporary scientists to develop an approach called *community-based participatory research*, or CBPR. This is an approach in which the community is to benefit from the *process* of the research as well as the outcome. It calls for the community to be involved in every phase of the research: identifying the topic, defining the research question, developing the protocol, conducting the study, and analyzing and disseminating the results.

CBPR virtually requires the COD process as a prerequisite; without this process, "the community" is undefined. In practice, some version of COD is likely to have already taken place and there may be a community organization or coalition with which the research team can partner. But it is important to identify an organization or coalition that truly does represent the population of potential research participants; a public agency or charitable foundation whose staff does not live in the community is unlikely, by itself, to be such an organization.

CBPR researchers have developed principles for conducting research in the community. In fact, many sets of principles have been published (Ahmed & Palermo, 2010; Green et al., 1995; Israel, Schulz, Parker, & Becker, 1998). Probably the most frequently cited are those formulated by Israel et al. (1998).

1. CBPR acknowledges community as a unit of identity.
2. CBPR builds on strengths and resources within the community.
3. CBPR facilitates a collaborative, equitable partnership in all phases of research, involving an empowering and power-sharing process that attends to social inequalities.
4. CBPR fosters colearning and capacity building among all partners.
5. CBPR integrates and achieves a balance between knowledge generation and intervention for the mutual benefit of all partners.
6. CBPR focuses on the local relevance of public health problems and on ecological perspectives that attend to the multiple determinants of health.
7. CBPR involves systems development using a cyclical and iterative process.

8. CBPR disseminates results to all partners and involves them in the wider dissemination of results.
9. CBPR involves a long-term process and commitment to sustainability.

The overlap with the "general partnership principles" listed earlier in this chapter is obvious, but the CBPR principles are directed particularly at altering the research process so that it provides benefits to the community as well as to the researchers.

CBPR presents a number of unique challenges. The first, as in any community partnership, is defining the community. It may be difficult to recruit a sufficient number of participants for a research project from a small, geographically defined community. On the other hand, a large community that is not defined by geography (for instance, "the African American Community") may be too diffuse to enter into a meaningful partnership. The COD process can help solve the problem; one can, for instance, organize a community coalition that incorporates a number of contiguous geographically defined communities. Alternatively—or in addition—investigators and their community partners can recruit as many participants as possible from the defined community, then reach outside it for others.

Identifying community representatives that truly represent the community and its interests is a second challenge. Staff of social service or public health agencies that often sit on "advisory boards" may not actually live in the community. Elected officials are often seen as beholden to special interests rather than representative of the grass roots. Ideally, most community representatives will be community leaders who have broad-based support and a sincere interest in health research.

Involving community representatives in every aspect of the research presents another set of problems. For instance, the topic to be researched may be determined more by the focus of the funding agency (e.g., the National Cancer Institute only funds cancer research) or the expertise of the lead professor than by the priorities of the community. Compromise may be the solution: If the community accepts the research proposed by the academic team, that team also needs to make a good-faith effort to identify faculty with the expertise to respond to community priorities and a funding agency that can provide the required resources.

Academics doing CBPR face their own set of issues. They often complain that institutional review boards do not understand this type of research and create barriers, such as requiring extensive consent documents for seemingly minimal-risk research. In addition, the time to publication may be longer for a CBPR project than for more traditional research. The partnership-building process itself may take a year or more. This means that CBPR faculty on the typical academic timetable for promotion and tenure may be at a disadvantage.

In addition, faculty engaged in CBPR may face criticism from both traditional research scientists and from fellow CBPR practitioners. From the former may come the criticism that the research in CBPR is not sufficiently rigorous: that attending to community needs and priorities has superseded the requirements of good research methodology. From CBPR colleagues may come the criticism that the project was not sufficiently participatory: that attending to the rigor of the research has superseded the needs and priorities of the community.

Despite the challenges, faculty conducting research in the context of a community partnership need to strive to adhere to the principles of CBPR. To do otherwise is to undermine the partnership, to the detriment of both the community and the academic institution.

SUSTAINABILITY

The sustainability of a partnership is at particular risk when the partnership is created specifically to carry out a grant-funded research project. Grants, whether offered by a federal agency, a foundation, or a corporation, are time-limited—typically 1 to 3 years and almost never more than 5 years—and when the grant comes to an end, the academic–community partnership is likely to come to an end as well. It is perhaps for this reason that commitment to sustainability is included in the CBPR principles listed earlier, while the list of general partnership principles near the beginning of this chapter does not mention sustainability (but, ironically, does address the dissolution of a partnership).

An academic institution that initiates a community partnership for the purpose of conducting a grant-funded research project and then abandons the community when the grant expires should be seen as particularly exploitative. In any grant-funded project, the university almost always commands the majority of the funding and controls the project. If, after reaping these benefits, the university walks away, the community gatekeepers may understandably feel deceived and forsaken—and will be unlikely to cooperate when the next researcher from the university proposes a partnership.

Ideally, an academic–community research partnership will be created before applying for a grant. This provides the best opportunity to adhere to CBPR principles: Community priorities can guide the grant-seeking process. In practice, however, this occurs relatively rarely. More often, it is the opportunity to secure a grant—or even a grant that is already in hand—that motivates the university to seek a liaison with a community. In this case, a commitment to continue the partnership beyond the lifespan of the grant, regardless of the status of grant funding, should be fundamental to the university's understanding with the community.

There are two principal ways in which the university can participate in the partnership in the absence of funding. First, of course, the partners can continue to work together to seek funding. Second, the university can provide services to the community: health education and promotion, tutoring or mentoring for children and youth, health fairs, and more. Faculty often balk at the idea of time-consuming involvement of this sort in the absence of compensation. But that is the nature of genuine partnership. It is well to remember that in most partnerships, the community participants are not compensated for their time. Moreover, continuing partnership activities in the absence of funding can be viewed as an investment: groundwork is being laid for the next grant.

EDUCATIONAL PARTNERSHIPS

Academic institutions usually require extramural funding (grants) to conduct research, but the cost of educating their students is supported with institutional funds, derived from tuition, state appropriations (in the case of a public university), endowment income, and donations. For this reason, academic–community partnerships created for educational purposes have the potential to be more stable than research partnerships, which are threatened whenever a grant expires.

Community-based education usually takes the form of *service-learning*, an activity that has become popular at levels ranging from elementary school to graduate and professional school. Typically, a student or group of students is assigned to a community agency to assist agency staff in carrying out their responsibilities. The agency benefits from the student's labors, and the student learns about the community needs addressed by the agency.

Service-learning is promoted by the federal government, and the Community Service Act of 1990, which authorized the Learn and Serve America grant program, defines service-learning as:

> A method under which students or participants learn and develop through active participation in thoughtfully organized service that is conducted in and meets the needs of a community; is coordinated with an elementary school, secondary school, institution of higher education, or community service program, and with the community; and helps foster civic responsibility; and that is integrated into and enhances the academic curriculum of the students, or the educational components of the community service program in which the participants are enrolled; and provides structured time for the students or participants to reflect on the service experience.

Service-learning is usually characterized as having the following components:

■ *Curricular connections:* Integrating learning into a service project is key. Academic ties should be clear and build upon existing disciplinary skills.

■ *Student voice:* Beyond being actively engaged in the project itself, students have the opportunity to select, design, implement, and evaluate their service activity, encouraging relevancy and sustained interest (http://en.wikipedia.org/wiki/Youth_voice).
■ *Reflection:* Structured opportunities are created to think, talk, and write about the service experience.
■ *Community partnerships:* Partnerships with community agencies are used to identify genuine needs, provide mentorship, and contribute assets toward completing a project. In a successful partnership, both sides will give to and benefit from the project.
■ *Authentic community needs:* Local community members or service recipients are involved in determining the significance and depth of the service activities involved.
■ *Assessment:* Well-structured assessment instruments with constructive feedback through reflection provide valuable information regarding the positive "reciprocal learning" and serving outcomes for sustainability and replication.

The website of the National Service-Learning Clearinghouse provides a good set of examples of what service-learning is *not*:

■ An episodic volunteer program
■ An add-on to an existing school or college curriculum
■ Logging a set number of community service hours in order to graduate
■ Compensatory service assigned as a form of punishment by the courts or by school administrators
■ Only for high school or college students
■ One-sided; benefiting only students or only the community

Ideally, a service-learning program will occur in the context of an active partnership, one in which the academic and community collaborators work to ensure that community organization and development takes place. At the other end of the spectrum from the ideal is a program in which the community agency merely considers students to be free labor, and the supervising professor merely considers the agency a place to send students in lieu of having to give a lecture.

A public agency or charitable program such as a health department or a homeless shelter may not represent the community well since it is often the case that none of the staff live in the community served. The agency may be an important part of the community and should be represented in any community coalition but other representatives should be part of the coalition as well. A service-learning program in this context can teach the participating students about the community and about community development while at the same time helping to advance the interests of the community. A partnership with an agency, however, should not be confused with a partnership with a community.

SERVICE PARTNERSHIPS

As mentioned earlier, "service" at an academic institution can mean service on a university committee or service to the profession. But it can also mean service to the community. At a health professions school, this will usually be in the form of patient care (for clinical faculty) or community health promotion (for public health or other nonclinical faculty).

Clinical care at a medical school is usually provided in an academic faculty practice or at a public hospital, and neither of these constitutes a community partnership. However, some of the most successful academic–community partnerships have been based on clinical service. The original Community Health Centers (CHCs) at Columbia Point in Boston and Mound Bayou, Mississippi, were developed through a partnership with Tufts University School of Medicine in the mid-1960s. Similarly, the Matthew Walker Health Center in Nashville, Tennessee—one of the early CHCs—was developed through a partnership with Meharry Medical College.

Each CHC (and similar "Federally Qualified Health Centers," or FQHCs) is overseen by a community board of directors that often could serve as a model for the sort of community board created through the COD process. A number of examples of medical school–CHC partnerships exist currently. A few diverse examples include the Robert Wood Johnson School of Medicine in New Brunswick, New Jersey, and the Eric B. Chandler Health Center; Albert Einstein College of Medicine and the Martin Luther King Jr. Health Center in the Bronx, New York; Quillen School of Medicine at East Tennessee University School of Medicine and the Johnson Country Health Center in Mountain City, Tennessee; and the A.T. Still School of Osteopathic Medicine in Phoenix, Arizona, and a dozen or more CHCs around the United States.

But these partnerships are sustained in large part by the clinical income generated by the CHCs, the federal subsidies that enable the CHCs to care for the poor and the uninsured, and the referrals from the CHCs to the specialists at the academic medical centers. The CHCs also are often part of the teaching program of the academic medical center, so that these service partnerships may become educational partnerships—service-learning for clinical students.

A greater challenge, then, is the creation and sustainability of academic–community partnerships that exist solely for the purpose of nonclinical community service. In fact, there are relatively few of these; when they exist, they are usually dependent on federal, state, or local grants that are awarded for the purpose of providing health promotion services to the community. The academic center may have to compete for these grants with other providers of the services, such as health departments or community hospitals.

Another challenge to this type of partnership is the fact that faculty involved in the partnership may get no credit for their activities from their academic employer. Faculty are rewarded for conducting research and publishing, for teaching, and (for clinicians) for generating clinical income. Faculty are not generally rewarded for providing community service.

One approach to addressing this challenge is to regard community service for nonclinicians as equivalent to clinical service for clinicians. Just as a physician faculty member might have, for instance, 50% of her time assigned to patient care in a clinical setting, a nonphysician faculty member might have 50% of his time assigned to community service in the form of health promotion activities in a community partnership. The difference, of course, is that the clinician can charge the patient or the patient's insurance company for clinical services, but the community generally cannot pay for health promotion services. For this reason, the nonclinician is obliged to seek out grants. At the time of faculty evaluation, the nonclinician is assessed in the same way that he would be if he were providing clinical services, on the grounds that "the community is our patient."

Thus, we have come full circle. Near the beginning of this chapter, we described how the concept of "the community as patient" could support our thinking about working with communities, and now we see that it can also serve as a model in promotion and tenure decisions about faculty. Adopting this perspective throughout the academic health center may facilitate the process of engaging communities in genuine, trusting, and committed partnerships.

Case Study Exercises

Individually, or as a group, review the following case study and respond to the questions posed at the end of the study, as appropriate. Be sure to focus on the why, how, and what emphasized in each exercise. Your professor/instructor will provide you with specific guidance on how you are to report your findings for the class.

Case Study 5.1: The Tuskegee Syphilis Study

From 1932 until 1972, the U.S. Public Health Service studied 399 men with syphilis who lived in and around the town of Tuskegee, Alabama, to better understand the natural history of the disease. The men were not told that they were the subjects of a research study; rather, they were falsely told that they were being treated. At the time the study was initiated, there was no good treatment for syphilis but when penicillin became generally available after World War II, the scientists directing the study made special efforts to ensure that the study subjects did not receive any, either for their syphilis or for other unrelated infections that they might develop, such as pneumonia. The project was not conducted in secret; the local medical society signed off on the study and Tuskegee Institute (now Tuskegee University) was heavily involved. A number of papers about the project were published while it was underway.

In 1972, a journalist named Jean Heller wrote an exposé in the *Washington Star* condemning the study's ethical violations. Literally overnight, the Tuskegee Syphilis Study became the poster child for unethical research. Dr. Merlin Duval, the assistant secretary for health in the Department of Health, Education, and Welfare, ordered the study stopped immediately. Twenty-five years later, President Bill Clinton issued an apology to the men who were still alive and directed that federal funds be awarded to Tuskegee University to establish a bioethics center.

The Tuskegee Study illustrates a number of the important points of this chapter. In terms of data gathering, the study was very well organized, and there was very little attrition. The community as often defined by academe was quite involved in the research. "The community" in this case included the health department, the medical society, and the local educational institution. It did not, however, include any representatives of the men who were the subjects of the research. It would have been difficult to say who those representatives should have been—the community was not organized. If there had been an organization of the poor farmers and share-croppers who were the research subjects, and if that organization had been represented at the meetings at which the research had been planned, the project surely would not have taken place.

Study Exercises

1. What credible approach could have been used by the research institution to partner with the community to conduct this study?
2. Describe how a public health practitioner can help to build "trust" between community and institutional partnerships before, during, and after research or intervention efforts are begun.
3. Who should be at the table when research and intervention efforts are conducted at the community level?
4. Describe the pros and cons of conducting community research and interventions such as the Tuskegee Study.

REFERENCES

Ahmed, S. M., & Palermo, A. S. (2010). Community engagement in research: Frameworks for education and peer review. *American Journal of Public Health,* *100*(8), 1380–1387.

Blumenthal, D. S. (2009). Clinical community health: The community as patient revisited (online). *Education for Health, 9,* 234. Retrieved from http://educationforhealth.net/publishedarticles/article_print_234.pdf

Community-campus partnerships for health: Partnership perspectives (2000, Summer). I(II).

Gamble, V. N. (1997). Under the shadow of Tuskegee: African Americans and health care. *American Journal of Public Health, 87*(11), 1773–1778.

Green, L. W., George, M. A., Daniel, M., Frankish, C. J., Herbert, C. P., Bowie, W. R., & O'Neill, M. (1995). *Guidelines and categories for classifying participatory research projects in health promotion.* Study of Participatory Research in Health Promotion. Ottawa, ON: Royal Society of Canada, pp. 43–50. Retrieved July 13, 2010, from http://www.lgreen.net/guidelines.html

http://www.servicelearning.org/what_is_service-learning/characteristics/index.php

Israel, B. A., Schulz, A. J., Parker, E. A., & Becker, A. B. (1998). Review of community-based research: Assessing partnership approaches to improve public health. *Annual Review of Public Health, 19,* 173–202.

Shapiro, F. R. (2006). *Yale book of quotations* (p. 825). New Haven, CT: Yale University Press, quoting *Frederick (MD) News,* 1976.

Viswanathan, M., Ammerman, A., Eng, E., Gartlehner, G., Lohr, K. N., Griffith, D., . . . Whitener, L. (2004, July). *Community-based participatory research: Assessing the evidence.* Evidence Report/Technology Assessment No. 99 (Prepared by RTI—University of North Carolina Evidence-based Practice Center under Contract No. 290–02-0016). AHRQ Publication 04-E022–2. Rockville, MD: Agency for Healthcare Research and Quality.

6

Engaging the Faith-Based Community in the CEOD Process

Rueben C. Warren, Sandy D. Maclin, Jr., Darryl Scriven, and Frederick G. Murphy

The Most sacred place isn't the Church, the Mosque or the Temple, it is the temple of the body. That's where Spirit lives.
Susan Taylor, in Essence Magazine

LEARNING OBJECTIVES

What you can learn by studying this chapter:

- How to apply principles of community-based participatory research methodologies to interfaith and community-based organization partnerships
- How to differentiate between *faith-based* and *faith-placed* organizations
- How to describe, differentiate, and demonstrate cultural competencies among the varying types of communities
- What to discuss and how to respect the influence of culture and faith within community settings
- How to apply the methodology described in the Authentic Culturecology Model to enhance interaction with faith- and community-based organizations
- To identify the differences among religiosity, faith, and spirituality

The goal of this chapter is to review how to effectively and ethically engage faith-based communities in the community organization, development process, and propose a model to work efficaciously in diverse faith-based communities (Holmes, 2007). This chapter focuses on health as an example of a salient issue in all communities, because health impacts at every level, in each life stage of the human experience. In this chapter, health is described as "a relationship, a dynamic interplay between the physical, social, psychological, and spiritual well-being of the individual and the group and their interaction with the physical and social environment." Describing health in this manner highlights several constructs such as the importance of relationships for human health; the group, as well as the individual, being essential for human health; spirituality and its relationship to human health; and the physical and social environment as critical influences on human health (Warren, Lockett, & Zulfiqar, 2002). Health, in this chapter, is viewed as a journey, not the destination. Tremendous health disparities continue to persist in the United States and throughout the world. Health disparities are targeted by many community-based organizations, including faith-based communities. To target health as a focus of the chapter, we will provide the opportunity to review several cogent theories and discuss how to apply those theories to the community origination and development process.

Inherent in any effort to organize and/or develop communities is a definition of community, which, operationally, can be defined in many ways (Fellin, 2001; Hunter, 1975; Parker et al., 2001). For the purpose of this chapter, community is defined as: "individuals who share certain commonalities, be they cultural or geographic, social or political" (De La Cancela, Chin, & Jenkins, 1998). In this context, community refers to faith-based communities, of which there are many. Yet, all faith-based communities reference some vertical relationship with something or someone beyond themselves. Some faith-based communities belong to specific religious or spiritual groups that share one or more metaphysical tenets (Warren et al., 2002). The requisite for working within faith-based communities must first be to understand both vertical and horizontal faith.

To whom is faith entrusted? Vertical faith relates to something beyond humankind or human capacity—God, Allah, Buddha, Yahweh, and so on. For some, it is the ancestors with whom their faith is entrusted. For others, it is both a Supreme Being and the Ancestors in whom they have faith. Horizontal faith is trust in other individuals (McKim, 1996). Often vertical and horizontal faiths are consistent with religious affiliation, but not always. Religion, in many instances, is intermingled and sometimes confused with culture. Yet, if properly understood, culture and religion are complementary and can be used synergistically to enhance community organization and development.

Religion is "ritual, social, and ethical elements combined with belief in an unseen world and often with a deity" (McKim, 1996, p. 243). Culture is a "functional, internally consistent system of beliefs, attitudes, values, expectations, and norms/patterns of conduct" (King, 2002, p. 102). Religion and culture have cross-cutting influence on and in communities. Comparing and contrasting these two constructs will be addressed later in the chapter.

The conceptual framework for the chapter is based on the Authentic Culturecology Model developed by Lewis M. King, PhD, former Executive Director of the Fanon Research Center and Professor of Human Development at the Charles R. Drew University of Medicine and Science in Los Angeles, California. The model presupposes a cultural framework for people of color, particularly in relationship to health. The authors are

African American and therefore write from that cultural context. However, the chapter is based on the universal principles previously listed that may have cross-cultural, interfaith, and ecumenical application.

AN ALTERNATIVE VIEW OF PUBLIC HEALTH AS THE HEALTH OF RELATIONSHIPS

Minkler, Wallerstein, and Wilson (2002), in their book chapter titled "Improving Health Through Community Organization and Community Building," propose several key concepts in community organization and community building by cross-tabulating the terms: concepts, definitions, and application along the x-axis (horizontal), and empowerment, critical consciousness, community capacity, social capital, issue selection, and participation along the y-axis (vertical). This theoretical construction provides a generic way to innumerate the essential elements in organizing and developing diverse communities. The authors acknowledge that "no single unified model of community organization or community building exists, but some key concepts are central to the most widely used models." Still, the elements listed in their theoretical construction are relevant to any effort to work with communities.

In this chapter, various monotheistic and polytheistic traditions are presented to underscore that faith-based communities are constructed from all types of religious traditions. In order to build successful and self-sustaining organizations, the underlying orientations and tenets of some of the largest religions must be understood. Thus, the first section of this chapter discusses the differences among spirituality, faith, and religion in context, so the reader will know that the three concept may overlap but are not the same. The second section reviews some of the differences between religion and ethics, as well as how ethics, as a discipline, can be utilized to mediate between faith-based organizations when religion reaches its limitations. The third section distinguishes between religion and culture. Acknowledging the symbiotic relationship between the two entities, this section suggests that mutual respect among cultures is a functional tool to transform disjointed, faith-based community organizations into interfaith, ecumenical coalitions and partnerships. The fourth section addresses an approach to a community-based participatory research process that seeks to fully engage community, in this case the faith-based communities, as full participants in its organization and development. The fifth section, because the focus is on health, targets education for health. The last section further explores King's model of Authentic Culturecology by demonstrating operational constructs to include cultural framing, primary assumptions, principles, methodology, basic procedural steps, and conclusion. The chapter ends by discussing how the model applied to faith-based communities can enhance community organization and development.

This is illustrated by three case studies that model recommendations for moving forward.

CONCEPTS OF SPIRITUALITY, FAITH, AND RELIGION

Increased attention has been given in recent times to leaders of faith-based organizations for the purpose of improving individual and group health. Faith institutions are expected to assume meaningful roles in health promotion and protection, disease prevention, and cures, which may sometimes be inappropriate, for example, flu vaccination campaigns, HIV prevention and testing, and Medicare prescription rallies (Warren, 2007). The public policy discourse concerning faith-based communities may, however, focus on constitutional separation of church and state or the intrusive role of government in relation to programs and policies (Baker, 2009). Nevertheless, engaging the faith-based community in the community organization and development process is quintessential in improving health in the U.S. population.

Faith-based organizations seek to improve and strengthen the same populations as existing nonfaith-based prevention programs (Barry, Sutherland, & Harris, 2006). The development process of faith-based community engagement in providing health-related programs is necessary in improving access to care for the 43 million nonelderly, uninsured adults residing in the United States (DeHaven, Hunter, Wilder, Walton, & Berry, 2004). However, there are challenges when considering spirituality, faith, and religion as part of the U.S. health landscape (Warren & Tarver, 2010). The challenge lies with the lack of understanding of key terms and the misappropriation of their utility. The previously indicated terms are often synonymously linked to organizations that are "faith-based" without fully exploring their utilization in the overall organization. For example, the term faith-based is used liberally without clarifying its role and impact in usage. Thus, the term often fails to embrace the socioreligious factors that are culturally rooted in the context, leading resources ultimately to be *faith-placed* and not faith-based.

The term faith-based community is many times used as a catch-all reference to health programming designed, conducted, or supported by affiliated groups with or based in nonsecular settings (DeHaven et al., 2004). However, the interface with the metaphysical concepts of spirituality, faith, and religion, and their synergistic relationship to science and medicine are essential in improving the human condition and, if understood, can be helpful in improving health (Warren & Tarver, 2010). Faith-based groups can execute provisional initiatives that improve health through community organization and community building. These key concepts will be explored later in the chapter.

According to Tillich (1958), "there is hardly a word in the religious language, both theological and popular, which is subject to more misunderstandings, distortions and questionable definitions than the word *faith*."

To include spirituality and religion into the conversation creates additional confusion. Warren and Tarver (2010) write that spirituality, faith, and religion are terms that are often misunderstood and used interchangeably. Spirituality is one of the most complex terms to define and constructs to understand. In postmodern times, the relationship between religion and science is being revisited and the term spirituality is the bridge that renews this relationship. Often spirituality is described merely as a "quality of being spiritual" (Warren, 2006).

So, what is spiritual and spirituality? Spirituality is presented as the human search for meaning (Walter, 2002). If the vision is to improve the health of individuals and groups, then spirituality must be included in the approach toward how health and well-being are socially constructed (Warren & Tarver, 2010). Spirituality, faith, and religion may overlap, but they are different.

Faith has primarily been associated with religion in modern times; however, faith is social as well. In fact, faith covers all of reality, secular and sacred (Hopkins, 1999). To have faith does not require a person or group to be religious. Fowler (1981) in his book titled *Stages of Faith* writes, "Faith is not always religious in its content or context." Faith is a way of finding coherence in and giving meaning to the multiple forces and relationships that make up people's lives (Warren & Tarver, 2010). The relational aspect of faith is through the shared experiences that cultivate beliefs. Seeing oneself in relationship to others against a background of shared meaning and purpose is, in essence, faith.

Religion, or the religious dimension, consists of the encounter of human beings with the "sacred" or "divine" (Lincoln & Mamiya, 1990). For the majority of human beings, the expression of faith is equated with religion (Al Farugi & Sopher, 1974). Religion converges upon faith in something that transcends the human existence (Warren et al., 2002). Transcendent, derived from the Latin word *transcendere*, is to "climb over," "to surpass." Philosophically, transcendent is that which stands beyond all limits of human experience or knowledge. In the religion of Christianity and others, God is described as transcendent (McKim, 1996). However, religion is a social phenomenon, a shared group experience that has shaped and influenced the cultural screens of human communication and interpretation (Durkheim, 1965). Religion and religious institutions are an integral part of the lives of many residing in the United States (Isaac, Rowland, & Blackwell, 2007).

RELIGION AND ETHICS

Religion is defined as "ritual, social, and ethical elements combined with belief in the unseen world and often a deity" (McKim, 1996, p. 235). To speak of why one ought to love one's neighbor as oneself is, at once, to speak both of the religious and social. In fact, in such contexts, it is difficult to tell the difference between the two. Moreover, the social element of religion is prescriptive in that it tells the adherent what it means to live successfully and in good faith within a societal framework. The ethical element of religion can tell practitioners how they ought to treat others, both inside and outside the religious group. As well, it conveys the criteria for what counts as *right* action and what practices ought to be preferred over others.

Yet, there is still a need to make a fundamental distinction between religion and ethics. Whereas religion contains ethical elements, religion need not operate under the methodology of an ethical system. Ethics is foremost a rational enterprise that seeks to determine *the good* based upon reason and/or empirical information. Ethics is a branch of philosophy and, as such, addresses questions of good and bad, right and wrong, virtue and vice, and justice and injustice. While religion may do this as well, it does so privileging the religious methodology over the ethical. This means that religion could employ ethical language and pursue ethical ends without committing to the rational standard of noncontradictory rules within the religious framework (Aristotle, 1941). This phenomenon is partially explained by divine command theory, which states that a principle or action is right solely because the deity says it is right, and wrong otherwise. In this schema, pronouncements of goodness or the correctness of action are absolutely at the discretion of the enunciating deity. Thus, substantive efforts at critique or disagreement with the ethical defensibility of codified behaviors and concepts is rendered impossible or, at least, frustrated.

Religion performs a profound function in society by providing a narrative environment in which our moral imaginations can be stretched. It re-enacts ubiquitous stories, layered in a way that facilitates our ability to interpret and derive meaning in connection with our maturity and life experience. Ethics stands back from the fray and allows each to seek *the good* without privileging any worldview, including the religious. This *non-privileging of worldviews* is sometimes viewed antagonistically as a slight against religion. But, perhaps a more appropriate way to view the distinction is as one of checks and balances, particularly where faith-based community organizations around issues that disproportionately affect vulnerable populations are concerned.

As an example, the process of informed consent is foundational to conducting research ethically; yet, voluntariness on the part of the prospective study participants precedes that process. To achieve favorable reception of their aims, many researchers have relied heavily on the influence of clergy to solicit participation in biomedical research. Authority figures like pastors, imams, and rabbis have been instrumental in recruiting their congregants for clinical studies across ethnic lines. When this is done, it is presumed that participation is voluntary and that potential study participants are knowledgeable about the proposed research to the degree that they are able to make an informed decision regarding both consent and participation. While these elements constitute the gold standard for practical implementation and respecting individual autonomy, the scientific literature is sparse regarding the extent to which consent and participation are measurably voluntary. Participation involves decision making and decision making can be heavily influenced by those who have vested interest in the research. Thus, the worry arises that consent and participation in biomedical research solicited in religious contexts may not be wholly voluntary or entirely free from soft coercion.

This is a case of potential ethical violations that could occur within the context of religion. The discipline of bioethics was designed to address these very cases. If enlisted religious leaders, regardless of their faith traditions, are not properly informed or trained in the mechanisms and necessary standards of consent, the guarded willingness of the congregants could be abused if a stalwart notion of consent is weakened or overridden because religious authority figures make the request for participation.

Given the well-documented atrocities against the most defenseless persons in American society that were often justified on religious grounds (Scriven, 2007), an ethical analysis that did not privilege prejudicial tenets derived from how a particular religion was practiced would have been helpful to produce just social theories, leading to actual justice. These safeguards are necessary precisely because of the influence that religion continues to wield in the lives of many people. Religious communities are community organizations. With this understanding, they must be developed in accordance with the highest standards and most effective tools for self-governance to fulfill their mission on behalf of the people they represent. So, the distinction between religion and ethics is really one of methodology and presupposition. However, within a religious community organization, religion is a given and ethics is a functional necessity. If we consider the above discussion on informed consent, the issues of faith and medicine are inextricably linked in a religious community and greatly benefit from ethical mediation.

Regarding faith, the structure of most religious communities lends itself to their leaders holding vast amounts of authority to shape the theology of the laity. This sway extends not only to the interpretation of sacred texts, but also to being the arbiter of the will of deity for the lives of individual congregants. Questions of social association, mate selection, sexual practices, employment choices, political allegiances, and philanthropic expression all fall under the domain of clergy influence and are vital areas of concern for a large segment of the population.

Medically, many religious leaders enjoy the privilege of articulating what they understand to be God's desires concerning how followers should eat, whether or not they should seek medical attention, and if they should follow the directions of medical professionals *as a matter of faith*. In some faith traditions, avoiding physicians is seen as an act of devotion to

God and a demonstration that one trusts God to heal sickness and disease. Likewise, some religious communities do not believe in blood transfusions or invasive surgery, even to save the life of a child or family member. The extent to which congregants hold these views is often related to the perspective, teachings, and interpretation of sacred texts emanating from faith leaders.

What things ought to be done and how those actions are determined lie within the clerical domain for many as well. But, it is not clear that when these issues are determined solely on religious grounds (textually or invoking divine command theory), fairness and justice are consistent primary outcomes. Issues of liberty, acceptable life choices, end of life decisions, pregnancy terminations, contraception, and who should have access to social goods are some of the questions that arise in this context. Of real concern is the way the ethical and medical often overlap in faith communities, making these environments highly susceptible to bioethical, biomedical, and clerical infractions based upon abuses of authority and an absence of mechanisms to govern power differentials among religious leaders, researchers, physicians, and congregants.

RELIGION AND CULTURE

King defines culture as a functional, internally consistent system of beliefs, attitudes, values, expectations, and norms/patterns of conduct (King, 2002). Because cultures are forms of social interaction accepted by discrete communities within time and place, they evoke worldviews and historical experiences that mark our humanity and inhumanity (Townes, 1998). All groups have culture and, thereby, participate in culture creation. Yet, often the culture of a group is so closely linked to religious practices that the two appear identical. As an exemplar of this phenomenon in action, consider the links and overlap between African American culture(s), faith-based community organizations, and religious orientation as they relate to health and health outcomes.

At one point in American history, it was argued that African Americans had no culture because their ancestral connections and historical memories as a group had been damaged by slavery. But culture is an amalgam of past and present life activities, both passed on and newly created, that define social activity. Again, every group possesses and creates culture. In fact, with variation on certain ingredients, certain groups may participate in subcultures that are distinct and somewhat separate. It is therefore unnecessary and unwarranted to debate assumptions as to whether African Americans have culture. Douglass (Speech at Rochester, July 5, 1852, quoted from Woodson, 1969) is also helpful here. When responding to the charge that Black people lacked critical capacities Douglass retorted, "Where all is plain, there is nothing to be argued" (Woodson, 1969). For

Douglass (Speech at Rochester, July 5, 1852, quoted from Woodson, 1969), prohibitions against developing African American capacities *presupposed* those very capacities. Likewise, the claim asserting nonexistence of African American culture requires no argument to refute it, because it is false by both definition and fact. However, the evidence does suggest that African Americans are disproportionately impacted by excess morbidity and mortality. Thus, the subject of specific cultural practices must be centralized and interrogated when engaging in communal health dialogue pertaining to the elimination of racial and ethnic health disparities.

The Pew Forum on Religious and Public Life conducted a survey in 2007 with results indicating that African Americans are more religious than others in the United States (Pew Forum on Religion and Public Life, 2009). Dennis, Hicks, Banerjee, and Dennis (2005) write that, according to Martin and Martin, spirituality supersedes and overarches religiosity for most African Americans. Spirituality is at the heart of the African American community, whether the view is explored through religion or not, it is foundational to faith. As noted previously, Lincoln and Mamiya (1990, p. 7) write that "culture is the form of religion and religion is at the heart of culture."

It is important to understand that many persons of African descent believe that a Supreme Being, or God, exists and is present in all things, both the inner and outer universes, and that a person's life experiences evolve around a world filled with spirituality (Holloway, 1990). Black persons' affirmation of their faith is in the god of freedom and is closely related to spirituality. The Black Christians who formed the historic Black churches also knew implicitly that their understanding of Christianity, which was premised on the rock of antiracial discrimination, was more authentic than the Christianity practiced in racialized churches (Lincoln & Mamiya, 1990). The key to understanding and engaging Black churches compared to non-Hispanic White churches is to know that they are not the same theologically, socially, psychologically, and even spiritually.

Isaac et al. (2007) write that "the belief and faith that one can rise above the personal struggles, adversity, racism, and poverty is a familiar refrain that echoes throughout the African American church today." The belief and faith to affirm one's social condition are beyond religion, but ultimately spiritual concerns. Ancient African views of spirituality "allow every individual to go within and focus on one's personal spark of the CREATOR and attune it to the higher power that cannot be described adequately due to human limitations, but can be experienced as the individual resonates with it" (Chissell, 1993, p. 43). In order for individuals and groups of African descent to resonate in community participatory approaches toward the improvement of health, one must understand the cultural context of spirituality, faith, and religion for social relevancy prior to communal engagement. For the fact is that over time, African Americans have developed a set of values, beliefs, meanings, and practices—and, by extension, a way of health (King, 2002).

The dynamics of personal life are vertical faith as relational to God and horizontal as the relationships persons have with other human beings. These relationships present metaphysical and social dynamics that can pose some faith and identity concerns. Faith is an act of the personality as a whole; it participates in the dynamics of personal life (Tillich, 1958). The actions and practices are indicators of a pragmatic functionality of faith. The functionality of faith in health is based upon trust. The faith and identity concerns, however, extend to the experiences of the African American population in the United States. According to King (2002), "the experiences are extended to the United States where the relationship between African Americans, the health establishment, and the community and social environment is not an isolated phenomena, as scientific rationalism would have one believe, but the product of a history of relationships." Health is a relationship that extends vertically (relational to God) and horizontally (relational to others human beings), based on one's personal perceptions of dimensions of faith (Warren et al., 2002); issues that surround decisions about physical and mental health are initially technical, "the experiences are extended to the United States where the relationship between African Americans, the health establishment, and the community and social environment is not an isolated phenomena, as scientific rationalism would have one believe, but the product of a history of relationships." but they are ultimately ethical concerns; and issues of health and illness are theological and spiritual issues (Epperly, 1997), and how one takes care of themselves—body, mind, and spirit—is a matter of faith and unfaith (Warren, 2006).

COMMUNITY-BASED PARTICIPATORY RESEARCH

In reaching faith-based communities there must be a systemic, authentic approach that ensures trust. The public health community has embraced an approach that appears to have measurable efficacy. That approach is called community-based participatory research (CBPR) and focuses on social, structural, and physical environmental inequities through active involvement of community members, organizational representativeness, and researchers in all aspects of the research process (Israel, Schulz, Parker, & Becker, 1998). The CBPR process is scientific inquiry that is conducted as a partnership between a traditionally trained practitioner(s) and lay-participants. In this instance, the lay-participants are representatives of faith-based organizations committed to organizing and developing their specific organization. The research effort is process or translational research and asks the empowering question, *how do we organize and develop*? Faith-based community members must participate fully in all aspects of the process, and seeking and honoring their views, concerns, and interests are fundamental in building trust. Not only are their views, concerns, and interests important, their approach to identifying strategies, answers, and solutions must also be authentically considered.

The work in the CBPR process combines three activities: investigation, learning, and action. It is a method of social investigation of problems, involving participation in problem formulation and resolution. It is a learning process for analyzing the structural causes of problems through collective discussion, analysis, and interaction. Finally, the process engages all stakeholders in concerted action, both short and long term (Merzel & D'afflitti, 2003). The direct link between research and action is a unique aspect of participatory research. Environmental justice principles provide a rich example of the utility of the CBPR process. In fact, the definition of environmental justice includes the "... meaningful involvement of all people ..." (EPA, 1998). This approach is instructive in determining and overcoming the challenges in organizing and developing faith-based communities. Adopting a CBPR approach will ensure that the faith community is involved from the beginning to the end in organizing and developing their organization. Health, used as an example and described broadly, is the major challenge confronting many faith-based organizations. As indicted earlier, many of these groups host a variety of health-related services that appear to be effective, but there is little evidence of measurable individual, group, or community health benefits. But, what benefits are expected and how should they be measured? One strategy is education and, in this instance, it is education for health.

EDUCATION FOR HEALTH

Health, if described broadly, is the major challenge confronting many faith-based organizations. As indicted earlier, many of these groups host a variety of health-related services that appear to be effective, but there is little evidence of measurable individual, group, or community health benefits. But what benefits are expected and how should they be measured? One strategy is education and, in this instance, it is education for health. The United States purports to be the richest country in the world, spends the most money on health, and has the most developed and technologically advanced health delivery system in the world (Walker, Mays, & Warren, 2004). Yet, the United States ranks low in the overall health status of its people. Faith-based communities and others have relied on health professionals to guide, direct, and counsel on salient matters related to individual, group, and community health (Campbell, 1995). In more recent times, consumers and community-based groups have taken greater responsibility for their health and health care. This shift has placed a greater role on health literacy and health education (Warren, 1992). Ironically, for many years health educators have known the importance of health education and have engaged in applied research to know what works and what does not.

As far back as 1970, Young writes, "Health education includes all those experiences of an individual or community that influences beliefs, attitudes and behaviors with respect to health, as well as processes and efforts of producing change when it is necessary for optimal health." However, it is difficult to plan, implement, and evaluate health education interventions without first conceptualizing and understanding the community in which the interventions are planned. The essential strategies for community organizing and development are critical if the health education effort is to succeed (Warren, 1992). Over the years, selected theories and practices of heath education and behavioral change have been studied, implemented, and evaluated; yet, the health of those in greatest need still lags far behind the general population (Warren, 2006). There have also been efforts to organize the faith community to promote heath and prevent disease among the people they serve (Resnicow et al., 2004). While much has been attempted, little has been rigorously evaluated in understanding the process of organizing and developing faith-based community efforts (Warren, 2006). The faith community health fairs, health screening, nutrition, and weight loss programs continue. The mental and emotional health counseling is ongoing, yet objective measures remain elusive (Wimberly, 2001).

The authors of this chapter argue that faith-based communities are an essential part of the U.S. landscape and must be considered as unique and diverse cultural groups. The notion that health is narrowly defined as physical, or even mental health, has resulted in a false separation of mind, soul, and body. This myopic view has often resulting in minimizing the role and influence of faith leaders and thus by-passed an essential stakeholder in the health and well-being of the population. Over 50% of the people in the United States claim some religious tradition and even for those who do not, there is some faith and/or spiritual tradition that they respect. If engaging any of these faith communities to promote health or any other life-sustaining quality is viewed as important, one must also seriously and rigorously consider systematic, if not scientific, methods to organize and develop these important subcultures of the complex "American" population. Shifting the order from *health education* to *education for health* opens the conversation about knowing that being healthy is essential to *Be-ing (w)hole* and complete in a universe that is large and abundant enough to celebrate all of its creatures.

As previously mentioned, King's Authentic Culturecology Model has a clear utility for faith-based communities because it provides a structured approach to integrate religious constructs in the cultural context.

DIMENSIONS OF CULTURAL FRAMING: AUTHENTIC CULTURECOLOGY

There are also several applications within the cultural framework according to King's model that should be described. One is cultural framing, which is the idea that the individual's health is a relational event that can be best understood as a situationally bound unit of relationships. These relationships may be organic, psychological, family, social, political, and/ or spiritual in which culture is the unifying unit (King, 2002). A culturally framed event is another term that is important to the model. This term describes its reality, system of values, and ways of knowing (King, 2002).

In adapting King's model to faith-based organizations, one dimension of cultural framing attends to the group as "community." In this instance, community refers to the specific faith-based community in which the organizing effort is targeted. The basis of the group's identity may be religious, faith, or spiritual, or any combination of the three. In this instance, they may be bound by specific tenets, rituals, litany, and/or practices in their faith-context, which have influence on their culture. Many faith-based communities are culturally distinct groups of people based on their specific denomination, but perhaps very different in the praxis. In terms of the monotheistic religions, "All Jews, Christians or Muslims are not the same." For example, the Pew Foundation documents that African Americans, regardless of denomination, are the most "religious" population in the United States (Pew Forum on Religion and Public Life, 2009). More than 75% of Hispanics in the United States are Catholic and the influence of Catholicism in Hispanic/Latino culture is well documented (Delgado, 1997).

The second consideration is group identification. Different faith-based communities hold different beliefs and practices related to health. For example, Seventh Day Adventists, in large part, engage in health practices, particularly related to diet, consistent with their theological/religious beliefs and belief systems. This faith-based group reports better health statistics than the general U.S. population (Montgomery et al., 2007). Muslims avoid eating pork based on writings in the Quran, their sacred text. A tenet of Judaism requires kosher food preparation. In this instance, it is difficult, and maybe unnecessary, to separate religion from culture. It is also difficult to separate religious and cultural practices and beliefs from race/ethnicity.

Medicine and modern public health practice have adopted and reflect the culture of modern medicine (King & Nobles, 1996). The medicinal model is the dominant paradigm of modern medicine, which focuses on the individual. Therefore, the emphasis of modern public health is on the individual *at risk*, or identifying biological intrapersonal factors (weak organ systems), or psychological intrapersonal factors (beliefs, cognitions, attitude, intentions, skills) as determinants of health outcomes (King, 2002). Many faith-based communities focus attention on those in greatest need as well. However, much of their work is population based and addresses systemic problems, sometimes called *systemic sin*. While much of the work is mission-driven, focusing on food, clothing, and shelter, organizing themselves to reframe challenging circumstances for the people they serve is also part of many of their missions. Culture places in context historical values and meanings so that people are better able to adapt to stresses and life's adversities in rapidly changing society (King, 2002).

Another dimension in King's (2002) model spotlights the environment as context—political, ecological, economic, and spiritual. In other words, another dimension of culture is context, the web of relationships between the public and social reality (King, 2002). Culture is the mediating construct in the web of relationships (King & Nobles, 1996), and the force that maintains unity and coherence of the web of relationships (King, 2002).

PRIMARY ASSUMPTIONS OF THE MODEL

According to King and Nobles (1996), there are four primary assumptions of an Authentic Culturecology Model. The first assumption is that public health is a cultural phenomenon. The basis for all phenomena is relationship, or a person nested in a triadic set of relationships known as a web of relationships, which consists of the person, their community, and their environment (Haslam, 1994). In the case of this chapter, the community is faith-based. Culture can be defined as the sum of relationships (unit or web of relationships) of any phenomenon; culture is the defining substance of all human action (Carruthers, 1995; Hilliard, 1976). Culture is functional, internally consistent beliefs, attitudes, values, expectations, and norms/patterns of conduct (King, 2002). In the personal dimension, culture directs the person's level of autonomous capacity for self-organization, as well as that of self-restoration (King, 2002). In the community dimension, culture directs the level of social and economic support and the balance in relation to ecology and faith (King, 2002).

The second assumption is that bonds are the dimensions internal to culture. A bond is a historical–cognitive emotional structure (connection) that has clear functions in everyday functioning of a unit of relationships (King, 2002). The web of relationships reflects bonds to personal, conventional, social, and spiritual order (King, 2002). If culture represents the structure of a system in unity, then bonds represent or are forms of "glue" that maintain the ties or attachments, and therefore the function or dysfunction of the web of relationships (King, 2002). The ties that bind people of faith together define their essential nature as a historically and culturally distinct group within the context of the dynamics of the faith-based community, which provides the *cultural key* for organizing with and for them. Cultural framing prompts the articulation of the organic set of bonds as the defining reality at any given moment for any given relationship (King, 2002).

The third assumption is that there are four primary bonds (Fiske, 1993). According to King (2002), these bonds can be conceptualized as follows:

- *Affinity bonds:* The need for collective belonging, or solidarity, and intimacy based on memory. These bonds grow from the memory of childhood (feeding, comfort, protection) and are based on the need for security and trust.

■ *Obligation bonds:* The drive to establish rules according to status markers, such as deeds (good or bad), age, skill, knowledge, class, social position, and race. These bonds are based on the meaning of power, order, and control, and grow from the spirit or nature of relationships and the need for accountability, duty, responsibility, and moral commitment.

■ *Assurance bonds:* Bonds based on the organization of common sets of values of exchange, such as vocation, production, money, goods, materials, or intellectual work. The emphasis is on good return on investment or time. Social transaction is based on costs and benefits. Assurance bonds are based on the search or need for competence, mastery, and autonomy.

■ *Harmony bonds:* These are the bonds governed by the search for fairness and rhythm. They are the ties organizing the construction and interpretation of relationships in strictly impartial terms. An example of this is the search for equity (King & Nobles, 1996). These focus on reciprocity, fairness as primary values. Such bonds are based on the motivation for justice, fairness, and balance.

Every relationship can be defined by these bonds (King, 2002). Bonds are present or absent (King, 2002). When they are present, they are either strong or weak, health-enhancing or health-compromising (King, 2002). Bonds characterize the nature of the event (King, 2002).

The fourth and final assumption is that the essence of an event/phenomenon is not the phenomenon itself, but in its web of relationships (King, 2002). This implies that the unit of analysis in the examination of any public health occurrence must be the web of health relationships in that event (King, 2002). Fundamental to understanding the event as a relationship is the nature of the bonds in the culturally framed web (King, 2002). Bonds constitute the essence (King, 2002). It is within the framework that the person's (family's, community's) bond to a larger reality factors (psychological, social, ecological, spiritual) centrally in setting the stage for modifying the bonds and therefore conditions for behavior change occur (King, 2002).

PRINCIPLES OF THE MODEL

According to King (2002), there are three principles of the Authentic Culturecology Model. The first principle is that the presence of strong health-enhancing bonds in all four bonding domains is necessary for optimum health and the prevention of illness (King, 2002). For the person, the stronger the health-enhancing bonds, the stronger the formation of a collective self-identity, as a part of community. Therefore, it is less likely that the person will engage in relationships that involve risk factors for a host of negative health outcomes. The second principle is that the same statement is true and can be applied to the family and the community/ society (King, 2002). The third principle is that the presence of health-compromising bonds, or the absence or weakness of autonomous bonds (to personal, spiritual, and conventional social order), predict a greater likelihood of the person engaging in risk factors for a host of negative outcomes for self, community, or society (King, 2002). In the context of the African American experience, King and Nobles argue that African American health relations are significantly compromised by a society that has historically negated [Maafa] (Ani, 1994) African American bonds to society (conventional social order). What allows the African American to survive is the positive [Maafa] (Ani, 1994) remnants of historical bonds to cultural history (spiritual connections) (King, 2002). This may be applicable to other vulnerable populations as well.

METHODOLOGY OF THE AUTHENTIC CULTURECOLOGY MODEL

The methodology of the Authentic Culturecology Model focuses on the web of relationships as the unit of analysis and the subject for exploration with culture as the unifying link (King, 2002). The model suggests that the first step of design of intervention always begins with careful work in identifying or locating the smallest web of relationship or cultural event of the whole person in whole contexts (King, 2002). The second step is cultural framing, which requires both cultural sensitivity and competence (King, 2002). The frame consists of the representation of the types, strength, and valence of bonds present in the web of relationships (King, 2002). The central methodology for the discovery of bonds with cultural framing is the use of narrative (Fluker, 1998). The third step is the participation of the subject in change, recognizing that what is to be changed is the nature of bonds within the web of relations, which maintain outcomes that are health compromising (King, 2002).

BASIC PROCEDURAL STEPS FOR THE FRAMEWORK

The first task is always to undertake a critical study of the nature and epidemiology of the basic units of relationships that produce high-risk behaviors and the converse of relationships that preserve health and well-being (King, 2002). The critical search for the relationship must be consistent with seeing the relationship in the context (political, ecological, economic, and social) of the larger web of relationships (King, 2002).

The second intervention task begins with selecting and specifying the set of relationships, the relationship of primary focus (as subject) that produces the behavior leading to the outcome (as object) (King, 2002). Careful research must be undertaken to identify and define this basic unit of study, intervention, or discourse (King, 2002). Having specified the key relationship of interest, the task then becomes the thorough exploration in this dominant attribute of interest, the bonds that maintain both health indicators and the relative risk indicators (King, 2002).

The third task is one of strategic goal setting. The health approach always must seek to formulate goals and strategic direction for intervention in conjunction with the other relationship (national and community policies, and priorities for prevention and health promotion) in which the primary relations are embedded. This unit must be embedded in the community. The strategic direction should guide the development of goals for health promotion, health protection, prevention services, or clinical intervention (King, 2002).

The fourth task is to develop a culturecological intervention program appropriate to, and in conjunction with, the subject population (King, 2002). This development is the cultural framing that should guide the intervention to include timing (primary, secondary, and tertiary prevention; level of personal relations, family relations, community relations, and so on) and desired outcomes. The desired outcome usually falls into one of three categories: changing the existing relational complex, establishing a new relational context, or both (King, 2002).

King's fifth task is to situate the entire enterprise in a research-based context to inform all relationships within and between units, and put in place intervention, implementation, and evaluation protocols to include:

a. Process research
b. Pilot research
c. Efficacy trial
d. Effectiveness trial
e. Data analysis and dissemination

CONCLUSION ABOUT THE FRAMEWORK

The Authentic Culturecology Model asserts that the public health approach should move away from its emphasis on individuals, scientific rationalism, and knowledge gained from objects, but rather focus on the study of relationships. The framework promotes a continuous critique to validate the importance of cultural understanding in the promotion of health, in its broader context.

SUMMARY

Most persons in the United States pursuing the "American Dream" are deeply imbedded in there own cultural and religious customs and traditions. These religious beliefs and cultural customs are intermingled, making these groups very resistant to lifestyle change. Especially in inner city communities, these groups live and work in very close proximity to each other, making standardized approaches to community health efforts difficult and time consuming. Attempts to impact on these communities with positive health reform and practices by faith-based organizations have failed, primarily because these organizations have not understood the "how to" of approaching these communities.

For the most part, inner city communities are diverse groups of sub-cultures, with various residents, which are defined by their own individual leadership and infrastructure. These communities trust their *own* and tend to be very suspicious and cautious in cultivating new relationships. Just because a health initiative is a faith-based one does not ensure that an immediate trusting relationship is guaranteed, or will ever be realized. So, then the fundamentals for community entry for a faith-based organization are the same as with any other institution. Trust building takes time and ongoing engagement in the community targeted. Effective faith-based health initiatives call for *hands-on* approaches to building trust, which demands that practitioners commit to immersing themselves in the cultural rhythm of the community. It requires accommodation and the ongoing respect for residents and leaders in the community.

Successful faith-based health efforts, as with any others, will require elbow grease. It will require patience on the part of the leadership. There is no quick fix to addressing disparities in communities, not even for religious leadership. Community Engagement, Organization and Development (CEOD) is a complex and time-consuming process that calls for foundational principles of the process to be put in place. Even then there may not be solutions to the health problems existing in communities; however, this does not mean efforts should not be made to address these problems. This is where, over time, true or weak commitment of faith-based leadership will manifest itself.

Case Study Exercises

Individually, or as a group, review the following case studies and respond to the questions posed at the end of the study, as appropriate. Be sure to focus on the why, how, and what emphasized in each question. Your professor/instructor will provide you with specific guidance on how you are to report your findings for the class.

Case Study 6.1: Overcoming Interfaith Conflict to Save Marriages

According to a March 26, 2006, article in the *Washington Post*, marriage rates in America have been in steady decline since the 1960s (Jones, 2006). At that time, 91% of White households were headed by married couples, while the number was 67% for Black households. However, in 2000, marriage rates in White households had dropped to 80%, while Black households had a steep drop to 48% (Jones, 2006). By 2007, 69% of African American children were born to unwed mothers and the numbers are increasing (African American Healthy Marriage Initiative, 2010). Marriage is a sacrament in many faith traditions that impacts the rearing of children and the stability of community for generations. Thus, it is natural that community, faith-based organizations would form to address the crisis of declining marriage rates, particularly in the African and the American faith community.

Background

Two African American, faith-based community organizations form to take on this pressing issue: one Christian and one Muslim. While they both agree on the sanctity and social utility of marriage, they have different conceptions of marriage that hinders cooperation between the groups. The Christian idea is that marriage is a monogamous relationship between one man and one woman. The Muslim idea is that marriage can be monogamous, but can also be a polygamous relationship between one man and multiple wives. Even though polygamy is prohibited by law in American society, as a permissible Islamic practice, it is part of the thought that shapes the Muslim approach to marital solutions, particularly when the idea of arranged marriages is introduced.

The differing conceptions of marriage are simultaneously religious as well as cultural, since both contexts are involved and influence the construction of the other. Both organizations realize that the issue of African American marriage is critical to both American society and their respective faith traditions, but they have legitimate concerns about building a faith coalition that is religious, cultural, and ethical in complex ways. Yet, because of the gravity of the situation, the two groups are committed to finding meaningful ways to work together toward ameliorating the problem of African American marriage rate decline.

Formulating Strategies for Solutions

Notice that the issues raised in the discussion section did not begin to address the problem of the decline in African American marriage rates. Instead, the emphasis of the exercise concerns the building blocks involved in forming and sustaining meaningful faith-based community organizations. Often those things that threaten cooperation are parochial idiosyncrasies that may have very little to do with the obvious objective. That being said, one helpful strategy is to revisit King's assumption in his culturecology framework for bonds: affinity bonds, obligation bonds, assurance bonds, and harmony for us. To convince one group or the other to relinquish their theological or cultural position on marriage may be fruitless. But to recognize that all community organizations require the development of certain bonds to be effective and remain viable is imperative.

Developing these bonds allows for the kind of cultural reciprocity and interfaith dialogue necessary to focus the new coalition on the issue of declining African American marriage rates.

Study Questions

1. What are the spiritual/faith/religious factors and perspectives involved?
2. What are some relevant cultural considerations that influence this discussion?
3. What are the ethical dilemmas arising in the context of this effort?
4. How do these concerns overlap in ways that are difficult to distinguish?
5. How can community members and churches spend time more productively working together to solve the problem individually?

Case Study 6.2: Horizontal and Vertical Faith and the Beguiled System of Justice

Oral tradition is a key form of information dissemination in many cultures. African American families throughout the African Diaspora in the United States are aware of the human subject research and experimentation on persons of African descent. Below is an issue that outlines historical injustices in biomedical research where African Americans experienced horrific exploitation and later received an apology from the President of the United States, acknowledging the intentional negligence and abuse. Imagine engaging a community-organizing effort where *faith–trust* relationships may pose some limitations in your efforts to organize a segment of the Black community. You work for the Centers for Disease Control and Prevention and are responsible for convincing young Black women to participate in a clinical trials research project focused on HIV vaccines.

Apologies have repeatedly been made in response to unjust practices in the United States related to Black people. One of the most noted apologies was offered on May 16, 1997, by former President William Jefferson Clinton, who apologized for the U.S. Public Health Syphilis Study at Tuskegee. The U.S. Public Health Service physicians conducted unethical research from 1932 through 1972, on 600 Black men in rural Macon County, Alabama. Moreover, in the 1950s, these men were denied treatment for syphilis even when effective treatment (penicillin) was discovered and available. Instead, the unethical practice of telling the men that they were being treated for *bad blood* continued. The very painful lumbar punctures and nontherapeutic, basic medical check-ups also continued; leaving the primary disease to follow its natural progression until the men died and were ready for autopsy (Warren & Tarver, 2010).

Another recorded occurrence of such "experiments" was conducted by J. Marion Sims, MD, who is considered by some as the *Father of American*

Gynecology. Dr. Sims recorded hundreds of surgical experiments on enslaved women in his backyard clinic from 1845 to 1849. He performed unanaesthetized surgeries in the genital areas of dozens of enslaved Black women in an attempt to correct vaginal fistulas (Townes, 1998). These and other unauthorized experimental practices that under-gird the delivery of health care in the United States for women have established a historical distrust of health practitioners by African Americans, particularly for Black women.

The American Medical Association (AMA) on July 10, 2008, acknowledged historical and systemic transgressions by apologizing to the nation's Black physicians, citing a century of *past wrongs* (Washington, 2008). Following this, on July 29, 2008, the United States House of Representatives passed a resolution apologizing for American chattel slavery and for Jim Crow laws (Fears, 2008). Though each response is considered to be a formal apology, the long-term effects or results of the apologies to Black people can only be measured over time. However, data indicate that since federal health record-keeping began more than 100 years ago, Black people have experienced statistically significant health disparities compared to other groups in the United States (Warren, 1992).

Study Questions

1. What are the historical problematic variables that have impacted minority health?
2. What is the value of an apology without resources, particularly if the injustices continue?
3. How has multidisciplinary, systemic negligence and policy contributed to the issue?
4. Does the African American cultural experience justify distrust? If so, how and why?

REFERENCES

African American Healthy Marriage Initiative. (2010). Retrieved December 22, 2010, from www.aahmi.net/focus.html#stats

Al Farugi, I. R., & Sopher, D. E. (1974). *Historical atlas of the religions of the world.* New York, NY: Macmillan.

Ani, M. (1994). *An African-centered critiqe of European cultural thought and behavior.* New York, NY: African World Press.

Aristotle. (1941). *The basic works of Aristotle.* New York, NY: Random House.

Baker, J. (2009). Faith-based inefficiency: The follies of Bush's initiatives [Review of the book *Faith-based inefficiency: The follies of Bush's initiatives*]. *Sociology of Religion, 70*(2), 196–197.

Barry, A. E., Sutherland, M. S., & Harris, G. J. (2006). Faith-based prevention model: A rural African-American case study. *American Journal of Health Studies, 21*(3/4), 148–157.

Campbell, A. (1995). *Health is liberation.* Cleveland, OH: Pilgrim Press.

Carruthers, J. (1995). *MDW NTR divine speech: A historical reflection of African deep thought from the time of the Pharaohs to the present Red Press.* London: Karnak House.

Chissell, J. T. (1993). *Pyramids of power! An ancient African centered approach to optimal health.* Baltimore, MD: Positive Perceptions Publications.

De La Cancela, V., Chin, J. L., & Jenkins, Y. M. (1998). *Community health psychology . . . empowerment for diverse communities.* New York, NY: Routledge, p. 2.

DeHaven, M. J., Hunter, I. B., Wilder, L., Walton, J. W., & Berry, J. (2004). Health programs in faith-based organizations: Are they effective? *American Journal of Public Health, 94*(6), 1030–1036.

Delgado, J. (1997). *Salud: A Latino's guide to total health—Body, mind, and spirit.* New York, NY: Harper Collins.

Dennis, D. L., Hicks, T., Banerjee, P., & Dennis, B. G. (2005). Spirituality among a predominately African American college college student population. *American Journal of Health Studies, 20*(3/4), 135–142.

Durkheim, E. (1965). *The elementary forms of the religious life.* New York, NY: Free Press.

Environmental Protection Agency. (1998). *Final guidance for incorporating environmental justice concerns in EPA's NEPA compliance analyses.* Washington, DC: U.S. Governmental Printing Office.

Epperly, B. G. (1997). *Spirituality & health, health & spirituality: A new journey of spirit, mind, and body.* Mystic, CT: Twenty-Third Publications.

Fears, D. (2008, July 30). *Politics: The house issues an apology for slavery.* Retrieved September 14, 2010, from *The Washington Post* website www.washingtonpost.com/wp-dyn/content/article/2008/07/29/AR2008072902279.html

Fellin, P. (2001). *Understanding American communities.* In J. Rothman, J. Erlich, & J. Tropman (Eds.), *Strategies of community interventions* (5th ed.). Itasca, IL: Peacock.

Fiske, A. P. (1993). *Structures of social life: The four elementary-forms of relations.* New York, NY: Free Press.

Fluker, W. E. (1998). Introduction: The failure of ethical leadership. In W. E. Fluker (Ed.), *The stones that the builders rejected: The development of ethical leadership from the Black church tradition* (pp. 1–22). Harrisburgh, PA: Trinity Press International.

Fowler, J. W. (1981). *Stages of faith: The psychology of human development and the quest for meaning* (1st ed.). San Francisco, CA: Harper & Row.

Haslam, N. (1994). Categories of social relationships. *Cognition, 53,* 59–90.

Hilliard, A. G. (1976). *Free your mind: Return to the source.* San Francisco, CA: Urban Institute Publication.

Holloway, J. E. (1990). *Africanisms in American culture.* Bloomington, IN: Indiana University Press.

Holmes, E. (2007). *The science of the mind.* Radford, VA: Wilder Publications.

Hopkins, D. N. (1999). *Black faith and public talk: Critical essays on James H. Cone's Black theology and black power.* Maryknoll, NY: Orbis Books.

Hunter, A. (1975). The loss of community: An empirical test through replication. *American Sociology Review, 40*(5), 537–552.

Isaac, E. P., Rowland, M. L., & Blackwell, L. E. (2007). Fighting health disparities: The educational role of the African American church. *Cross Currents, 57*(2), 261–265.

Israel, B., Schulz, A., Parker, E., & Becker, A. (1998). Review of community-based research: Assessing partnership approaches to improve public health. *Annual Review of Public Health, 19*(1), 173–202.

Jones, J. (2006, March 26). *Washington Post.* Retrieved December 22, 2010, from www.washingtonpost.com/wp-dyn/content/article/2006/03/25/AR2006032500029_2.html

King, L. M. (2002). Development of authenticity in public health: A culturecology model as a culture critique. In J. C. Chunn (Ed.), *The health behavioral change imperative: Theory, education, and practice in diverse populations* (pp. 91–111). New York, NY: Kluwer Academic/Plenum.

King, L. M., & Nobles, W. (1996). *Science, culture, church, and community: An authentic prevention model for non-insulin dependent diabetes in African American women.* Center for Disease Control. Atlanta, GA: United States Department of Health and Human Services.

Lincoln, C. E., & Mamiya, L. H. (1990). *The Black church in the African-American experience.* Durham: Duke University Press.

McKim, D. K. (1996). *Westminster dictionary of theological terms* (1st ed.). Louisville, KY: Westminster John Knox Press.

Merzel, C., & D'afflitti, J. (2003). Reconsidering community-based health promotion: Promise, performance, and potential. *American Journal of Public Health, 93*(4), 557.

Minkler, M., Wallerstein, N., & Wilson, N. (2002). Improving health through community organization and community building. In K. Glanz, B. K. Rimer, & K. Viswanath (Eds.), *Health behavior and health education.* San Francisco, CA: Jossey-Bass.

Montgomery, S., Herring, P., Beeson, L., Butler, T., Sabate, J., Chan, J., ... Preston-Martin, S. (2007). Comparing self-reported disease outcomes, diet, and lifestyles in a national cohort of Black and White Seventh-Day Adventists. *Preventing Chronic Disease, 4*(3), A62.

Parker, E. A., et al. (2001). Disentangling measures of individual perceptions of community social dynamics: Results of a community survey. *Health Education Behavior, 28*(4), 462–486.

Pew Forum on Religion & Public Life. (2009). *A religious portrait of African Americans.* Washington, DC: Author.

Resnicow, K., Cambell, M. K., Carr, C., McCarty, F., Wang, T., Periasamy, S.,...Stables, G. (2004). Body and soul: A dietary intervention conducted through African-American churches. *The American Journal of Preventative Medicine, 27*(2), 97–105.

Scriven, D. (2007). *A dealer of old clothes: Philosophical conversations with David Walker.* Lanham, MD: Lexington Books.

Tillich, P. (1958). *Dynamics of faith.* New York, NY: Harper & Row.

Townes, E. M. (1998). *Breaking the fine rain of death: African American health issues and a womanist ethic of care.* New York, NY: Continuum.

Walker, B., Mays, V. M., & Warren, R. (2004). The changing landscape for the elimination of racial/ethnic health status disparities. *Journal of Health Care Poor Underserved, 15*(4), 506–521.

Walter, T. (2002). Spirituality in palliative care: Opportunity or burden? *Palliative Medicine, 16*(2), 133–139.

Warren, C. L. (2006). *A quantitative analysis of the synergy among self-reported faith, health and health care practices of black baptists: A culturecology perspective.* Pittsburgh, PA: University of Pittsburgh.

Warren, R. (1992). *Health education and Black health status.* In R. Braithwaite & S. Taylor (Eds.), *Health issues in the Black community.* San Francisco, CA: Jossey-Bass.

Warren, R. C. (2007, Spring). The impact of horizontal and vertical dimensions of faith on health and health care. *Journal of the Interdenominational Theological Center, 34,* 71–85.

Warren, R. C., Lockett, H. C., & Zulfiqar, A. A. (2002). The social context for faith and health. In J. C. Chunn (Ed.), *The health behavioral change imperative: Theory, education, and practice in diverse populations* (pp. 127–151). New York, NY: Kluwer Academic/Plenum.

Warren, R. C., & Tarver, W. L. (2010). A foundation for public health ethics at Tuskegee University in the 21st century. *Journal of Health Care Poor Underserved, 21*(Suppl. 3), 46–56.

Washington, H. A. (2008, July 29). *Health views: Essay, apology shines light on racial schism in medicine.* Retrieved September 14, 2010, from *The New York Times* website www.nytimes.com/2008/07/29/health/views/29essa.html

Wimberly, A. (2001). The role of Black faith in fostering health. In R. L. Braithewaite & S. E. Taylor (Eds.), *Health issues in the Black community* (2nd ed.). Nashville, TN: Jossey-Bass.

Woodson, C. (Ed.). (1969). *Negro orators and their orations* (pp. 207–208). New York: Russell & Russell.

Young, M.A.C. (1970). Dental education: An overview of selected concepts and principles relevant to programming planning. *International Journal of Health Education, 13*(1), 1–26.

7

Capacity Building and the Role of Community Health Workers in CEOD

Robert M. Mayberry, Robina Josiah Willock, and
Pamela V. Daniels

LEARNING OBJECTIVES

What you can learn by studying this chapter:

- What "community capacity" and capacity building is and how best to engage community members in this participatory process
- The role of community health workers (CHWs) and their potential effectiveness as representatives of the community
- The relationship between community action, community-based participatory research, and community engagement
- The leadership role of CHWs in community engagement
- Core competencies and content training for CHWs
- How the application of a conceptual model based on the social capital theory can help to understand the value of CHWs in capacity building
- How the application of a conceptual model based on the social capital theory can help to increased social capital leading to sustainable community intervention(s) and policy change

Community capacity is the development of the skills, knowledge, and infrastructure to effectively promote health, prevent disease, improve the quality of life, and engage local communities in self-determined activities for desired change to an undesirable social condition. The concept of "community capacity" is one that has gained currency over the past decade and overlaps with the concept of "community empowerment." Both concepts recognize the transforming ability of education and skills enhancement to enable even the less well-professionally trained community members to take on the task of changing the structures of society.

In this chapter, we explore the role of the CHWs in building community capacity for change. We perceive CHWs as well-trained community members and an integral part of the community's capacity to address its health and social concerns. An obvious role of CHWs in this context is as paid employees of community-based organizations (CBOs), community clinics, academic institutions, or other health and human services agencies. CHWs are also independent public health practitioners who would be excellent collaborators with CBOs and community stakeholders.

Because community capacity building often focuses on faith-based organizations and CBOs, CHWs may be particularly effective in enhancing the capacity of CBOs. The CBOs' capacity may be defined as the ability to deliver education and prevention programs (Hawe, Noort, King, & Jordens, 1997; Roper, Baker, Dyal, & Nicola, 1992; Sobeck & Agius, 2007). It also involves knowledge, skills, and willingness of individuals; the academic, health, or social service partners; and the funding agency to collaborate to establish common goals, articulate technical assistance needs, and develop agreed upon and appropriate responses to the community health concerns (Eng & Parker, 1994; Raczynski et al., 2001). CHWs are positioned to strengthen the capacity of CBOs as well as bridge the gap in collaborations among the community, CBOs, academic, health, and social services partners.

THE PUBLIC HEALTH ROLE OF CBOs

The HIV/AIDS pandemic, the increasing prevalence of obesity, the recalcitrance of chronic diseases, and new and reemerging public health threats have elevated the status of CBOs as a basic component of the public health infrastructure. CBOs are a core component of national strategies to disease prevention and to address other public health challenges. The engagement of CBOs also plays a key role in helping public health professionals to better understand social, behavioral, and other community determinants of health and provide guidance for local community disease-prevention activities. This essential participatory role of CBOs, their community-level expertise, and community credibility establish the cornerstone of intervention planning and implementation aimed at eliminating racial, ethnic, and socioeconomic health disparities and achieving health equity. Furthermore, the involvement of CBOs in promoting health, preventing disease, and addressing the ill-health burden in local communities acknowledges our limited understanding of sociocultural and contextual factors which are unique to local communities. It also recognizes the CBOs as both experts and influential stakeholders.

THE CAPACITY OF CBOs: THE PRESUMED ROLE OF COMMUNITY MEMBERS

While the participatory role of CBOs to promote and sustain health, prevent disease, and address health disparities in local communities is well recognized, the measurable effectiveness of CBOs is yet to be realized. Many CBOs lack the capacity to plan and implement appropriate community interventions (Richter et al., 2000). Most CBOs are yet to develop beyond a foundational infrastructure of coalition building, general planning, and limited action plan development. In our yearning for evidence-based practices, CBOs may be perceived as having limited effectiveness or an effectiveness that is yet undeterminable (Richter et al., 2000).

In some of our previous work with 24 established, small- to mid-size CBOs to provide HIV/AIDS education and prevention programs to multicultural, rural, and urban communities throughout nine states of the southern region of the United States, we found limited organizations' intervention capacity in several areas: (1) evaluation to measure program success, (2) qualitative and quantitative methods to measure change, (3) data-collection tools development, (4) protocol development for consistent data collection, management, and analysis, (5) data management, and (6) logic model development to delineate the path of program planning (Mayberry et al., 2008). Our collaborations with the CBOs strengthened significantly their abilities for community intervention planning and implementation. Community volunteers were an integral part of the CBOs' infrastructure as were community advisory committees and volunteer and paid peer educators. Presumably, these community representatives significantly contributed to the enhanced capacity of the CBOs observed in a relatively short period (less than 2 years; Mayberry et al., 2008).

THE ROLE OF CHWs

The role of the community member in capacity building is exemplified by the CHW. CHWs are primarily lay people trained to deliver important health care information and provide social support and advice within the community setting. CHWs have played effective roles in many settings, interventions, and health outcomes. Also known as lay health advisors, community health representatives, promotores de salud, patient navigators, and outreach workers (and a growing list of names as the CHW's role expands), CHWs are advocates who bridge structural, cultural, and social gaps between providers of health and social services and the community members they serve. They provide culturally relevant education, counseling, social support, and may be trained to deliver clinical support services such as teaching a patient the proper technique of taking blood pressure, patient follow-up, peer counseling and education, social support, and care coordination. CHWs also facilitate access to care, promote continuity of care, optimize the appropriate use of health care services, facilitate the adoption of self-care and management skills to disease management, and enhance treatment adherence. The role and effectiveness of CHWs are indicated in the selected areas below.

Diabetes In diabetes care, CHWs have facilitated improvements in disease knowledge, self-care behavior, keeping appointments, and patient satisfaction. In interventions that utilized CHWs, positive behavioral changes were noted in diet and managing blood pressure, increased physical activity levels, self-monitoring of blood glucose, HbA$_{1c}$, and provider standards of care. Several interventions, using CHWs, have demonstrated an increase in diabetes knowledge and self-management behaviors, commonly, in 6 to 12 months of following-up intervention (Norris et al., 2006).

Hypertension: CHWs have also contributed to improved blood pressure management and control. In a study of urban African Americans, CHWs trained in hypertension management were able to increase the percentage of participants with controlled blood pressure by 12% to 14% at the final follow-up of 40 months (Levine et al., 2002). In this case, the CHWs provided educational, counseling, referral, and social support at home visits. Studies that have employed a nurse–CHW–physician intervention for blood pressure control have also shown a significant difference in control rates for the intervention group compared to the standard care group (Hill et al., 1999, 2003). A CHW-led counseling intervention also showed significant improvement in blood pressure control (a 13% increase to a 46% control rate) at 6 months and sustained at 12 months, a statistically significant higher sustained control rate compared to usual care (Morisky et al., 2002).

Medication Adherence: Previous randomized controlled trials which used CHWs in interventions focused on medication adherence have demonstrated significant improvements (Brownstein et al., 2007; Norris et al., 2006; Hovell et al., 1984 [abstract only]; Becker et al., 2005; Hill et al., 2003). The results of a randomized control trial of hypertensive urban, low socioeconomic African American men, which used a CHW as part of the nurse–CHW–physician team, demonstrated an increase in the proportion of men on antihypertensive medication from 35% at baseline to 91% in a 36-month period of intervention follow-up of hypertension education, telephone call reminders every 6 months, and an annual home visit by the CHW. This increase in medication use was significantly greater than the increase observed for the control group (35%–69%) who received only community referrals for hypertension care and did not receive home visits by the CHW. Other studies of African American patients have demonstrated significant medications use in a 1-year intervention period (Becker et al., 2005).

Bridging the Health Care Divide: One of the main functions of CHWs is to serve as "'vital links' or bridges" between the community members they serve and the health care system. However, the roles and responsibilities of lay health advisors have not been consistently defined across studies that utilized them. Instead, what constitutes a CHW varies widely according to the needs and designs of the intervention. What has been consistent, however, is that once trained, CHWs provide an effective, community-directed, service to disadvantaged populations that complement the formal health care system. In some studies, such as blood pressure control, for example, CHWs operated in similar roles as nurses; they also achieved similar successes in blood pressure control compared to those achieved by the nurses.

CHWs are more likely to establish rapport more quickly with clients and may foster the relationship, which better facilitate discussions regarding where the patient is, where he or she would like to be, what he or she sees as challenges or enabling factors of health behavior change. This level of effectiveness may be achievable because the CHW is accepted as a community representative or a peer, or has the community's trust and cultural credibility.

THE COMMUNITY ACTION MODEL AND COMMUNITY-BASED PARTICIPATORY RESEARCH

The role of CHWs matches well with the conceptual framework of the Community Action Model (CAM). The CAM is asset-based and builds on the strengths or capacity of a community to create change from within. The CAM focuses on mobilizing community members and agencies to change environmental factors that promote economic and environmental inequalities. The CAM is an advocacy model that encourages communities to mobilize themselves to impact public policy, thus increasing community social capital. The goal of the CAM is to work in collaboration with communities and provide a framework for community members to acquire the skills and resources to investigate the health of the place where they live and then plan, implement, and evaluate actions that change the environment to promote and improve health.

Increasing social capital can lead to comprehensive community changes around health, as well as economic and civic well-being. Fundamental elements of CAM are shown in Figure 7.1.

The community action model is an interactive five-step process designed to address the fundamental determinants of population health through a community-based participatory process. The model was initially designed to address the social determinants of tobacco-related health disparities through grassroots efforts focused on policy and organizational practices and is applicable to other community issues.

The steps of CAM are as follows: *Step 1*—Dialogue of Concern and Issues/Skill-Based Training; *Step 2*—Community Diagnosis; *Step 3*—Analysis; *Step 4*—Plan and Implement Action/Activity; and *Step 5*—Sustaining Action/Activity and Evaluate Action. The role of CHWs can be easily defined within the CAM.

Step 1—Dialogue of Concern and Issues/Skill-Based Training: In this initial step, CHWs, in collaboration with community members and stakeholders, engage local communities on issues of concern. Some local communities may have established community coalition boards (CCBs). CHWs could work with CCB to engage community residents to serve as CCB members or CHWs could serve as CCB members themselves. The important aspect of Step 1 is community engagement to identify, understand, and focus actions on specific community concerns and issues. Specific skill-based

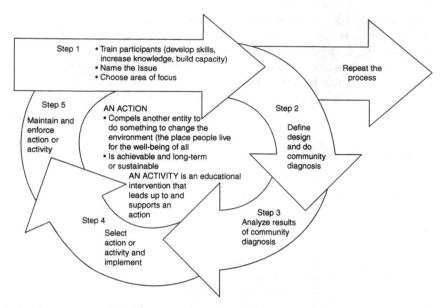

FIGURE 7.1   The five steps of the Community Action Model process.
Source: Lavery et al. (2005).

training is implemented to equip community members with skills to identify and describe health concerns or develop skills to fundamentally impact problems of concern to the local community. This is a first step of capacity building.

Step 2—Community Diagnosis: In collaboration with academic partners and other stakeholders, the CHW serves as a unique knowledge base and as a community representative to better understand the significant disparities in the local community through qualitative and quantitative data capture. The CHW is expected to actively participate in the review of multiple sources of preexisting data related to the disease burden, prevention, and health disparities. The CHW could also work closely with the academic, social services, or health agency partner to qualitatively capture perspectives on the community at large, through focus group discussions, one-on-one interviews, and impromptu street-level observations and key informant interviews.

Step 3—Analysis: In addition to data input and analyzes the CHWs, in applying a unique perspective in interpreting the collected data and integrating these findings into proposed action plans, are crucial to the intervention development process. The assistance that CHWs could give in determining how to address the local area information gaps should not be underestimated. As important is the role of the CHW as the community advocate in presenting findings to the broad base of stakeholders and interested parties to make a compelling case for needed action.

Step 4—Intervention Design: The CHW can provide invaluable expertise to help set specific priorities amenable to change and identify strategies for change that are culturally relevant, community acceptable, and more easily implementable. An extended role of the CHW is that of spearheading adoption and implementation of programs to promote continuous community involvement in selected priority areas.

Step 5—Sustaining Action/Activity and Evaluate Action: Sustainability of identified actions needs community acceptance, the omnipresent face of the community, and a champion for change. The integration of evaluation into community intervention conceptualization, planning, and implementation, and regular monitoring of activities likewise necessitate the role of the CHW being intertwined throughout this repeated cycle of sustaining long-term efforts to address local communities, concerns.

The CAM shares attributes with the community-based participatory research approach and helps to further shape and define the CHW's role. "Community-based participatory research" is a collaborative process of research involving researchers and community representatives. It engages community members, employs local knowledge in the understanding of health problems and the design of interventions, and invests community members in the processes and products of research. In addition, community members are invested in the dissemination and use of research findings and ultimately in the reduction of health disparities (Agency for Healthcare Research and Quality [AHRQ]).

Previous work has extensively defined the community-based participatory research (CBPR) approach and calls for researchers to (1) learn the "community ecology" before entering the community, (2) establish relationships with community gatekeepers, (3) build credibility before proceeding, (4) develop a CCB, (5) work with the CCB to conduct a health needs assessment, and (6) collaborate with the board to develop and implement one or more health-promotion interventions (Braithwaite et al., 1989). Less acknowledged, but equally as important, is the participatory role of the community in all stages of the evaluation process. The CHW then becomes the liaison to the community for this comprehensive approach to community-level action for desired change.

THE CHW AS LEADER OF COMMUNITY ENGAGEMENT

It is now well acknowledged that when people get involved in their community and work together for a common benefit, long-term improvements in social conditions and health and other concerns can be achieved. The CHW's role of liaison between the community members and the highly structured health care system, driven largely by an acute care modality of treatment, would suggest that they are, or should be, lynchpins in health-related community engagement efforts. Community engagement as a cornerstone of effective public health practice suggests a broader, yet leadership role for CHWs. Their involvement in every phase of the community engagement process can reduce the significant number of health initiatives that are often short term that, for this reason, are not of enduring value to the community, and are vulnerable to commandeering by counterproductive personal or political interests.

The definition of "community engagement" varies considerably depending on the context of the program or perspective of the one who seeks to define it. A central theme that remains constant in authentic community engagement is the desire to facilitate right input at the right time, which accurately represents the needs and wishes of a community and which ultimately facilitates community self-determination. It is a community-wide process by which organizations, individuals, and institutions are mobilized to identify challenges, and propose and execute solutions to their common concerns.

Several models of community engagement exist. We choose here to highlight what one author labels "the cycle of community engagement." This community engagement cycle is defined as a process of: (1) coming together (planning), (2) moving forward (engagement), and (3) sustaining momentum (evaluation and feedback), while being guided by the basic principles (i.e., clear purpose, community knowledge, trusting and respectful relationships, community self-determination, and long-term commitment; Minnesota Department of Health, Office of Performance Improvement, 1999).

Community engagement is not simply consulting with a community before executing or imposing a health intervention. It is a combination of "informing, consulting with, involving, collaborating with, and empowering the community" (Wilcox, 1994). Each of these activities is an area of prospective opportunities for CHWs to exert leadership to make tangible and invaluable contributions to the process of engaging communities.

Informing

In the informing phase of community engagement, CHWs serve as conduits of information from the academic, civic, or commercial stakeholders to their communities. They bring credibility to the motives and mission of the external stakeholder as information conduits, bridging the roles and interests of the diverse stakeholders. At this stage, their value lies primarily in their willingness and skills to authenticate the external stakeholder's long-term commitment to improving the community's health and related public health efforts. They primarily execute this function by disseminating information through printed materials, teaching, and promotion. This early process serves to sensitize the community to the potential for working collaboratively and more specifically generate buy-in for using the community engagement process.

Consulting: A second area that holds much promise for the CHWs is the consulting phase. Consulting begins the two-way dialogue that eventually leads to problem solving. A cadre of trained CHWs can serve as mediators to ensure that the values, history, priorities, and concerns of the community are not lost in translation. Their experience and versatility in operating both in the community and within the health care and social services systems makes them a key resource in helping to delineate the responsibilities and account- ability of each research partner. They are also invaluable to the ongoing com- munication of the research team by helping to articulate the experiential and codified knowledge of the community members, researchers, and other community stakeholders. In this capacity, they primarily become resource persons and fiduciary agents of the community and are able to provide information and facilitate data gathering in myriad forms on a formal and informal basis. A well-documented advantage of utilizing CHWs in this regard is their commonality of culture, value/beliefs systems, language, life experiences, and expectations with the communities they serve.

Involving

Substantively involving community members and stakeholders in miti- gating or resolving the community's concerns necessitates moving beyond the conversation of consultations. This is a critical step in the community- engagement process subsequent to the conversations between external stakeholders and the community. This begins a more formal process of conceptualizing activities and solutions, which fully takes into account community needs, priorities, and capacity. There is often bound to be diver- gent priorities at the outset; however, CHWs involved at this point in the process can find a role in identifying and soliciting broad-based support and resources (financial, tangible, intangible) from the community with the goal of securing the active participation of the community members. The CHWs should be competent in problem solving and demonstrate an acumen for the level of negotiation needed to facilitate the group's efforts to create new solutions and methodologies reflective of the communities priorities, resources, and expectations. In its ideal configuration, commu- nity involvement in the context of community engagement imbues the community with the mandate to "decide" which solutions are acceptable and actively contribute to solutions based on their strengths, not simply to serve as facilitators acquiescent to an imposed "greater good."

Collaborating

In the community-engagement process, CHWs serve as key facilita- tors of collaborative activities. They will be acutely aware of the need to engage with the formal, informal, and hidden representatives and interest groups of the community. This level of collaboration engages the commu- nity partners and stakeholders in all aspects of the research process with shared authority. As previously mentioned, this includes an iterative pro- cess of identifying and defining problems and priorities; identifying local, expert, and external knowledge bases; harnessing community capacity to implement solutions; and creating opportunities for learning and dissemination of findings. Collaboration with the community is also an important precursor to sustainability. There are great opportunities to create synergies in capacity building, cost reduction, and overall effectiveness of solutions implemented. The interdependent decision-making systems, shared authority and formalized linkages, roles, and accountability attendant to collaboration lay the groundwork for activities that are self-sustaining over the long term. CHWs can play a critical role in identifying, building, and, most importantly, managing the networks of long-term and newly created relationships and communication. In the process of community-based collaboration, there are typically numerous opportunities to use and develop community leaders, trainers, facilitators, and evaluators, any number of which a CHW can reasonably fill.

Empowering

Community empowerment is one of the most important components of community engagement. Empowerment refers to the process by which people gain control over the factors and decisions that shape their lives. It is the process by which they increase their assets and attributes and build capacities to gain access, partners, networks, and/or a voice, in order to gain control (Labonté & Laverack, 2008). CHWs are designated to be champions and advocates for community self-determination, particularly in areas of disease prevention and health promotion. Their presence in the community can minimize the stagnation and regression to status quo that is more likely to occur over time. It is important that at this point of the community-engagement process, external stakeholders are primarily facilitators, incorporating CHWs as consultants in various roles as previously discussed. CHWs may remain indistinguishable from the community they represent, while bridging the gap between the community and those who provide external resources. Additionally, a group of vested CHWs can serve as an enduring repository of knowledge and skills accessible to the community for highlighting new issues and spearheading future efforts.

There are numerous opportunities for well-trained CHWs to significantly impact the community-engagement process. The starting point is recognition of the unique perspective and leadership contributions they can offer beyond the traditional health educator role.

CORE COMPETENCIES AND TRAINING ISSUES FOR CHWs

Training and educational opportunities for CHWs on a national level are best described as disjointed. In recent years, however, the expansion of CHWs' utilization and responsibilities has stimulated a concurrent increased interest in CHW training, standardized curricula, certification, and other types of formal credentialing. The evolution of standardized training has been largely initiated by CHW advocacy organizations and local and regional stakeholders. Until recently, the training of CHWs was primarily structured as on-the-job training, largely defined by the specific nature of the CHWs' roles and responsibilities related to a project. Training was also specifically designed to enhance generic CHW competencies, such as patient care, health education, communication, patient advocacy, and program-specific knowledge.

Within recent years, however, trends in CHW training have included formal college-based training opportunities, as well as state-sponsored or state-supported certification programs. In addition to widespread standardization of CHW training, the shifting responsibility for training to the formal education system also has the potential to reduce the training burden traditionally placed on community-based programs, health and social services agencies, and employers. Training programs currently focus on health outreach, health promotion and education, health services access, specialized health services access, individual and community advocacy, or community capacity building, with a goal to formalize ongoing unorganized activities of CHW across a diverse range of community health concerns, stakeholders, and community context (Berthold, Miller, & Avila-Esparza, 2009). In lieu of formal CHW training, some programs, such as the Texas CHW credential program, recognize equivalent experience (in this case, at least 1,000 hours of CHW activities within the most recent 6 years). Many programs also recognize that well-established ties to the local community are a highly desirable prerequisite for formal training.

While well-recognized career pathways, skill sets, and training standards do not exist, reputable CHW education and training are now generally guided by a modifiable set of core competencies, knowledge, and transferrable skills. The 1998 National Community Health Advisor Study (Rosenthal et al., 1998) identified eight core CHW competencies: communication skills, interpersonal skills, service coordination skills, capacity-building skills, advocacy skills, teaching skills, organizational skills, and content knowledge of specific health issues (U.S. HRSA, 2007). Additional skills and competencies include computer literacy, data-collection skills, and confidentiality and protecting health information.

The integration of adult learning principles into CHW training is also an important characteristic of recognized training programs. In this regard, it is recognized that the CHW learns better when the material is presented in ways that support the CHW and in an environment that is supportive and encouraging. The learning environment must also allow the CHW to build on past experiences to supplement what he or she already knows, help the CHW make self-directed choices about what and how much he or she willing to learn, and allow the CHW to participate in interactive learning bidirectional feedback. Furthermore, the learning environment must allow the CHW to use what he or she learns in the community and workplace and highlight the opportunities for personal and professional growth and development (Knowles, Holton, & Swanson, 1998). Continuing education or refresher training is as important as initial training. Skills and knowledge acquired in initial training can be quickly lost if regular refresher training is not available (World Health Organization, 2007).

Training and certification of CHWs serves several distinct purposes representing the vested interests of the health care system, the community, and the CHW. For the health care system, training and certification codify the work of the CHW and increases the potential for better quality assurance, reimbursement potential, and access to the health care services the CHW provides. For community members, the training of the CHW represents an increased social capital, the dissemination of more diverse health education and promotion resources, and an improved health services system. By taking advantage of standardized training and credentialing opportunities, CHWs are exposed to better career opportunities, professional recognition, and professional and personal growth. They also become better community resource persons, more valuable assets to their communities, and can demand remuneration commensurate with their abilities and experience.

CHWs AS SOCIAL CAPITAL: A THEORETICAL FRAMEWORK OF CAPACITY BUILDING

We view trained CHWs as a critical component of social capital. Social capital, in turn, is a key component of community capacity building. Through the use of CHWs for capacity building, the concepts of several theories such as the Health Belief Model (HBM), Self-Determination Theory (SDT), Transtheoretical Model (TTM), and self-efficacy are all taking place at different stages when community members interact with CHWs for extended periods of time. This interaction forges relationships and bonds of trust that lead to social support, social networks, and continuous capacity building within the community and, subsequently, increased social capital. The increased social capital within a community leads to improved health status of individuals and healthier communities.

Depending on the academic discipline, the definition of social capital varies. Social capital is defined as "not a single entity," but a variety of different entities having two characteristics in common: (1) They all consist of some aspect of social structure, and (2) they facilitate certain actions of individuals who are within the structure (Coleman, 1990). Communities who are fortunate enough to have CHWs possess both characteristics. The community is the social structure and the CHW facilitates specific actions of the community members through social support (whether it be informational, instrumental, emotional, or appraisal), education, and providing resources to clients/patients within the community.

In the perspective of public health, both social cohesion and social networks are prominent features of social capital. The school of social cohesion posits that social capital is a group attribute and not an individual one. CHWs, although they work with individuals to educate, empower, and facilitate change in behavior, are actually creating social ties within the community (Kawachi et al., 2008). The information that is shared with individuals is often shared by word-of-mouth to family members, friends, church members, and other community members. Although the information is shared on the individual level, the community as a whole has the opportunity to benefit from information sharing. Through the education process, the CHW is increasing the knowledge, abilities, and skills of the community members to manage and control their health. The CHW is shaping the health beliefs of the participant, empowering and motivating the individual to take control of his or her health, and encouraging behavior change to promote a healthy lifestyle. Through this process, the CHW is the "group attribute" that is building capacity on the community level.

Social networks are another aspect of the social capital theory. Social networks are centered on resources within the community. These resources include social support systems, social service agencies, faith-based organizations, food banks, and social credentials of individuals within the community (i.e., pastors, doctors, lawyers, teachers, business owners, etc.)—all are embedded within an individual's social network (Lin, 1999). Social networks are often measured on both the individual and group level. The CHW develops both individual social networks and group networks. At the basic level, the individual bonds that the CHW develops with each individual are networks for that involved individual. On the group level, as the CHW introduces the community member to different community resources, networks develop and continue to expand and grow. These social networks that are developed and developing have the power to mobilize communities to promote policy changes, increase social capital, and build community capacity.

As social capital is being developed within a given community through the use of CHWs, several other theories can be applied to explain the work of CHWs that lead to capacity building. These include the HBM, SDT, TTM, and self-efficacy.

Health Belief Model

The HBM assesses and identifies factors in tailoring both the CHW's training and the education/skills-development sessions with community members. The HBM has been a primary sociocognitive framework used to explain individuals' decisions to take preventive action with respect to maintaining health, adherence to medical regimens, physical activity, health checkups, and self-management of diagnosed disease. The HBM posits that preventive behavior change is a function of several factors: perceived severity, perceived vulnerability, perceived self-efficacy, benefits, barriers, and cues to action. The model maintains that the motivation to engage in a positive health behavior depends upon one's perceived vulnerability to the threat of illness and one's perceptions of the severity of the illness (Glanz et al., 2008). The course of action one takes depends upon a cost/benefit analysis of the psychological, physiological, and financial barriers and benefits associated with the behavior. If the barriers outweigh the benefits, one is less likely to engage in the positive behavior and vice versa. "Cues" refer to internal or external catalysts for behavior change and have been suggested as an effective addition to the model when used in conjunction with perceived vulnerability and self-efficacy (i.e., one's perception of their ability to perform the behavior; Glanz et al., 2008). Providing individuals with ongoing cues related to their health via feedback is one mechanism for influencing preventive behavior. Other methods include increasing their knowledge of disease-related severity, heightening their perception of vulnerability for disease-related complications, improving self-efficacy, and reducing barriers while emphasizing benefits of behavior change. CHWs are trained (increasing their knowledge and shaping their health beliefs) to educate the community member on the risk and benefits of desired action. The CHW also connects the individual or patient to other resources, such as diabetes self-management classes, information on medication assistance programs, and social service organizations that provide transportation, child care, food pantries, and other community resources.

Self-Determination Theory

SDT is a theory that is based on four minitheories: cognitive evaluation theory, basic need theory, organismic integration theory, and causality orientations theory. SDT assumes that individuals are naturally motivated to grow and improve their own well-being. The constructs for SDT are similar to stages of change (Prochaska, DiClemente, & Norcross, 1992) and social learning theory. SDT has four forms of motivation: intrinsic motivation, self-determined extrinsic motivation, nonself determined extrinsic motivation, and amotivation. All humans have three psychological needs: autonomy (volition), competence (feelings to be able to accomplish a goal), and relatedness (positive relationship with others). When all three needs are met, individuals will be able to engage in behaviors that are of personal value to them, rather than a forced behavioral change. SDT is not based on reinforcements (rewards or punishments) that can cause an individual to revert back to his or her old behavior once the incentives are gone. It is based on autonomous self-regulation and perceived competence. Individuals are autonomously motivated because they have volition and choice. The CHW acts as motivator or cheerleader, in a sense, to encourage, empower, and self-motivate individuals to participate in self-management classes, control their health issues, and improve their quality of life through lifestyle changes.

Transtheoretical Model

Change theory, and in particular, the TTM of intentional behavioral change, is the cornerstone of the work that is performed by CHWs. One of the main goals in public health research is to increase knowledge, promote

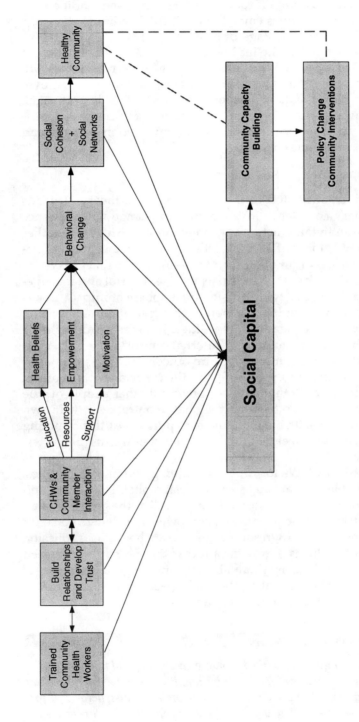

FIGURE 7.2 Conceptual Model: Social capital and capacity building through the use of community health workers.

positive attitudes, increase self-efficacy, locus of control, and readiness for change, which are all constructs embedded in TTM. Readiness to change is captured by the concept of stage of change in TTM. TTM posits five discrete stages, which reflect the individual's interest and motivation to alter an undesirable behavior. When modifying behavior, individuals will move through these five stages, or a series of gradual steps, on their own or through a formal intervention: precontemplation (not ready to change), contemplation (aware of problem, but ambivalent about change), preparation (intend to act in the near future), action (involved in change), and maintenance (sustaining the change).

Self-Efficacy

It is a concept often attributed to the social cognitive theory. It posits that an individual's confidence in the ability to change will influence the behavior the individual actually engages in consistently. Another theoretical concept is locus of control. This theory operates in conjunction with the constructs of confidence and self-efficacy so that CHWs are able to identify and work with individuals who see control and management of their health issue as lying outside their sphere of impact. Locus of control refers to an individual's generalized expectations concerning where control over subsequent events resides. In other words, who or what is responsible for what happens. "Internal control" is the term used to describe the belief that control of future outcomes resides primarily in oneself, while "external control" refers to the expectancy that control is outside oneself, either in the hands of powerful other people or due to fate or chance. Those who feel that they have control over their own health and value their health are more likely to pursue health-promoting behaviors than those who feel that their health is contingent upon external factors.

Through the use of CHWs for capacity building within communities, the community is able to obtain and sustain social capital. This social capital is developed on both the individual level as well as the group or community level. CHWs are able to educate, empower, and change behavior through the use of community resources that create both social cohesion and social networks. This is a growing process that promotes increased community capacity and that is sustainable over time. Figure 7.2 illustrates a conceptual model of how social capital and capacity building are developed through the use of community health workers.

Case Study Exercises

Individually, or as a group, review the following case study and follow the exercises found at the end of the study, as appropriate. Be sure to focus on the why, how, and what emphasized in each exercise. Your professor/instructor will provide you specific guidance on how you are to report your findings for the class.

Case Study 7.1: iADAPT—A CHW Intervention to Evidence-Based Medication Adherence Among Adults With Type 2 Diabetes

In our ongoing research, we use a CHW intervention model to increase medication knowledge and awareness, increase patient communication with the primary care provider regarding medication use, improve adherence to evidence-based prescribed medication use, and facilitate self-motivation to improve self-management among adults with type 2 diabetes. The project (iADAPT) is funded by the Agency for Healthcare Research and Quality (grant number R18HS019259) and is conducted in collaboration with a local community health center.

The Problem: Adults with type 2 diabetes are often unable to effectively manage their condition through adherence to prescribed medication, self–care, and lifestyle changes.

The Issues of Medication Adherences and Self-Care: We do not know for sure why it is difficult for persons with diabetes to keep their blood glucose under control, but failure to control glycemia is probably best explained by inadequate self-care and ineffective medical management. The benefits of glycemic control in persons with type 2 diabetes are well established. Controlling glycemia (i.e., reducing high blood glucose to normal range) can delay microvascular complications of the eye, kidney, and nerves and the severe long-term sequelae of blindness, kidney failure, and lower-extremity amputations.

Oral or insulin medication is the primary focus of type 2 diabetes treatment, concurrent with lifestyle modifications, including healthy eating and regular exercise. And, while there are many effective medications to control glycemia, choosing among antidiabetes medications and adherence to prescribed medications along with lifestyle modifications challenge providers and patients in glycemic control.

There are many individual psychosocial and behavioral barriers to adherence to medication, choice of medication, and intent or desire to use medication as prescribed. Among these are the patient's understanding of how to take medication and knowledge of effect of medication on the body, medication side effects, the consequences of not taking medications, regimen complexity of more than one drug or more than one dose daily, depression, and patient–provider communication. A patient's desire or ability to adhere to medical treatment and self-care best practices, however, seems to be grounded in psychological and motivational factors rather than solely education factors. The time typically allotted to routine diabetes care during a clinic visit represents only a small fraction of the time that a patient with diabetes needs to be actively supported.

A Solution: A CHW's Approach to Medication Adherence and Self-Care: We use a CHW model with the innovation of motivational interviewing (MI) to improve adherence to evidence-based antidiabetes medication and self-care among adults with type 2 diabetes. The CHW intervention is delivered according to the psychosocial needs and stage of readiness for change of the person with diabetes and for the purpose of facilitating motivation for adherence to prescribed medications. CHWs are well-integrated into the multiple components of the intervention, including audit and feedback discussion of patient follow-up and missed appointments, attendance at diabetes self-management education (DSME) classes, medication adherence problems, and patient–provider communication issues during the monthly 1-hour "Lunch and Learn" sessions with physician, nurses, and diabetes educators.

Recruitment and Selection of CHWs: We identified and recruited CHWs through networks and organizations with which we have collegial relationships: the state CHW network, an academic prevention research center, a federally qualified community health center, and other CBOs that utilize CHWs located in the targeted community. Eligible CHWs had at least a high school diploma. They had to be fluent in written and spoken English; Spanish as second language was an added advantage. Selected CHWs had moderate to extensive experience in community-based activities, health education, or health promotion in diabetes, stroke, asthma, hypertension, cancer, or other chronic disease management.

CHW Training: All CHWs received training in the eight core competencies recommended by the 1998 National Community Health Advisor Study, human subject protection, and Health Insurance Portability and Accountability Act (HIPPA). CHWs were also trained in the six standard content areas of DSME as recommended by the American Diabetes Association by an experienced, certified diabetes educator. CHWs also received training in MI by a certified MI trainer. (MI is a proven patient-centered, directive counseling approach to sustainable behavioral change.)

Delivery of the CHW Intervention: The CHWs are randomly assigned to and provide ongoing counseling sessions to as many as 60 adults with type 2 diabetes. The MI-trained CHWs provide monthly one-on-one in-person and phone-administered counseling sessions over the 12-month intervention period. The counseling sessions last for 20 to 30 minutes. The CHW intervention is aimed at improving diabetes care, follow-up visits, knowledge and awareness of evidence-based medication use, patient communication, medication adherence, and participation in DSME classes where medication adherence will be reinforced.

Anticipated Effectiveness of CHWs: The CHW intervention model is expected to increase evidence-based medication knowledge and awareness, increase patient communication with the provider, reduce medication problems, and improve adherence to prescribed medication. "We have already seen a reduction in A1c in our patient population and an increase in patient participation in DSME classes," the health center medical director.

Study Exercises

1. List problems associated with type 2 diabetes self-care.
2. What strategy would you use to recruit CHWs appropriate for community work?
3. What training strategies would you recommend for CHWs before they enter the community?
4. Outline a diabetes intervention program that would increase community awareness and adherence to prescribed medication practices.
5. How can CHWs play an even greater role in adherence?
6. Provide a brief outline of how you would evaluate effectiveness to your program.

REFERENCES

Becker, D. M., Yanek, L. R., Johnson, W. R., Garrett, D., Moy, T. F., Reynolds, S. S., ... Becker, L. C. (2005). Impact of a community-based multiple risk factor intervention on cardiovascular risk in Black families with a history of premature coronary disease. *Circulation, 111*(10), 1298–1304.

Berthold, T., Miller, J., & Avila-Esparza, A. (2009). *Foundations for community health workers*. San Francisco, CA: Jossey-Bass.

Braithwaite, R. L., & Lythcott, N. (1989). Community empowerment as a strategy for health promotion for black and other minority populations. *Journal of the American Medical Association, 1261*(2), 282–283.

Brownstein, J. N., Chowdhury, F. M., Norris, S. L., Horsley, T., Jack, L., Zhang, X., & Satterfield, D. (2007). Effectiveness of community health workers in the care of people with hypertension. *American Journal of Preventive Medicine, 32*(5), 435–447.

Coleman, J. S. (1990). *Foundations of social theory*. Cambridge, MA: Harvard University Press.

Eng, E., & Parker, E. (1994). Measuring community competence in the Mississippi Delta: The interface between program evaluation and empowerment. *Health Education Quarterly, 21*, 199–200.

Glanz, K., Rimer, B. K., & Viswanath, K. (2008). *Health behavior and health education: Theory, research, and practice* (4th ed.). San Francisco, CA: Jossey-Bass.

Goodman, R. M., Speers, M. A., McLeroy, K., Fawcett, S., Kegler, M., Parker, E., ... Wallerstein, N. (1998). Identifying and defining the dimensions of community capacity to provide a basis for measurement. *Health Education & Behavior, 25*(3), 258–278.

Hawe, P., Noort, M., King, L., & Jordens, C. (1997). Multiplying in health gains: The critical role of capacity-building within health promotion programs. *Health Policy, 39*, 29–42.

Hill, M. N., Bone, L. R., Kim, M. T., Miller, D. J., Dennison, C. R., & Levine, D. M. (1999). Barriers to hypertension care and control in young urban black men. *American Journal of Hypertension, 12*(10), 951–958.

Hill, M., Han, H. R., Dennison, C. R., Kim, M. T., Roary, M. C., Blumenthal, R. S., ... Post, W. S. (2003). Hypertension care and control in underserved urban African American men: Behavioral and physiologic outcomes at 36 months. *American Journal of Hypertension, 16*(11), 906–913.

Hovell, M., Geary, D. C., Black, D. R., Kamachi, K., & Kirk, R. (1984). The effects of lay counseling on medication adherence and blood pressure: Adjunctive treatment for hypertension. *Patient Education and Counseling, 6*(2), 91–94.

Kawachi, I., Subramanian, S. V., & Kim, D. (2008). *Social capital and health.* New York, NY: Springer.

Knowles, M. S., Holton, E. F., III, & Swanson, R. A. (1998). *The adult learner: The definitive classic in adult education and human resource development.* Houston, TX: Elsevier.

Labonté, R., & Laverack, G. (2008). *Health promotion in action: From local to global empowerment.* London: Palgrave Macmillan.

Lavery, S. H., Smith, M. L., Esparza, A. A., Hrushow, A., Moore, M., & Reed, D. F. (2005). The Community Action Model: A community-driven model designed to address disparities in health. *American Journal of Public Health, 95*(4), 611–616.

Levine, D. M., Bone, L. R., Hill, M. N., Stallings, R., Gelber, A. C., Barker, A., ... Clark, J. M. (2003). The effectiveness of a community/academic health center partnership in decreasing the level of blood pressure in an urban African-American population. *Ethnicity and Disease, 13*(3), 354–361.

Lin, N. (1999). Building a network theory of social capital. *Connections, 22*(1), 28–51.

Mayberry, R. M., Daniels, P., Henry, A. T., Yancey, E. M., Berry, J., & Clark, N. (2008). Community-based organizations' capacity to plan, implement, and evaluate success. *Journal of Community Health, 33*(5), 285–290.

Minnesota Department of Health, Office of Performance Improvement. (1999). *Strategies for public health: A compendium of ideas, experience and research from Minnesota's public health professionals* (Vol. 2). Retrieved from www.health.state.mn.us/strategies/intro.pdf

Morisky, D. E., Lees, N. B., Sharif, B. A., et al. (2002). Reducing disparities in hypertension control: A community-based Hypertension Control Project (Chip) for a low income minority population. *Health Promotion and Practice, 3,* 267–278.

Norris, S. L., Chowdhury, F. M., Let, K. V., Brownstein, J. N., Zhang, X., Jack, L., & Satterfield, D. W. (2006). Effectiveness of community health workers in the care of persons with diabetes. *Diabetic Medicine, 23,* 544–556.

Prochaska, J. O., DiClemente, C. C., & Norcross, J. C. (1992). In search of how people change: Applications to addictive behaviors. *American Psychologist, 47*(9), 1102–1114.

Raczynski, J. M., Cornell, C. E., Stalker, V., Phillips, M., Dignan, M., Pulley, L., & Leviton, L. (2001). A multi-project systems approach to developing community trust and building capacity. *Journal of Public Health Management and Practice, 7*(2), 10–20.

Richter, D., Prince, M., Potts, L., Reininger, B., Thompson, M., Fraser, J., & Fulmer, S. L. (2000). Assessing the HIV prevention capacity building needs of community-based organizations. *Journal of Public Health Management and Practice, 6*(4), 86–97.

Roper, W., Baker, E., Dyal, W., & Nicola, R. (1992). Strengthening the public health system. *Public Health Reports, 107*(6), 609–615.

Rosenthal, E. L., Wiggins, N., Brownstein, J. N., Johnson, S., Borbon, I. A., Rael, R., . . . Blondet, L. (1998). *The final report of the National Community Health Advisor Study: Weaving the future.* Tuscan, AZ: University of Arizona.

Sobeck, J., & Agius, E. (2007). Organizational capacity building: addressing a research and practice gap. *Evaluation and Program Planning, 30*(3), 237–246.

U.S. Department of Health and Human Services, Health Resources and Services Administration, & Bureau of Health Professions. (2007). *Community health workers National Workforce Study.* Rockville, MD: HRSA.

Wilcox, D. (1994). *The guide to effective participation.* London: Partnership Book.

World Health Organization. (2007). *Community health workers: What do we know about them? The state of the evidence on programmes, activities, costs and impact on health outcomes of using community health workers.* Retrieved July 21, 2011, from www.who.int/healthsystems/round9_7.pdf

8

Engaging and Organizing Rural Communities for Public Health Practice

Lynda Murphy-Freeman and Frederick G. Murphy

LEARNING OBJECTIVES

What you can learn by studying this chapter:

- How to define the meaning of "rural"
- How to identify methods in which to determine the needs of rural communities
- How to identify steps for organizing a rural network
- Description strategies for implementing rural health interventions
- How goals and objectives should be formed
- Why it is important to build trust within the rural community
- The definitions of the types of evaluation and their importance
- To identify the approaches of marketing
- To identify the types of sustainability and explain ways to sustain a program

Various definitions exist for the term "rural." According to the Rural Assistance Center (n.d.a), the U.S. Census Bureau, the Office of Management and Budget, and the Economic Research Service of the U.S. Department of Agriculture (USDA) are three government agencies that provide definitions of what rural is. Because rural is an inexact term that can mean different things to different people, it is important to understand what the "official" definition is, especially when it comes to determining eligibility for federal grant programs. The Census Bureau's definition is viewed as the "official" definition because it is the only federal definition that applies the term "rural" in an official, statistical capacity (Rural Assistance Center, n.d.a).

The Rural Assistance Center further explains:

> The U.S. Census Bureau initially defines specific urban entities. An Urbanized Area (UA) has an urban nucleus of 50,000 or more people. Individual cities with a population of 50,000 may or may not be contained in these UAs. Urbanized Areas have a core (one or more

contiguous census block groups or BGs) with a total land area less than two square miles and a population density of 1,000 persons per square mile. They may contain adjoining territory with at minimum 500 persons per square mile and encompass a population of at least 50,000 people. An Urban Cluster (UC) also has a core as identified above with a total land area of less than two square miles and a population density of 1,000 persons per square mile. They may contain adjoining territory with at minimum 500 persons per square mile and encompass a population of at least 2,500 but less than 50,000 persons. The Census Bureau's classification of "rural" consists of all territory, population, and housing units located outside of UAs and UCs.

To summarize the definition above: *Urbanized Areas* (UAs) have 50,000 or more people; *Urban Clusters* (UCs) have at least 2,500 and less than 50,000 people. *"Rural"* encompasses all population, housing, and territory not included within UAs or UCs (U.S. Census Bureau, 2010).

DETERMINING NEEDS OF RURAL COMMUNITIES

Research on rural health issues is also plagued by the research and institutional structure and bias that favors urban areas. Yet, there is a substantial need for research efforts to identify and analyze significant rural health problems.

Research is needed on attitudes about family planning among adolescents and young adults, access to health care for rural Medicaid populations, the health of rural homeless families, and incidence and management of domestic violence and mental health disorders. It is also important to develop and monitor health policies that take consequences for rural communities into account. At the beginning of the 21st century, much health policy activity revolved around cost-containment issues rather than access to services. Access is, of course, a crucial issue for rural communities and needs to be addressed. The policy implications of ongoing and future demographic changes—such as the increase in rural elderly residents and minority populations and the frequency of chronic diseases, which place significant stresses on rural health systems—also require attention. Policy development will need to address the emergence and increase of diseases such as HIV/AIDS, sexually transmitted diseases, drug-resistant tuberculosis, and substance abuse in rural populations. Effective environmental interventions in farms, including the allocation of more resources to farm safety programs and a revision of current farm safety legislation, are also necessary (Sumaya, 2002).

Though the majority of U.S. population resides in urban areas, rural communities still face the same public health challenges and concerns as metropolitan areas; furthermore, these challenges and concerns are magnified in rural settings, thus placing these communities at an even greater risk for diseases and health disorders. Economic factors, cultural and social differences, educational shortcomings, lack of recognition by legislators, and geographic characteristics all contribute to health disparities in these communities (National Rural Health Association, n.d.). So then, what are some of the basic items for which one gathers information when initially approaching a rural community to conduct ongoing health-related activities? Here is a listing of several:

1. Identify priority community concerns and health issues
2. Identify target population
3. Identify service organizations
    a. Resources and services
4. Meet with key representatives of organizations
5. Gather community support (meet with key community entities [churches, YMCA, etc.])
6. Map out services to provide
7. Assign duties
8. Assign coordinator to provide necessary coordination of activities
9. Create and review necessary forms for health fairs (i.e., sign-in sheets, biographical data, health status data, etc.)
10. Choose accessible venues
11. Order supplies/equipment
12. Schedule meetings to keep track (weekly or biweekly or monthly)
13. Advertise (radio, newspaper, flyers, church bulletins, etc.)
14. Participate in existing community activities
15. Plan how to sustain program/intervention
16. Continue to look for opportunities and partnerships

Let's briefly discuss some of the methods that can be used to gather some of the items listed above.

Needs Assessment

A *needs assessment* will allow the community-based organization to identify concerns of residents and begin to set an agenda to address these concerns. According to Moore (2009), the assessment is the beginning of the strategic planning process. Moore (2009) also stated that, "Community assessments can and should be more than just a gathering and analyzing of data, they can also be a basis for creating change.... It can provide important community information as to who may be working on issues and where gaps in community services lie."

Some data-identifying community needs may already exist. Local and state health departments are a valuable resource in the process of identifying health disparities within target communities. Utilizing this information properly will allow organizations to be effective in their outreach efforts. Health priorities differ from community to community; therefore, program design should reflect the priorities unique to each community. For example, organizations should not make HIV testing a priority if complications due to diabetes accounts for 95% of the deaths in the community and HIV accounts for only 1%; this is not to say that the HIV testing and education should not take place in the community, but it should not be the top priority. Whatever the primary health issue may be, organizations should aim to improve health outcomes, improve health behaviors, and prevent/reduce further complications if applicable. The needs assessment can greatly assist in completing this task.

Access to Health Care

In a study conducted by the USDA, it was found that "the accessibility of health care resources generally declines as geographic isolation increases." Lack of access to health care and lack of health insurance are major disparities that affect rural communities. Unfortunately, some rely on emergency care as their primary source for health care. The rural care model focuses on providing primary care locally, as well as emergency care since small volumes of patients will not support a hospital. The model also refers these patients to regional health care centers, which are often distant, resulting in rural residents incurring higher travel-time costs compared to urban residents. These factors also may result in patients substituting a local general practitioner or a specialist, or reducing their usage of health care (Jones, Parker, Ahearn, Mishra, & Variyam, 2009).

Costs to treat patients without access to providers and/or health insurance result in increased visits to the emergency department. The federal agency's analysis also found that rates of emergency department visits were 39% higher for Americans living in rural areas compared to those living in urban areas (515 visits vs. 372 visits per 1,000 adults). Cardiac conditions and diabetes were among the most frequent chronic conditions seen in the emergency department (Owens & Mutter, 2010).

According to the National Rural Health Association (n.d.), only about 10% of physicians practice in rural America despite the fact that nearly one-fourth of the population lives in these areas. To help supplement the lack of health care providers, some organizations that serve rural communities will provide free health screenings to meet the basic medical needs of the community. These screenings can include testing for hypertension, cholesterol, diabetes, and HIV, and can also include eye exams, dental exams, and body mass index readings. The tests and exams are provided depending on the organization's ability, and the needs of the population. For example, some programs target diabetes and its risk factors, so you will find hypertension, glucose, and cholesterol testing, but you will not find HIV testing at their screenings. On the other hand, others will solely focus on HIV testing and HIV/AIDS education.

Identifying and Organizing a Rural Network

In rural communities, it is imperative to identify organizations that are well respected. Whether it is the local YMCA or a university, the organization must identify community partners to help implement the screening programs. With different populations, this may not be an easy task; here are some fundamental ways this can be achieved.

Collaboration and Networking

Collaborating with other community organizations can allow a sharing of expertise and resources, thus improving the effectiveness of service delivery. Creating meaningful and effective partnerships create new opportunities to serve the community. Sharing education, technology, supplies, manpower, and so on can potentially enhance the service program, thus benefiting the communities they serve. The collaboration or network should be centered on providing holistic health for individuals and communities. During planning, participating organizations should focus on improving access and availability of health care services, while improving the quality of life for rural residents (Kelly, 2002). Program development should create opportunities for resource sharing while avoiding duplication. It is important to have the pulse of the community. A way to do that is to add a lay community member on the program planning committee. This will prove valuable during the planning process, especially if dealing with unfamiliar populations.

The rural network should also possess *cultural competence*—having the capacity to effectively function and provide services that are sensitive and responsive to cultural differences presented by the target population. Being aware of the impact of culture and being able to respond appropriately to unique cultural differences will increase the quality of services; thereby producing better outcomes (Rural Assistance Center, n.d.b).

Defining Roles and Responsibilities

Kelly (2002) also emphasized that identifying leaders (formal and informal), and establishing and defining roles of partners should be done early in the collaboration process to ensure success. Clearly identifying the responsibility of each organization will establish accountability; however, the responsibilities should not be a burden or add too much to the existing workloads, but it should complement the partner organizations. This may be more difficult for rural areas because in most rural communities, health care providers are limited in number and most belong to the same health care agencies that service the same target populations. These providers also belong to many of the same community groups and organizations, and thus there can easily be routine "network overlap" and "scheduling conflicts" when planning and scheduling rural health interventions and screening events. In addition, providers can suffer from "burn out" and they can "over book" when they are continually called upon to participate in each other's community programs, health and nonhealth related.

Provider Planning Meetings

It is important to continue to meet after roles are established. Meeting regularly will present opportunities to exchange ideas and information, while also developing relationships with partners and their staff. It is important to recognize the natural leaders in the program development process, and recognize the strengths each partner possesses (Kelly, 2002).

Identification of Potential Barriers

Collaborating and forming networks is not always a simple process. The Rural Assistance Center (n.d.c) highlights barriers that organizations may face while trying to create partnerships:

- Racial disparities
- Poverty
- Lack of communication
- Turf issues
- Federal grant programs that discourage collaboration
- History of conflict and mistrust
- Isolation
- Poor access due to road conditions and/or severe weather conditions
- Absence of public transportation
- Small population base
- Limited pool of professional talent including leadership capabilities

Strategies for Implementing Rural Health Interventions

Among other elements, prevention is a desired outcome for most organizations utilizing health screenings. The World Health Organization (WHO, 2002) describes primary and secondary prevention. *Primary prevention* can protect susceptible individuals from developing a condition. Let's use diabetes, a chronic condition, as an example. A health-screening program that includes health education can provide diabetes awareness to susceptible groups and promote modifications to behavior (such as improvements in diet and increased physical activity). Screening programs can also provide *secondary prevention*—prevention of immediate and long-term consequences. Secondary prevention includes early detection, prevention, and treatment. For example, a diabetes health screening provides opportunities for participants to have their blood glucose tested. Detection of elevated blood glucose and referrals to health care providers for treatment can lead to control of blood glucose (through behavior change and/or medication), which can substantially reduce complications of diabetes (WHO, 2002).

WHO (2002) also discussed the type of costs that can occur due to diabetes complications, such as costs for medicine, increased payments for insurance, and hospital stays. In 2008, stays in rural hospitals were more likely to be preventable when compared to urban hospitals. Rural hospitals had 15.9% preventable stays, 8.9% had potentially preventable chronic conditions, and 7.0% had preventable acute conditions. Urban hospitals had 9.2% preventable stays: 5.8% were potentially preventable chronic conditions and 3.4% potentially preventable acute conditions (Stranges & Stocks, 2010).

Identifying Target Populations

Health screenings should be provided when the community's health needs are clearly identified (as discussed in *Determining the Need of Rural Communities*) and the target population has been selected. There are various populations that an organization can target within a community (i.e., elderly, children, adults, minorities, etc.), and specific subpopulations (i.e., elderly women, Hispanic men, African American women, etc.). Populations can also differ based on educational level, gender, income, geographic location, race, culture, and so on. The organization should select the particular group of individuals intended to be identified and served through its service program. This group is also known as the *target population* (Bureau of Justice Assistance Center, n.d.). This group will be those within the community who are most at risk for the health indicator that the organization has chosen to target. The identification of a target population is a key component in designing an effective program.

Goals and Objectives

Once the health problem and target population have been identified, and partnerships are formed, the services can be designed to fit the community. Goals and objectives for the health-screening program should be established. Whether it is disease control, health education, or disease prevention, the program activities (types of tests, educational information provided, etc.) should reflect the goals and objectives set in place. For example, the CDC (2009) emphasized that objectives should be *SMART*, which is defined as follows:

Specific: persons/population doing the action and the action/activity
Measurable: how much change is expected
Achievable: attainable given the time frame and available resources
Realistic: reasonable steps to address problems and help achieve the
    program goal

Time-phased: provides a timeline for the objective to be met
   Here's an example of *SMART* goals and objectives:

Goals: Improve health outcomes of County B Hispanic/Latino farm workers with hypertension; increase healthy lifestyle behaviors among Hispanic/Latino farm workers in County B

Objectives: In 1 year, a total of at least six health screenings will be conducted for Hispanic health workers at County B chicken farm

- Increase the workers' knowledge of hypertension (contributing risk factors, preventive measures, and self-management of hypertension).
- At least 50% of the Hispanic/Latino farm workers will report that they have changed their behaviors to improve their health status.

Building Trust

Trust is a key ingredient to successfully conduct health programs in rural communities. However, it does not take place in and of itself. True trusting relationships must be built. They occur with time and effort, with ongoing engagement and involvement, and by the sweat of one's brow. One of the most important aspects of building trusting relationships is to constantly reach out to and consult with community gatekeepers or community leaders living in the community. In the context of rural communities, this may mean approaching church leaders (i.e., pastors, nuns, farmers, etc.). If an organization does not have existing relationships, or has problems establishing new relationships, many times it can use the state and/or local health department as a resource for obtaining community contacts. For example, an organization may have problems reaching the Hispanic/Latino population or African American population; if so, it can contact the state Office of Minority Health for assistance.

Another important component of the building trust effort is the "where in accessibility" or the site location of health programs when they are implemented. Organizations should be mindful of the barriers rural communities face, such as lack of access to health care, so providing screenings at sites that are familiar and accessible to residents will enhance the success of the service programs.

Community workers must be careful not to dismiss distrust as unwarranted or as a misperception that should be addressed by trying to change members of the community and their attitudes. Disparities in the quality of health care are real, and ongoing concerns exist about how the community members are informed and involved. Trust and distrust must be manifested by the provider, making the matter of trustworthiness as one that evolves from the provider agency or institution (Wynia & Gamble, 2006).

Viewing the problem from the perspective of provider trustworthiness, rather than community distrust, opens the door to potential solutions. Most importantly, ownership of the health efforts must belong to both the rural health providers and communities. Each should feel equal partnership in this regard.

In order to effectively reach rural communities and to nurture trusting relationships in these communities, health intervention and screening programs many times must be conducted in settings that are *not typical* when compared to traditional urban settings. Settings in rural communities where programs can be implemented are, in most instances, dictated by where the target population can be "accessed" in meaningful and productive ways. These settings may include migrant worker farms, small churches, trailer parks, and so on.

The identification and development of culturally appropriate recruitment materials, as well as the engagement of staff and assistants with similar racial and cultural backgrounds as the subject population, can help provide accurate information and reduce distrust in many rural community residents. Additionally, the establishment of community organizations or advisory boards, which provide feedback at all stages of the health effort, has been another means to ensure that community members take ownership of the effort and help to protect the interests the community targeted, thus reducing distrust.

EVALUATION

Organizations must start thinking about evaluation once the primary issue and target population are identified. It is important for organizations to create and/or obtain the necessary forms/documents (i.e., sign-in sheets, demographic data, health status data, satisfaction surveys, etc.) that will capture data reflecting the network's goals and objectives in order to successfully evaluate their program. Evaluation is a step that must be kept in mind from the beginning stages of the planning process. The program-evaluation process is important because it provides an opportunity for organizations to reflect on the process, influence policy makers and funders, build capacity and engage community, share what works and what doesn't work with other communities, and ensure funding and sustainability. The Center for the Advancement of Community-Based Public Health (CBPH, 2000) defines *program evaluation* as "the systematic collection, analysis, and reporting of information about a program to assist in decision making." *What have we done? How well have we done it? Who did we do it to? How effective has our program been? What could we do differently?* are all questions that organizations may answer by conducting program evaluation.

Process evaluation focuses more on how the program is being implemented, and how its outcomes are being achieved. It also tracks the strengths and weaknesses of the program. Process evaluation answers questions such as "Is the program being implemented as planned? How is the program achieving its objectives? What activities were conducted? What materials or services did participants receive? What did people experience? How is our coalition working? Do we have the 'right' stake-holders?" (CBPH, 2000).

SOCIAL MARKETING

To promote their health-screening programs in rural communities, networks should utilize social marketing. *Social marketing* is different from commercial marketing, but utilizes some of its strategies (i.e., audience orientation, audience segmentation, influencing behavior, competition, exchange, and marketing mix). Social marketing involves having a systematic and strategic plan for influencing voluntary behavioral change and promotes an end goal of improved personal welfare and improved welfare of society (CDC, 2007).

According to Turning Point (n.d.), social marketing is:

- A social or behavioral change strategy
- Most effective when it activates people
- Targeted to those who have a reason to care and who are ready for change
- Strategic, and requires efficient use of resources
- Integrated, and works on the "installment plan"

Social marketing is not:

- Just advertising
- A clever slogan or messaging strategy
- Reaching everyone through a media blitz
- An image campaign
- Done in a vacuum
- A quick process

Organizations must find ways to advertise and promote their programs and remember that communities have different methods of communication, especially rural communities. They should reach out to the "voices" of the community, such as churches, newspaper, radio, senior centers, and so on, to help promote the program. Each community is unique and has to be approached in a manner that will specifically meet the needs and reach the culture of the particular community. A marketing strategy that may work in one community may not necessarily work in another.

SUSTAINABILITY

Organizations should seek ways to find *sustainability*, which is to continue community health or quality of life benefits over time (Center for Civic Partnerships, 2001). Retaining networks or collaborations, gaining new partners, and seeking additional funding are all ways to help sustain the health interventions and screening program. There are two types of sustainability to consider (CDC, n.d.):

1. *Program Sustainability:* refers to the likelihood of the program continuing despite various factors (changes in management, available funding, etc.)
2. *Behavior Sustainability:* focuses on how easy or difficult it will be for the target population to continue their new behavior(s) once the program ends.

The Center for Civic Partnerships (2001) provides ten steps to maintaining community improvements:

1. Create shared understanding of sustainability
2. Position yourself to increase your sustainability odds
3. Create a plan to work through the process
4. Look at the current picture and pending items
5. Develop criteria on what to continue
6. Decide what to continue and prioritize
7. Create options for maintaining your priority efforts (including funding issues)
8. Develop a sustainability plan
9. Implement your sustainability plan
10. Estimate your outcomes and revise as needed

Case Study Exercises

Individually, or as a group, review the following case study and respond to the questions posed at the end of the study, as appropriate. Be sure to focus on the why, how, and what emphasized in each question. Your professor/instructor will provide you specific guidance on how you are to report your findings for the class.

Case Study 8.1: Alarural

Alarural, a nonprofit organization in rural Alabama, has received funding to provide health education and health screenings to County X and County Y. Alarural has worked with various community organizations in the past, including churches, universities, schools, health departments, and recreational centers in both counties and will include these organizations as a part of its network. The organization has already conducted a needs assessment and has identified diabetes as the health concern that has greatly impacted both communities. Since the prevalence of diabetes is much higher in County X's African American population, it has chosen this group as its target population. On the other hand, diabetes is affecting the Hispanic/Latino population in County Y.

Alarual is more familiar with County X because that is where it is located and has implemented several programs over the years in this community; they are not as familiar with County Y. Alarural has decided to reach County Y using the same method strategies that it uses to reach the residents of County X. It has decided to take the lead in implementing the program in both counties, since it has the most experience conducting health screenings out of any of the partners in the network. After 6 months of implementing its health screening and health education program, it has been very successful in reaching residents of County X. Unfortunately, participation numbers in County Y has been very low; lower than anticipated.

Study Questions

1. What strategies of implementing a health screening should Alarural implement?
2. How is Alarural utilizing its network partnerships?
3. In what ways could it improve the use of the network?
4. What other strategies could be used by Alarural to increase community participation in County Y?

Case Study 8.2: Owen County Health Department

The rural Owen County Health Department knows that community participation is essential to bringing about meaningful change. This three-county area, population 52,000, has been implementing a planning and mobilization process to assess and address local community issues. Even in their framing of their local partnerships as related to "health and safety," they were thinking of what would attract the most community member involvement.

Health Department staff invited concerned community citizens and people from numerous sectors of the community to be involved with their assessment and improvement efforts. More than 60 people attended the first meeting to kick off their process, and included judges, field representatives for congressmen, representation from the local faith communities, the hospitals, primary care center, board of health members, chiropractors, police, mayors, judges, the school superintendents, family resource representatives, youth service representatives, adult education, EMS workers, and other concerned citizens. Although many area residents lack access to cable television or Internet connections, energetic and resourceful Health Department staff members were effectively able to engage people. They advertised in local newspapers, church bulletins, and through venues such as the county extension service, dentists' offices, pharmacies, local businesses, hospice, the county sheriff, jailors, banks, and area technical colleges. Staff shared that their ability to allocate funds in their budget for food was also very helpful for convening people (they met over the lunch hour over catered sandwiches). At the first meeting, their sign-in sheet allowed people to indicate interest in joining the partnership on health and safety, and then staff followed-up with those people (e.g., using postcards and phone calls). Health Department staff members have also gathered support and membership for the partnerships by going and making presentations to many local community groups, including the rotary club, chambers of commerce, the schools, and local faith groups.

Since that successful launch, the coalition has strategically engaged members and collaborated with other existing local partnerships. The coalition has worked within each county to identify top health concerns. They sent out local surveys asking county residents (which asked them to identify the three most important things for a healthy county, the three top risky behaviors, and the top three health concerns). The $100 gift cards served as incentives for participation and each of the four counties received responses ranging from 600 to 1,000 returned surveys. This community input identified unique priorities for each county, including reducing tobacco use, reducing obesity, decreasing motor vehicle fatalities, and increasing access to care, and has been essential for improvement planning efforts.

The health education staff of the Health Department facilitates the local health and safety partnerships in each of the four counties. This provides institutionalized support for ensuring the staff time needed to facilitate these important community-driven processes.

Study Questions

1. It is important to include community members in the process of bringing about change. Identify ways the Owen County Health Department sought community member engagement.
2. Inclusion and engagement also means that community members can contribute. How did the Owen County Health Department create space for community members to contribute to the process?
3. Buy-in by community partners increases the likelihood that they will stay engaged in the effort. What did the Owen County Health Department do that promoted partner buy-in?
4. How will they ensure meaningful opportunities for community members to be involved?

REFERENCES

Bureau of Justice Assistance Center for Program Evaluation and Performance Measurement. (n.d.). Retrieved from www.ojp.usdoj.gov/BJA/evaluation/glossary/glossary_t.htm
Center for Civic Partnerships, Public Health Institute. (2001). *Sustainability Toolkit: 10 steps to maintaining your community improvements.* Oakland, CA: Public

Health Institute. Retrieved from www.civicpartnerships.org/docs/tools_resources/sustainability.htm

Centers for Disease Control and Prevention. (2007). *Introduction to social marketing: Primer for managers.* CDCynergy: Social Marketing Edition, Version 2.0 Primer for Managers. Retrieved from www.orau.gov/cdcynergy/demo/Content/activeinformation/intro_primer_managers.htm

Centers for Disease Control and Prevention. (2009). *Writing SMART objectives.* Evaluation Briefs 3(b), 1–2. Retrieved from www.cdc.gov/healthyyouth/evaluation/pdf/brief3b.pdf

Centers for Disease Control and Prevention. (n.d.). *Course module phase 6: Implementation.* Retrieved from www.cdc.gov/nccdphp/dnpa/socialmarketing/training/pdf/course/Implementation_6.pdf

Jones, C. A., Parker, T. S., Ahearn, M., Mishra, A. K., & Variyam, J. N. (2009). *Health status and health care access of farm and rural populations.* Economic Research Series U.S. Department of Agriculture. Retrieved from www.ers.usda.gov/Publications/EIB57/EIB57_ReportSummary.pdf (need/access to health care)

Kelly, M. L. (2002). *Partnering with other service organizations.* Retrieved from www.nationalserviceresources.org/practices/17380 (collaboration/resources and services)

Moore, D. P. (2009). *Community needs toolkit, 2–3.* Retrieved from http://communityaction.org/files/HigherGround/Community_Needs_Assessment_Tool_Kit.pdf

National Rural Health Association. (n.d.). *What's different about rural health care?* Retrieved from www.ruralhealthweb.org/go/left/about-rural-health/whats-different-about-rural-health-care

Owens, P. L., & Mutter, R. (2010). *Emergency department visits abuse for adults in community hospitals, 2008.* HCUP Statistical Brief (100), 2. Retrieved from www.hcup-us.ahrq.gov/reports/statbriefs/sb100.pdf

Rural Assistance Center. (n.d.a). *Information guide: what is rural?* Retrieved from www.raconline.org/info_guides/ruraldef/ (What is rural)

Rural Assistance Center. (n.d.b). *Cultural competence and limited English proficiency.* Retrieved from www.raconline.org/info_guides/culture/culturalcompetencyfaq.php#what

Rural Assistance Center. (n.d.c). *Networking and collaboration.* Retrieved from www.raconline.org/info_guides/networking

Stranges, E., & Stocks, C. (2010). *Potentially preventable hospitalizations for acute and chronic conditions, 2008.* HCUP Statistical Brief (99), 2. Retrieved from www.hcup-us.ahrq.gov/reports/statbriefs/sb99.pdf.

Sumaya, C. V. (2002). *Rural public health.* Gale Encyclopedia of Public Heatlh. Retrieved from www.healthline.com/galecontent/rural-public-health#ruralpublichealth

The Center for the Advancement of Community Based Public Health. (2000). *An evaluation framework for community health programs, 10–11.* Retrieved from www.cdc.gov/eval/evalcbph.pdf

Turning Point. (n.d.). *The basics of social marketing, 5.* Retrieved from www.turningpointprogram.org/Pages/pdfs/social_market/smc_basics.pdf

U.S. Census Bureau. (2010). Census: Urban and rural classification. *Federal Register,* 75(63), 3–4. Retrieved from www.census.gov/geo/www/ua/urbanruralclass.html

World Health Organizaition. (2002). *Diabetes: The cost of diabetes.* Fact Sheet (236). Retrieved from www.who.int/mediacentre/factsheets/fs236/en/

Wynia, M. K., & Gamble, V. N. (2006). Mistrust among minorities and the trustworthiness of medicine [published online ahead of print May 30, 2006]. *PLoS Medicine, 3*(5), e244–e245.

ADDITIONAL STUDY RESOURCES—RURAL COMMUNITY BIBLIOGRAPHY

Calle, E. E., Flanders, W. D., Thun, M. J., & Martin, L. M. (1993). Demographic predictors of mammography and Pap smear screening in U.S. women. *American Journal of Public Health, 83*(1), 53–60.

Davis, K., & Stapleton, J. (1991). Migration to rural areas by HIV patients: Impact on HIV-related health care use. *Infection Control and Hospital Epidemiology, 12,* 540–543.

DeStefano, F., Eaker, E. D., Broste, S. K., Nordstrom, D. L., Peissig, P. L., Vierkant, R. A.,...Layde, P. M. (1996). Epidemiologic research in an integrated regional medical care system: The marshfield epidemiologic study area. *Journal of Clinical Epidemiology, 49*(6), 643–652.

First, R. J., Rife, J. C., & Toomey, B. G. (1994). Homelessness in rural areas: Causes, patterns, and trend. *Social Work, 39*(1), 97–108.

Flowe, K. M., Cunningham, P. R., & Foil, B. (1995). Rural trauma systems in evolution. *Surgery Annual, 27,* 29–39.

Gesler, W. M., & Ricketts, T. C. (Eds.). (1992). *Health in rural North America.* New Brunswick, NJ: Rutgers University Press.

Grossman, D. C., Kim, A., Macdonald, S. C., Klein, P., Copass, M. K., & Maier, R. V. (1997). Urban-rural differences in prehospital care of major trauma. *Journal Trauma: Injury, Infection, and Critical Care, 42*(4), 723–729.

Hahn, B., & Flood, A. (1995). No insurance, public insurance and private insurance: Do these options contribute to differences in general health? *Journal of Health Care for the Poor and Underserved, 6*(1), 41–59.

Lam, N. S., & Liu, K. B. (1994). Spread of AIDS in rural America, 1982–1990. *Journal of Acquired Immune Deficiency Syndromes, 7*(5), 485–490.

Monroe, A. C., Ricketts, T. C., & Savitz, L. A. (1992). Cancer in rural versus urban populations: A review. *Journal of Rural Health, 8*(3), 212–220.

Mueller, K. (1999). *Rural implications of the Balanced Budget Retirement Act of 1999.* Columbia, MO: Rural Policy Research Institute.

National Rural Health Association. (1992). *A rural health agenda for the future. Report to health resources and services administration.* Rockville, MD: Author.

No authors listed. (1990). Rural health: A challenge for medical education. In *Proceedings of the 1990 Invitational Symposium,* San Antonio, Texas, February 1–3. *Academic Medicine, 65*(12, Suppl.), S51–S53.

Nyman, J. A., Sen, A., Chan, B. Y., & Commins, P. P. (1991). Urban/rural differences in home health patients and services. *Gerontologist, 31*(4), 457–466.

Stevens, M., & Youells, F. (1995). Drug use prevalence in a rural school-age population: The New Hampshire Survey. *American Journal of Preventive Medicine, 11,* 105–113.

Stone, S. E., Bron, P. M., & Westcott, J. P. (1996). Nurse-Midwifery service in a rural setting. *Journal of Nurse-Midwifery, 41*(5), 377–382.

Swanson, L. L. (1996). *Racial/ethnic minorities in rural areas: Progress and stagnation, 1980–90.* Agricultural Economic Report No. 731. Washington, DC: U.S. Department of Agriculture.

The Community Tool Box is a service of the Work Group for Community at the University of Kansas, Copyright 2012 by the University of Kansas.

U.S. Department of Health and Human Services. (1992). *Vital and health statistics: Current estimates from the National Health Interview Survey, 1991.* Hyattsville, MD: Author.

9

Ensuring Environmental Health and Justice in Communities of Concern

Stephanie Miles-Richardson and Rueben C. Warren

LEARNING OBJECTIVES

What you can learn by studying this chapter:

- How to define environment
- How to describe environmental heath
- What are communities of concern
- To identify three chronic diseases and potential environmental contributors
- What are the components of a framework to address environmental health challenges in communities of concern
- To describe the relationship between this framework and community-based participatory research (CBPR)
- How to identify the aspect of this framework that likely contributes to its success

Before ensuring environmental health and justice in communities of concern, one must first have a thorough understanding of environmental health. This first requires an initial discourse and agreement on the concept of "health." The World Health Organization (WHO) defines health as the physical, social, and psychological well-being of the individual and not just the absence of disease (WHO, 2012). This definition suggests that health and disease are not simply two diametrically opposed concepts. Rather, health is a much more complex continuum with various inputs. A more encompassing definition that includes another input that is critical in communities of concern describes health as a "dynamic relationship; the synergistic interplay between physical, social, psychological, and spiritual elements that create the well-being of persons and/or groups in their physical and social environment" (Warren, Lockett, & Zulfiqar, 2002). Not only does this definition speak to psychosocial and spiritual elements of persons, it includes references to physical space or the environment that people occupy. Public health, in its broadest, is social justice—and social justice is inclusive of matters of environmental health and justice.

Environment, per se, is inclusive of the physical environment and how that physical nature impacts health outcome, as well as environmental stewardship practices such as waste management, recycling, and other means of environmental conservation. Historically, mainstream organizations focused on the environment were concerned with protecting the wilderness and endangered species. There is a long-term appreciation for the relationship between animals and their environment. However, we have been slow to recognize the direct impact of the environment on persons, although the impact on environmental resources has been clear. As such, many organizations were also concerned with clean air and clean water, and other activities related to conservation. Recent efforts have targeted environmental stewardship, particularly as the effects of greenhouse gases and climate change have become more embedded in day-to-day conversation. But for the purpose of this discussion, environment specifically refers to the impact on persons and communities. While environment simply describes the circumstances, objects, or conditions in which one is surrounded, it includes the complex interaction of physical factors (such as light or noise), chemical factors (such as hazardous waste), and biotic factors (such as climate, soil, and living things) that act upon individuals or communities. This interaction ultimately determines not only the form and survival of organisms, but also the health status and quality of life of persons.

A strategy to ensure environmental health is important since we know that environmental stressors can negatively impact a person's health. Such stressors may be physical, chemical, or biologic factors, which are external to a person. According to the WHO, approximately one-quarter of the global disease burden can be attributed to the modifiable environment. Also, it is estimated that 24% of the number of years of healthy life lost to disease, and 23% of mortality associated with disease is related to environmental causes (WHO, 2006). Similarly, social and cultural conditions that influence the life of an individual or community directly impact the quality of an individual's and/or community's environment. When such an impact is negative and disproportionately affects certain communities, it is considered to be an issue of environmental justice (EJ). According to the Environmental Protection Agency (EPA):

> Environmental Justice is the fair treatment and meaningful involvement of all people regardless of race, color, national origin, or income with respect to the development, implementation, and enforcement of environmental laws, regulations, and policies. EPA has this goal for all communities and persons across this Nation. It will be achieved when everyone enjoys the same degree of protection from environmental and health hazards and equal access to the decision-making process to have a healthy environment in which to live, learn, and work. (EPA, 2012)

It is important to note the context in which this definition emerged. The EJ movement was born out of communities rallying together against environmental stressors that threatened the environmental health of persons collectively. Early on, for some, the environment served as another struggle for justice, not unlike the civil rights movement. This was the case in Warren County, North Carolina, where the EJ movement began. In Warren County, a toxic landfill was placed in a small African American community even though the location was not the most scientifically suitable site for a landfill. Shortly thereafter, it became evident that pollution-producing facilities were more likely to be placed in certain communities. In the early 1980s, the Government Accounting Office (GAO) released a report that revealed that three of four hazardous waste sites in the southeastern United States were in African American communities (General Accounting Office, 1983). A landmark report titled "Toxic Wastes and Race in the United States" published by the Commission for Racial Justice of the United Church of Christ followed the GAO report and provided tangible evidence that demonstrated that toxic facilities were disproportionately sited in minority and/or low income communities (1987). Several cases and lawsuits against the EPA throughout the 1980s led to the establishment of the Environmental Equity Working group and ushered in the response of the federal government to the impact of environmental stressors on communities of concern. EJ advocates define the environment in a way that speaks specifically to the communities impacted: "where we work, live, play and worship" (1999). To attain environmental health is to have freedom from illness or injury related to exposure to toxic agents and other environmental conditions that are potentially detrimental to human health. Environmental health—like public health—is social justice and a right for all.

COMMUNITIES OF CONCERN

Communities of concern refer to communities in specific regions where racial and ethnic minorities and/or persons who lead a low-income life live and often work. Persons in these communities have high prevalence of disease and disabilities, have shorter life spans, have a lower quality of life, and also have disproportionately high levels of exposure to environmental stressors resulting in real or perceived adverse health effects. Additionally, persons in these communities may have limited access to health care and are often less educated; they may be politically disenfranchised, and they may be of low socioeconomic status (SES). This terminology, first introduced by the Institute of Medicine, 1999, is used to describe persons who often experience environmental stressors that can adversely influence health. Environmental stressors include chemicals, biologics, allergens, and traditional toxicants. Environmental stressors can also include light, noise, odors, and exposure to particulate matter. Historically, however, environmental stressors typically referred to the preponderance of landfill sitings and exposure to other hazardous substances in minority and low-income communities (Brown, 1995). For example, in 1977, Chemical Waste Management established a large commercial hazardous waste treatment, storage, and disposal facility that was sited in Emelle (Sumpter County), Alabama, where African Americans comprised 90% of the population. Additionally, African Americans represented 100% of the population below the poverty level (General Accounting Office, 1983). This was the largest landfill in the United States. It was found that the fourth largest landfill in the United States was in Scotlandville, Louisiana, which, at the time, was comprised of 93% African Americans. Hispanic residents of Kettleman City, California, comprised 78.4% of the population; this was the home of the fifth largest landfill in the United States. These three communities comprised an estimated 40% of the total national commercial hazardous waste landfill capacity of the United States. This report was updated 20 years later—in 2007. Cases of disproportionate landfill sitings and other evidence of environmental injustice remain (Bullard, Mohai, Saha, & Wright, 2007).

Health effects resulting from environmental exposure can be acute or chronic. Also, complications to preexisting medical problems can occur. Childhood asthma is increasing, particularly in urban neighborhoods, among children who are of a low SES (Hill, Graham, & Divgi, 2011; Weitzman, Gortmaker, Sobol, & Perrin, 1992). Neighborhoods that are low SES are disproportionately located near highways, industrial areas, and toxic waste sites, since land there is cheaper and political resistance to polluting is often less visible (Gan et al., 2011; Laumbach & Kipen, 2012; Rauh, Landrigan, & Claudio, 2008). In addition to asthma, proximity to hazardous waste can cause immune dysfunction, autoimmunity, allergies, cancers, cognitive deficits, mood changes, neurological diseases, changes in libido, reproductive dysfunction, and glucose dysregulation (Gee & Payne-Sturges, 2004).

Unfortunately, members of communities of concern often also bear the burden of health disparities. It is, in fact, difficult to separate experiences of environmental injustice from experiences of health disparities. Health disparities, historically, were articulated as excess deaths, a term used in the 1985 Report of the Secretary's Task Force of Black and Minority Health (United States Department of Health and Human Services, 1985). Excess deaths referred to the difference between the number of deaths observed in a racial/ethnic group and the number of deaths that would have occurred in that group if it had the same death rate as the non-Hispanic White population. In 1985, there were 60,000 excess deaths experienced by African Americans. The report focused on mortality data from 1979 to 1981 and identified six causes of death that together accounted for over 80% of the mortality observed among African Americans and other minorities. Those six causes of death were cancer, cardiovascular disease and stroke, cirrhosis, diabetes, homicides and accidents, and infant mortality (United States Department of Health and Human Services, 1985). By 1990, HIV/AIDS was estimated to be the sixth leading cause of death for African Americans (Smith, 1992). Sadly, those causes of death remain prominent contributors to health disparities even today. In 2005, excess deaths had risen to 83,000 (Satcher et al., 2005). This was even after the elimination of health disparities was articulated as one of the nation's two overarching goals in Healthy People 2010. Many of the chronic health conditions that continue to plague persons in communities of concern also have environmental contributors suggesting that health outcomes may be modified with environmental mitigation.

ENVIRONMENTAL CONTRIBUTORS TO CHRONIC DISEASE

Chronic disease is a particular burden for people who also experience health disparities. In the United States, cardiovascular disease, primarily heart disease and stroke, is the leading cause of death for both men and women of all racial and ethnic groups. This is particularly alarming in minority populations. Well-known risk factors for heart disease include smoking, decreased exercise, increased weight, and increased saturated fat in the diet. Social and economic stress can also serve as a risk factor (Warren-Findlow, 2006). Lesser known risk factors include exposure to air pollution, which has been associated with myocardial infarction, initiation of life-threatening arrhythmias, changes in cardiac rhythm and autonomic function, endothelial dysfunction, increased plasma viscosity, and increased C-reactive protein (Kampa & Castanas, 2008; Zanobetti, Baccarelli, & Schwartz, 2011). While underlying biological mechanisms are not clear, these findings provide possible pathways in which air pollutants, especially particulate matter, affect the incidence and death rate of heart disease and stroke (Zanobetti et al., 2011). Such information is of particular relevance in cities like Houston, Texas, where airborne emissions from various sources contribute to frequent episodes of elevated air pollution (Sexton, Linder, Marko, Bethel, & Lupo, 2007). In Houston, the primary culprit is exposure to environmental hazards near the ship channel. In fact, the highest cancer risk in Harris County, Texas, is concentrated along a corridor that flanks the channel. It is noted that social disadvantage and Hispanic ethnicity is also related to the increase in cancer risk burden (Sexton et al., 2007). In other urban centers, proximity to road traffic can lead to adverse cardiovascular outcomes (Gan et al., 2011). Blood lead and bone lead are associated with increased blood pressure and hypertension (Hassing et al., 2009), as well as behavioral effects in children (Dilworth-Bart & Moore, 2006). Lead causes an elevation of systolic blood pressure among adult males. Early myocardial responses to environmental toxicants cause altered calcium homeostasis, which may lead to reversible cardiac arrhythmia, or with prolonged stimuli, hypertrophy and irreversible cardiomyopathy (Hassing et al., 2009).

Cancer is a complex disease that can have plausible associations with numerous environmental chemicals such as persistent, bioaccumulative organochlorines; ubiquitous, lipophilic solvents; and ubiquitous, persistent metals (Apelberg, Buckley, & White, 2005; Golden & Kimbrough, 2009; Sarafanov et al., 2011; Wolff, Britton, & Wilson, 2003; Wolff et al., 2000). Epidemiologic studies of hormonal factors in breast cancer, as well as prostate cancer, and animal studies of both hormonal activity and carcinogenicity of certain synthetic chemicals suggest environmental pollutants as possible sources of risk. Much research has been conducted to determine the impact, if any, of organochlorines on breast cancer. While research has not demonstrated a causal relationship, additional work is needed to identify potential effects of polychlorinated biphenyls (PCBs) and to determine if certain populations are more vulnerable because of differing exposure patterns (Salehi et al., 2008).

The burden of diabetes on the nation is so great that nationwide screenings and community-based lifestyle interventions are being proposed. The goal is to not only prevent the onset of type 2 diabetes, but also to reduce health care costs over time. In addition to the effects on health care costs, diabetes is a major cause of blindness, renal failure, amputation, and cardiovascular disease. Additionally, it increases the risk of cancer and dementia (Fradkin, 2012; Zhuo et al., 2012). Diabetes has a large incidence rate in African American and other minority populations. Risk factors include genetics/inherited tendencies; medical risk factors, such as insulin resistance; and lifestyle risk factors, such as physical activity. While interventions to combat diabetes have a strong focus on lifestyle modifications, environmental contributors must not be overlooked. Epidemiologic data demonstrate that populations with high exposure to arsenic generally have an increase risk of type 2 diabetes. Arsenic is metabolized in vivo to trivalent arsenic. A trivalent arsenical, phenylarsine oxide, has adverse effects on the insulin receptor and glucose transport in in vitro experiments (Longnecker & Daniels, 2001a). Dioxin exposure has been associated with type 2 diabetes, hyperglycemia, or hyperinsulinemia (Longnecker & Daniels, 2001b; Remillard & Bunce, 2002). Additionally, bisphenol A, which is found in plastics and other products, may lead to insulin resistance and type 2 diabetes. The mechanism is believed to be an overactivation of pancreatic beta cells (Silver, O'Neill, Sowers, & Park, 2011). There is also evidence that environmental tobacco smoke exposure may be associated with type 2 diabetes (Cupul-Uicab et al., 2011; Cupul-Uicab, Ye, Skjaerven, Haug, & Longnecker, 2011; Ko et al., 2011). In recent years, researchers have also focused on the impact of the built food environment, specifically access to fresh foods, on type 2 diabetes (Lamichhane et al., 2012).

Asthma is another chronic disease that has specific associations with environmental exposures. For well over a decade, evidence that environmental air pollutants are associated with asthma has increased (Koren & Utell, 1997; Rauh et al., 2008; Weitzman et al., 1992; Wong, Von, Douwes, & Pearce, 2006). This is particularly significant for children in the United States and worldwide (Laumbach & Kipen, 2012) and it may be that other vulnerable populations are also at greater risk (Cakmak, Dales, Rubio, & Vidal, 2011). Early exposure to particulate matter is strongly associated with the development of asthma. Air pollutants of concern are particulate matter, ozone, and nitrogen dioxide. Chronic exposure to particulate matter has been associated with, in addition to asthma, an increased risk of cardiovascular disease, cancer, chronic obstructive pulmonary disease, and neurologic disease (Ji & Khurana Hershey, 2012). Additionally, the negative effects of particulate matter and other air pollutants on lung function place children at continued risk for pollutant-induced asthma exacerbation (Grigg, 2004; Tzivian, 2011). When children live in environments near traffic, negative health effects also occur (Boothe & Shendell, 2008; Dales, Wheeler, Mahmud, Frescura, & Liu, 2009). Air pollution is a preventable cause of respiratory disease for which persons in communities of concern may be particularly vulnerable due to environmental stressors (Laumbach, 2010).

These are some examples of diseases and disorders that can be influenced by environmental exposures. Beyond the scientific certainty and/or plausibility of health effects of environmental chemical exposure, it becomes necessary to also consider the psychosocial impact of living in an environment with known or suspected environmental hazards. Indeed, when calculating cumulative exposures, investigators should take into consideration the role of different types of stressors. For example, when evaluating health risks, cumulative risk assessment should consider both chemical and nonchemical stressors, such as SES and related psychosocial stress (Lewis, Sax, Wason, & Campleman, 2011). This consideration is particularly critical for persons in communities of color and/or communities comprised of persons of low SES. Such communities are disproportionately affected. The relationship among health, environment, and culture is intertwined; therefore, the cultural context of community is an important consideration (Bent, 2003). Research demonstrates the effect of long-term economic and social stress on chronic disease (Warren-Findlow, 2006). Indeed, communities of concern and communities of color often describe the same disproportionately impacted populations. Theoretical frameworks that integrate nonchemical stressors such as poverty and discrimination have been identified (Lewis et al., 2011; Linder & Sexton, 2011). Several models have been proposed: Social determinant models suggest that disparate health outcomes are due to structural inequalities, health disparity models consider the social and contextual factors that act through individual behaviors and biological mechanisms, and multiple stressor models consider environmental agents (Linder & Sexton, 2011). Psychosocial stress is clearly a factor with the potential to exacerbate the real or perceived threats of environmental hazards (Gee & Payne-Sturges, 2004). Until there is agreement on how best to conduct an all-inclusive risk assessment of environmental exposure, a framework to address the real and perceived environmental exposures must be identified.

A FRAMEWORK TO ADDRESS ENVIRONMENTAL HEALTH CHALLENGES

The typical response to environmental exposures is the risk-assessment process (EPA, 2011a). Risk assessment involves hazard identification—utilizing available scientific literature to identify types of toxic effects; dose–response assessment—a quantitative description of risk with associated uncertainties; and human exposure assessment—identification of the range of exposures being assessed. Finally, risk characterization describes the particular risks likely to be experienced by the population of interest under actual or expected exposure conditions. The risk-assessment process relies heavily on assigning causation to manage risks. But assigning causation is not critical to assessing the risks associated with human exposures to those environmental agents that are of immediate concern. The reliance of the risk-assessment process on proof of toxicity is problematic. Often, neither epidemiologic evidence nor the scientific literature provides such proof. This fact alone does not demonstrate that harm is unlikely. Even so, a formal assessment of the health risks from environmental stressors can serve as a tool for risk management, as well as to inform EJ policy. When risk is assessed and management decisions are made, there must also be careful consideration of economic issues, ethical and moral principles, legal precedents, political realities, cultural beliefs, societal values, and bureaucratic impediments (Lewis et al., 2011). Taken together, these factors can ensure that vulnerable populations are protected. An alternative approach to utilize environmental impact assessment is the precautionary principle (Cranor, 2004; Goldstein, 2006; Powell, 2010). This approach requires the proof of safety prior to use and subsequent exposure. As such, it is an approach that remains controversial and not universally used.

In communities of concern, utilizing a strategy that includes assessment, advocacy, coordination, and evaluation has proven most useful and most likely to lead to a speedy resolution. *Assessment* is the determination of what the situation is without placing any value on it. Often, in communities of concern, assessment requires that "listening sessions" occur with members of the community. In such forums, which occur in places designated by community members, residents' concerns and fears are heard, and when possible, questions are answered. But the outcome of the listening session is not to provide information, rather, it is to hear concerns and begin the process of building a trusting relationship with all stakeholders. Assessment also involves utilizing resources that are available, such as the Toxic Release Inventory (TRI) managed by the EPA (EPA, 2011b), as well as available scientific literature. Although information provided to the EPA by industry is voluntary, the TRI database can provide information for communities about toxic chemical releases in the environment. Completing a public health assessment, as established by the U.S. Agency for Toxic Substances and Disease Registry (ATSDR), is one strategy to determine the relationship between adverse, population-based, human health effects and toxic and hazardous waste (ATSDR, 2011). ATSDR's public health assessment process utilizes the identification of a complete exposure pathway to determine if a given environmental release is likely to cause harm to a local population. While this is a reasonable process, when it is not possible to determine a complete exposure pathway, yet a population still has evidence—or belief—of harm, the process becomes problematic. Regardless of the outcome of the public health assessment, *advocacy* follows, and can only occur when one is clear of the issue—that is, clear of the outcome of the assessment. Advocacy is based on the best science available. In the absence of valid and reliable science, advocacy still occurs scientifically, at best, and systematically, at worst, and leads to the design of a strategy to measure the impact of the intervention used. *Coordination*, the next step, utilizes public health agencies and other networks within the federal, state, local government, and nongovernment trusted agencies and organizations to coordinate what should be advocated for and implemented to address the environmental health issues facing the community. Primary care physicians and/or physicians trained in environmental medicine are critical at this stage. When community members are provided the opportunity to articulate their major concern, one will often find that it centers on health. This type of critical information can be gleaned during the listening session in the first step of the process. Since the main concern of affected community members is often health, health providers who are willing and able to speak about the potential or known effects of environmental exposures are critical. Community gatekeepers, advocates, and academic, civic, social, and faith-based individuals and organizations are essential to build a sustainable movement to fully address the issues, which often extend beyond the authority and resources of the public health community. For successful resolution of concerns, communities rooted in principles of faith must have their faith leaders present and engaged. It is not uncommon for a listening session to be held in a faith-based institution. Finally, *evaluation research* should occur to measure impact and to ensure that the process is repeatable.

This strategy for addressing environmental health and ensuring EJ in communities of concern is rooted in the principles of CBPR methods, which focus on social, structural, and physical environmental inequities through active involvement of community members, organizational representatives, and researchers in all aspects of the process. The CBPR process is scientific inquiry that is conducted as a partnership between traditionally trained practitioners and lay participants. In CBPR projects, the community participates fully in all aspects of the research process. The "expert" practitioner and the lay practitioner are coequal partners in a CBPR project. This method requires that the views, concerns, and interests of all participants are given equal weight in determining the focus of the research question, the approach employed to attempt to identify answers and solutions, and the use and significance of the products of the research endeavor. Community–university partnerships are particularly fruitful, providing resources for the community and opportunities for service and learning for academicians. For example, issues of environmental health and justice impacting a low-income community of color located along the fence line of a major oil refinery in Richmond, California, were explored using CBPR. The partnership led to the formation of a health survey that revealed positive feelings that the residents had about their neighborhood, but also their concerns about environmental stressors. An outcome of this partnership was the discovery that children and long-time residents had elevated asthma rates (Cohen, Lopez, Malloy, & Morello-Frosch, 2011). While variations on the CBPR model exist, the common theme is the partnership between the so-called expert and representatives of the affected community. While those with expertise are typically practitioners, graduate interns focused on environmental public health have also been effective using this approach (Close, Zokovitch Paben, & Foster, 2011).

Persons in communities of concern already experience health disparities and poorer health outcomes. Residential segregation may lead to differential experiences with stressors—including psychosocial and environmental (Gee & Payne-Sturges, 2004). Ultimately, in order to develop policy to address the disproportionate impact on communities of concern, it is necessary to develop a model that accurately takes into account the additive effect of multiple environmental and social stressors (Brody et al., 2009). Some models have been proposed. For example, the cumulative environmental hazard inequity index provides a means by which to incorporate environmental hazards and characteristics related to SES to assess inequities in cumulative risk (Su et al., 2009). Psychosocial stress, coupled with disproportionate exposure to environmental hazards, requires that public health practitioners engaged in environmental public health embrace an approach that will best serve impacted populations. Meanwhile, an approach that utilizes the framework described herein will serve to begin the process of rebuilding trust and mitigating harm.

Case Study Exercises

Individually, or as a group, review the following case study and respond to the questions posed at the end of the study, as appropriate. Be sure to focus on the why, how, and what emphasized in each question. Your professor/instructor will provide you specific guidance on how you are to report your findings for the class.

Case Study 9.1: Environmental Concerns in Corpus Christi, Texas

You are a public health practitioner in Texas who learns of a community in Corpus Christi with concerns regarding environmental contamination. After doing some research and visiting with some members of the community, you learn the following: The "Refinery Row" districts of Corpus Christi, Texas, are primarily low income, African American and Hispanic communities located very close to a large collection of industrial companies.

The residents are concerned about air and ground (water and soil) pollution caused by these industries. Through a community organization, residents have voiced their concerns, but perceive an apparent disregard by both the polluters and the city and state. Incidents such as ground water contamination, lead contamination of soil, accidents and explosions at plants, and various toxic clouds resulting in nausea of the residents on several occasions have provoked little or no actions by the state and the city. Complaints phoned in by the citizens are routinely ignored. City Hall has refused to hold special town meetings on the subject of environmental contamination, and has rebuffed citizens when they brought up the topic while attending council meetings. Residents generally feel that there is no concern for their health and well-being. Many have no additional schooling beyond high school—20% do not have a high school diploma. The residents have various ailments that they believe are related to the environmental contamination. Many do not have health insurance and cannot afford to go for medical care. Every Saturday, from 8:30 p.m. to 1 p.m., the free clinic opens up to provide care for those in need. However, many residents cannot get to the clinic because they work the night shift at one of the refineries or at the nearby poultry plant. The residents are frustrated and distrustful of most public officials. However, they trust you as a public health practitioner and seek your guidance for resolution.

Study Questions

1. What are the key issues sighted here?
2. What cultural concerns are evident in this case study?
3. How would describe disparity in this case study?
4. How will you advise the community to move to address their concerns?

REFERENCES

Agency for Toxic Substances and Disease Registry. (2011). *Public health assessment.* Retrieved from www.atsdr.cdc.gov/com/pha.html

Apelberg, B. J., Buckley, T. J., & White, R. H. (2005). Socioeconomic and racial disparities in cancer risk from air toxics in Maryland. *Environmental Health Perspectives, 113,* 693–699.

Bent, K. N. (2003). "The people know what they want": An empowerment process of sustainable, ecological community health. *ANS Advances in Nursing Science, 26,* 215–226.

Boothe, V. L., & Shendell, D. G. (2008). Potential health effects associated with residential proximity to freeways and primary roads: Review of scientific literature, 1999–2006. *Journal of Environmental Health, 70,* 33–36.

Brody, J. G., Morello-Frosch, R., Zota, A., Brown, P., Perez, C., & Rudel, R. A. (2009). Linking exposure assessment science with policy objectives for environmental justice and breast cancer advocacy: The northern California household exposure study. *American Journal of Public Health, 99*(Suppl. 3), S600–S609.

Brown, P. (1995). Race, class, and environmental health: A review and systematization of the literature. *Environmental Research, 69,* 15–30.

Bullard, R. D., Mohai, P., Saha, R., & Wright, B. (2007). *Toxic waste and race at twenty 1987–2007: Grassroots struggles to dismantle environmental racism in the United States.* Cleveland, OH: United Church of Christ Justice and Witness Ministries.

Cakmak, S., Dales, R. E., Rubio, M. A., & Vidal, C. B. (2011). The risk of dying on days of higher air pollution among the socially disadvantaged elderly. *Environmental Research, 111,* 388–393.

Close, F. T., Zokovitch Paben, J. M., & Foster, A. (2011). Community-based internships to address environmental issues: A model for effective partnerships. *Progress in Community Health Partnerships, 5,* 77–87.

Cohen, A., Lopez, A., Malloy, N., & Morello-Frosch, R. (2011). Our environment, our health: A community-based participatory environmental health survey in Richmond, California. *Health Education & Behavior, 39,* 198–209.

Cranor, C. F. (2004). Toward understanding aspects of the precautionary principle. *Journal of Medicine and Philosophy, 29,* 259–279.

Cupul-Uicab, L. A., Skjaerven, R., Haug, K., Melve, K. K., Engel, S. M., & Longnecker, M. P. (2011). In utero exposure to maternal tobacco smoke and subsequent obesity, hypertension, and gestational diabetes among women in the MoBa cohort. *Environmental Health Perspectives, 120,* 355–360.

Cupul-Uicab, L. A., Ye, X., Skjaerven, R., Haug, K., & Longnecker, M. P. (2011). Reproducibility of reported in utero exposure to tobacco smoke. *Annals of Epidemiology, 21,* 48–52.

Dales, R., Wheeler, A. J., Mahmud, M., Frescura, A. M., & Liu, L. (2009). The influence of neighborhood roadways on respiratory symptoms among elementary schoolchildren. *Journal of Occupational and Environmental Medicine, 51,* 654–660.

Dilworth-Bart, J. E., & Moore, C. F. (2006). Mercy mercy me: Social injustice and the prevention of environmental pollutant exposures among ethnic minority and poor children. *Child Development, 77,* 247–265.

Environmental Justice (EJ). (1999). *Toward environmental justice*. Retrieved from http://www.iom.edu/Reports/1999/Toward-Environmental-Justice-Research-Education-and-Health-Policy-Needs.aspx

Environmental Protection Agency. (2011a). *Risk assessment process* [Online]. Retrieved from http://epa.gov/riskassessment/health-risk.htm

Environmental Protection Agency. (2011b). *Toxic release inventory* [Online]. Retrieved from www.epa.gov/tri/

Environmental Protection Agency. (2012). *Online source*. Retrieved from http://www.epa.gov/environmentaljustice/

Fradkin, J. E. (2012). Confronting the urgent challenge of diabetes: An overview. *Health Affairs (Millwood)*, *31*, 12–19.

Gan, W. Q., Koehoorn, M., Davies, H. W., Demers, P. A., Tamburic, L., & Brauer, M. (2011). Long-term exposure to traffic-related air pollution and the risk of coronary heart disease hospitalization and mortality. *Environmental Health Perspectives*, *119*, 501–507.

Gee, G. C., & Payne-Sturges, D. C. (2004). Environmental health disparities: A framework integrating psychosocial and environmental concepts. *Environmental Health Perspectives*, *112*, 1645–1653.

General Accounting Office. (1983). *Siting of hazardous waste landfills and their correlation with racial and economic status of surrounding communities*. Washington, DC: U.S. Government Printing Office.

Golden, R., & Kimbrough, R. (2009). Weight of evidence evaluation of potential human cancer risks from exposure to polychlorinated biphenyls: An update based on studies published since 2003. *Critical Reviews in Toxicology*, *39*, 299–331.

Goldstein, B. D. (2006). The precautionary principle: Is it a threat to toxicological science? *International Journal of Toxicology*, *25*, 3–7.

Grigg, J. (2004). Environmental toxins; their impact on children's health. *Archives of Disease in Childhood*, *89*, 244–250.

Hassing, C., Twickler, M., Brunekreef, B., Cassee, F., Doevendans, P., Kastelein, J., Cramer, M. J. (2009). Particulate air pollution, coronary heart disease and individual risk assessment: A general overview. *European Journal of Cardiovascular Prevention and Rehabilitation*, *16*, 10–15.

Hill, T. D., Graham, L. M., & Divgi, V. (2011). Racial disparities in pediatric asthma: A review of the literature. *Current Allergy and Asthma Reports*, *11*, 85–90.

Institute of Medicine. (1999). *Toward environmental justice: Research, education, and health policy needs* [Online].

Ji, H., & Khurana Hershey, G. K. (2012). Genetic and epigenetic influence on the response to environmental particulate matter. *Journal of Allergy and Clinical Immunology*, *129*, 33–41.

Kampa, M., & Castanas, E. (2008). Human health effects of air pollution. *Environmental Pollution*, *151*, 362–367.

Ko, K. P., Min, H., Ahn, Y., Park, S. J., Kim, C. S., Park, J. K., & Kim, S. S. (2011). A prospective study investigating the association between environmental tobacco smoke exposure and the incidence of type 2 diabetes in never smokers. *Annals of Epidemiology*, *21*, 42–47.

Koren, H. S., & Utell, M. J. (1997). Asthma and the environment. *Environmental Health Perspectives*, *105*, 534–537.

Lamichhane, A. P., Mayer-Davis, E. J., Puett, R., Bottai, M., Porter, D. E., & Liese, A. D. (2012). Associations of built food environment with dietary intake among youth with diabetes. *Journal of Nutrition Education and Behavior.* Epub ahead of print.

Laumbach, R. J. (2010). Outdoor air pollutants and patient health. *American Family Physician, 81*, 175–180.

Laumbach, R. J., & Kipen, H. M. (2012). Respiratory health effects of air pollution: Update on biomass smoke and traffic pollution. *Journal of Allergy and Clinical Immunology, 129*, 3–11.

Lewis, A. S., Sax, S. N., Wason, S. C., & Campleman, S. L. (2011). Non-chemical stressors and cumulative risk assessment: An overview of current initiatives and potential air pollutant interactions. *International Journal of Environmental Research and Public Health, 8*, 2020–2073.

Linder, S. H., & Sexton, K. (2011). Conceptual models for cumulative risk assessment. *American Journal of Public Health, 101*(Suppl. 1), S74–S81.

Longnecker, M. P., & Daniels, J. L. (2001a). Environmental contaminants as etiologic factors for diabetes. *Environmental Health Perspectives, 109*(Suppl. 6), 871–876.

Longnecker, M. P., & Daniels, J. L. (2001b). Environmental contaminants as etiologic factors for diabetes. *Environmental Health Perspectives, 109*(Suppl. 6), 871–876.

Powell, R. (2010). What's the harm? An evolutionary theoretical critique of the precautionary principle. *Kennedy Institute of Ethics Journal, 20*, 181–206.

Rauh, V. A., Landrigan, P. J., & Claudio, L. (2008). Housing and health: intersection of poverty and environmental exposures. *Annals of the New York Academy of Sciences, 1136*, 276–288.

Remillard, R. B., & Bunce, N. J. (2002). Linking dioxins to diabetes: Epidemiology and biologic plausibility. *Environmental Health Perspectives, 110*, 853–858.

Salehi, F., Turner, M. C., Phillips, K. P., Wigle, D. T., Krewski, D., & Aronson, K. J. (2008). Review of the etiology of breast cancer with special attention to organochlorines as potential endocrine disruptors. *Journal of Toxicology and Environmental Health B Critical Reviews, 11*, 276–300.

Sarafanov, A. G., Todorov, T. I., Centeno, J. A., Macias, V., Gao, W., Liang, W. M.,...Kajdacsy-Balla, A. A. (2011). Prostate cancer outcome and tissue levels of metal ions. *Prostate, 71*, 1231–1238.

Satcher, D., Fryer, G. E., Jr., McCann, J., Troutman, A., Woolf, S. H., & Rust, G. (2005). What if we were equal? A comparison of the Black-White mortality gap in 1960 and 2000. *Health Affairs (Millwood), 24*, 459–464.

Sexton, K., Linder, S. H., Marko, D., Bethel, H., & Lupo, P. J. (2007). Comparative assessment of air pollution-related health risks in Houston. *Environmental Health Perspectives, 115*, 1388–1393.

Silver, M. K., O'Neill, M. S., Sowers, M. R., & Park, S. K. (2011). Urinary bisphenol A and type-2 diabetes in U.S. adults: Data from NHANES 2003–2008. *PLoS One, 6*, e26868.

Smith, D. K. (1992). HIV disease as a cause of death for African Americans in 1987 and 1990. *Journal of the National Medical Association, 84*, 481–487.

Su, J. G., Morello-Frosch, R., Jesdale, B. M., Kyle, A. D., Shamasunder, B., & Jerrett, M. (2009). An index for assessing demographic inequalities in cumulative environmental hazards with application to Los Angeles, California. *Environmental Science & Technology, 43,* 7626–7634.

Tzivian, L. (2011). Outdoor air pollution and asthma in children. *Journal of Asthma, 48,* 470–481.

United Church of Christ Commission for Racial Justice. (1987). *Toxic wastes and race in the United States.* New York, NY: Author.

United States Department of Health and Human Services. (1985). *Report of the Secretary's Task Force on Black and Minority Health: Volume I: Executive summary.* Washington, DC: Author.

Warren, R., Lockett, H. C. J., & Zulfiqar, A. A. (2002). The social context for faith and health. In J. C. Chunn (Ed.), *The health behavioral change imperative: Theory, education, and practice in diverse populations* (pp. 127–151). New York, NY: Springer.

Warren-Findlow, J. (2006). Weathering: Stress and heart disease in African American women living in Chicago. *Qualitative Health Research, 16,* 221–237.

Weitzman, M., Gortmaker, S. L., Sobol, A. M., & Perrin, J. M. (1992). Recent trends in the prevalence and severity of childhood asthma. *Journal of the American Medical Association, 268,* 2673–2677.

Wolff, M. S., Berkowitz, G. S., Brower, S., Senie, R., Bleiweiss, I. J., Tartter, P., . . . Weston, A. (2000). Organochlorine exposures and breast cancer risk in New York City women. *Environmental Research, 84,* 151–161.

Wolff, M. S., Britton, J. A., & Wilson, V. P. (2003). Environmental risk factors for breast cancer among African-American women. *Cancer, 97,* 289–310.

Wong, G. W., Von, M. E., Douwes, J., & Pearce, N. (2006). Environmental determinants associated with the development of asthma in childhood. *International Journal of Tuberculosis and Lung Disease, 10,* 242–251.

World Health Organization. (2006). *Almost a quarter of all disease caused by environmental exposure* [Online]. Retrieved from http://www.who.int/quantifying_ehimpacts/publications/preventingdisease7.pdf

World Health Organization. (2012). *About World Health Organization* [Online]. Retrieved from http://www.who.int/about/definition/en/print.html

Zanobetti, A., Baccarelli, A., & Schwartz, J. (2011). Gene-air pollution interaction and cardiovascular disease: A review. *Progress in Cardiovascular Disease, 53,* 344–352.

Zhuo, X., Zhang, P., Gregg, E. W., Barker, L., Hoerger, T. J., Tony, P., & Albright A. (2012). A nationwide community-based lifestyle program could delay or prevent type 2 diabetes cases and save $5.7 billion in 25 years. *Health Affairs (Millwood), 31,* 50–60.

10

Using Conceptual Frameworks in Health Policymaking: A Guide for CEOD

Monica Taylor-Jones

LEARNING OBJECTIVES

What you can learn by studying this chapter:

- What public policy is
- What health policy/health care policy/public health policy are
- What the relationship between the social determinants of health (SDH) and health policy is
- How ordinary citizens can use the SDH to frame an issue for policy
- What steps are involved in the policymaking process
- How frameworks that focus on policy theory can guide ordinary citizens through the policy process
- How political theory can be used to guide ordinary citizens through the policy process
- How policy theories can help to frame health policies (or health care policies) aimed to impact the SDH and ultimately health disparities

Health inequities call for policy action, especially when the most vulnerable members in societies suffer the most. Historically, persons in the lower socioeconomic strata have been systematically burdened by morbidity and mortality across both chronic and infectious diseases (Hofrichter, 2003; Hofrichter & Bhatia, 2010). The causes for health inequities and health disparities have been linked to a dearth in critical resources particularly in low-income communities (Marmot, Friel, Bell, Houweling, & Taylor, 2008). These resources include the SDH and comprise education, income, employment, access to proper nutrition, transportation, racism and discrimination, access to clean water, access to medical care, sanitation, standard housing, insurance, and environmental conditions (Beltran, McDavid, Hall, & Dean, 2011; Braveman, 2011; Labonte & Schrecker, 2006; Marmot, 2005; World Health Organization [WHO], 2008).

Policy can play a critical role at eliminating health inequities by increasing access to the SDH (Exworthy, 2008; Navarro, 2009; Marmot et al., 2008). Policies that address the social, political, and environmental factors can impact the availability and distribution of the SDH (Exworthy, 2008).

Examples of such policies include (but are not limited to) zoning regulations to restrict the number of fast-food outlets in low-income communities, planning policies to increase walking and bike trails and decrease food deserts (Chen & Florax, 2010; Liburd, 2009), tax policies that favor lower income groups, health care reform to increase access to health care, or extending unemployment insurance, just to name a few (Bernstein, McNichol, & Lyons, 2006).

While these aforementioned policies are indeed considered a step in the right direction, the notion of engaging in the process of policy formation may seem intangible or an abstract concept for some. For instance, one may hold strong beliefs about a lack of smoking regulations in public spaces or about toxic dumping in one's community, but may not necessarily have knowledge on how to correct this injustice. However, it is important to note that it does not take an expert in the field of public policy to engage in the political process. Participants in the policy process do not require a formal education, training, certifications, or even experience. A suitable phrase that gets at the core of any advocacy effort in the pursuit for justice comes from Earl Knightingale, "All you need is the plan, the roadmap, and the courage to press on to your destination" (1921–1989). For this reason, this chapter offers a roadmap, from start to finish, on how to engage in the policy process. This chapter provides its readers with knowledge about what is involved in the policymaking process and is grounded in political theory that describes how policies are developed, adopted, and implemented into society. Regardless of its theoretical component, this chapter is written with the intent to be clear, user-friendly, and appealing to those who are nonsavvy to political jargon.

The approaches presented in this chapter are timely in that they offer guidance on how to embark upon a policy agenda that deals with the inequitable distribution of the SDH. This agenda, to use the SDH as a platform to address disparate health conditions, has been endorsed by the World Health Organization (2008) and has been implemented as goals and objectives for Healthy People 2020 (Sharpe, Harrison, & Dean, 2010). This recent movement considers policy as a pathway to alter health inequities (Marmot, 2005). This chapter offers insight on how ordinary citizens, communities, or coalitions can use a policy approach to address deficiencies in the SDH in order to ameliorate injustices in population health, be it political, systematic, or environmental. If the goals are to advocate for new policies, enforce policies that increase access to the SDH, or block policies that deprive communities of critical SDH, consider this chapter as a starting point.

First, this chapter discusses the fundamentals of public policy, health policy, the stakeholders involved in policymaking, the role of SDH on health disparities, and, finally, an example of how to use political theory to guide advocacy and policy efforts to formulate health policies that target the SDH.

WHAT IS PUBLIC POLICY?

How can ordinary citizens, communities, or coalitions begin to engage in public policy? First, some formal knowledge about public policy is required. Public policy consists of a set of rules made by governments to establish and regulate behaviors that are judged to be morally unacceptable (Theodoulou & Cahn, 1995). Public policies also include decisions made by governments to execute programs for the well-being of society (Cochran & Malone, 1995). Policies are then adopted to solve a social problem as a means to protect members of society (Dye, 2001). The policy is intended to be the solution to the social problem. If the government fails to act on a given social problem, this is still considered a policy decision (Dye, 2001).

Health policy is a form of public policy and centers on government actions intended to improve the health of its members (Longest, 2010). Health policies have been established to protect the health of society's most vulnerable individuals, including the elderly and the poor (Soldo & Agree, 1988). Parallel to public policies, health policies can be enacted at the federal, state, and local levels (Longest, 2010). Some examples of health policies include: the Patient Protection and Affordable Care Act of 2010 enacted to expand health insurance access to low-income citizens (P.L. 111–148); the Social Security Act of 1965 adopted to provide insurance to the elderly and persons with disabilities (P.L. 89–97); the Breast and Cervical Cancer Mortality Act of 1991 to provide access to breast and cervical cancer screening for underinsured women (P.L. 106–354); New York City's regulation to phase out artificial transfat from foods prepared in public food service establishments (111–203); and New Jersey's Smoke Free Air Act (2005, c383) to ban smoking in public spaces and the workplace (Henry J. Kaiser Family Foundation, 2011).

OFFICIAL AND UNOFFICIAL ACTORS

There are two types of participants involved in public policymaking: official and unofficial actors (Birkland, 2005). The *official actors* are participants who have legal authority to make laws (legislative branch); enforce, veto, or implement laws (Executive Branch); and interpret laws (Judicial Branch) (Birkland, 2005; Longest, 2010). These actors can also appropriate money toward social programs aimed to improve the welfare of society (Teitelbaum & Wilensky, 2007). The official actors are decision makers at the federal, state, and local levels and consist of the president, Congress, judges, mayors, cabinet officials, agency heads, commissioners, governors, and state and local legislatures (Birkland, 2005; Teitelbaum & Wilensky, 2007).

Unofficial actors do not have the legal authority to implement policies; however, they have the right to be involved in the policy process to protect their own interests (Birkland, 2005; Teitelbaum & Wilensky, 2007). Unofficial actors include ordinary citizens, special interest groups, advocacy groups, political parties, lobbyists, media, academics, consultants, researchers, or think tanks (Birkland, 2005; Coffman, Hendricks, Masters, & Williams Kaye, 2007; Dye, 2001; Kingdon, 2011; Theodoulou & Cahn, 1995). Interest groups can influence the policymaking process (Teitelbaum & Wilensky, 2007). They can use research that supports their position to frame a persuasive argument to the public, media, and politicians to garner support (Coffman et al., 2007; Malena, 2009; Smith, 2010). Unofficial actors can also engage in other promising advocacy strategies to garner support such as grassroots organizing, media advocacy, holding rallies and marches, developing alliances and partnerships with key constituents, or collaborating with organizations that support their cause (Coffman et al., 2007). Social movements have emerged and have been successful in the passage of significant legislation to support their interests. These include, policies to protect citizens from drunk drivers (MADD, Mothers Against Drunk Drivers) and lawsuits and policies against tobacco companies to protect citizens from secondhand smoke; and the Civil Rights Act (American Nonsmokers' Rights Foundation, 2010; Birkland, 2005; P.L. 88–352). Unofficial actors with common interests can work together to advance their policy goals and, at times, compete against one another (Birkland, 2005).

THE PROBLEM: HEALTH DISPARITIES AND THE SDH

Health disparities occur when there are differences in the health status of one group relative to another group (Kawachi, Daniels, & Robinson, 2005). Health disparities are salient when there are higher incidence rates of morbidity and mortality across diseases among comparable groups, often according to race/ethnicity or socioeconomic status (Kawachi et al., 2005; Williams & Sternthal, 2010). Health disparities between racial and ethnic groups and socioeconomic status have been pervasive and are often compared (House & Williams, 2003). The marked differences in health status are most salient between the health of wealthy groups compared to other income groups, especially the lower income strata (Kim, Millen, Irwin, & Gersham, 2000; Marmot, 2005; Navarro, 2000). More specifically, higher income groups (including racial and ethnic groups) experience better health outcomes relative to lower income populations (House & Williams, 2003; Kim et al., 2000). Lower income groups experience lower life expectancy and higher morbidity rates across various diseases, including cancer, diabetes, and heart disease (House & Williams, 2003; Kim et al., 2000; Navarro, 2000). Health disparities among these groups widened during periods of economic gains in the United States, especially during the Bush eras (Bernstein et al., 2006; House & Williams, 2003). Health disparities are attributed to the rise in the number of uninsured Americans during this period, which grew from 38.7 million in 2000 to 46.3 million in 2008 (U.S. Census Bureau, 2000, 2008). The increase in the number of the uninsured population parallel the rising costs of health care premiums, which rose to nearly 80% during the Bush eras (Kaiser Family Foundation, 2001).

According to Raphael (2003), the SDH impacts whether people "stay healthy or become ill." To achieve equity in health outcomes for the most vulnerable populations requires an equitable distribution of the SDH (Daniels, Kennedy, & Kawachi, 1999). This requires action, particularly through political and economic policies to inherently make these resources more accessible (Labonte & Schrecker, 2006; WHO, 2008). Prior to public health's attention to the need to address the SDH through effective policies, much of the discourse on public health focused on individual risk factors and programs that aimed to promote behavior change (Valente & Pumpuang, 2007). Health policies have also evolved. Historically, the impetus for health policies concentrated on financing medical treatments to improve population health (McGinnis, Williams-Russo, & Knickman, 2002). However, health care costs, particularly in the United States, have not resulted in the most favorable health outcomes (Rampbell, 2009). United States, spending on health care ranks highest compared to other wealthier nations, but the United States still has the worst health outcomes (Rampbell, 2009). Concomitantly, behavior change promotions have not resulted in sustainable change or lessened health disparities (Hofrichter, 2003).

Political, economic, and social forces have perpetuated conditions that systematically limited access to the SDH in the physical environment, especially in disenfranchised communities (Bell & Standish, 2010; Labonte & Schrecker, 2006; Raphael, 2008; Wilkinson & Marmot, 2006; WHO, 2008). Historically, civic engagement has been absent and the needs of individuals in disenfranchised communities have not been represented in the political process (Hofrichter, 2003). To achieve health equity calls for a political and economic policy commitment to invest in public expenditures that protect the basic needs and public services of its citizens, which requires the availability of the SDH. WHO's commission on the SDH (2008) concluded that: "(The) toxic combination of bad policies, economics, and politics is, in large measure responsible for the fact that a majority of people in the world do not enjoy the good health that is biologically possible." Given this, political theories are discussed to provide guidance on how to develop, block, or enforce effective health policies that aim to eliminate the problem of health disparities based on a dearth in the SDH. Examples are provided to demonstrate how to integrate the political theory, the SDH, and health disparities in the pursuit for optimal population health, regardless of race or income status.

THE POLICY PROCESS: INTRODUCTION TO POLITICAL THEORIES

Political theories or conceptual frameworks are assumptions that offer a rationale for understanding the components that are instrumental in the policymaking process (Sabatier, 2007). The Stages Heuristics Model was one of the initial and the most prominent framework that emerged in the 1970s and 1980s to guide our knowledge on what occurs during the policymaking process (Jann & Wegrichand, 2007; May & Wildavsky, 1978). The Stages Heuristic Model separated the policy process into distinct stages to describe events that occurred during policymaking. These stages include issue definition, agenda setting, formulation, adoption, implementation, and evaluation. In the issue identification stage, a social issue is perceived as problematic by the public or the media (Jann & Wegrichand, 2007). When the issue grasps the attention of policy makers, then it is in the agenda-setting stage (Kingdon, 2011). As the issue gains more serious attention by policy makers, it rises to a higher level on the political agenda into the policy-formulation stage where a special committee considers the issue to be adopted into public policy (Jann & Wegrichand, 2007; Longest, 2010; Theodoulou & Cahn, 1995). The issue is then enacted and implemented into society by an assigned government agency (Jann & Wegrichand, 2007). Policy outcomes are then evaluated to determine if the goals of policy were met, especially by the target population (Jann & Wegrichand, 2007; Theodoulou & Cahn, 1995). During this stage, a policy can be terminated or the cycle (of the Stages Heuristics Model) may begin again if a new problem was identified and the policy has to be modified (Theodoulou & Cahn, 1995).

Scientists have contributed substantive research on various stages within the heuristics framework (Dery, 1984; Kingdon, 2011; Longest, 2010; Van Meter & Van Horn, 1975). This framework provided valuable insight into a complex process. However, it has also been noted for its inaccuracies including assumptions that the policymaking process was oversimplified, occurs linearly, is absent of explanations on how each stage progresses sequentially and for its concentration solely on policy enactment (Jann & Wegrichand, 2007; Sabatier, 2007).

Additional frameworks of the policy process have emerged to respond to the critiques of the Stages Heuristic Model (Birkland, 2005; Boushey, 2010; Jann & Wegrichand, 2007; Kingdon, 2011; Nakamura, 1987; Sabatier, 2007; Sabatier & Jenkins-Smith, 1993). These frameworks include (but are not limited to): Three Streams Approach, Advocacy Coalition Framework (ACF), Punctuated Equilibrium Theory, Institutional Rational Choice, Policy Diffusion Framework, and Network Models (Boushey, 2010; Jann & Wegrichand, 2007; Kingdon, 2011; Nakamura, 1987; Sabatier, 1991, 2007; Sabatier & Jenkins-Smith, 1993; True, Jones, & Baumgartner, 2007). These frameworks have advanced the discourse on understanding the policy process beyond the Stages Heuristic Model and considers that policy change can: occur incrementally, take 10 years before laws are passed, accounts for additional influences that may obstruct or delay the policy process such as political or economic factors, or takes into account the influential behaviors of actors and unofficial actors (Schlager & Blomquist, 1996).

The utility of political theory is emphasized and serves as a point of reference for laypersons who want to engage in the decision-making process. Given the range and scope of conceptual frameworks in the policy discourse, this chapter will discuss only one theory, Kingdon's Three Streams Approach, not to discount the others. The Three Streams Approach lends its focus to understanding why some public problems emerge to ultimately gain the attention of policy makers where laws are formulated to solve the problem, while other problems evolve and policy makers choose not to be responsive to those problems (Kingdon, 2011). Kingdon's framework is presented as a case study to explain the processes involved in policymaking in the context of a specific health disparity and how to incorporate critical resources in the process to improve population health.

This chapter uses Kingdon's conceptual frameworks to demonstrate how to propose, adopt, or enforce policies that address the unequal distribution of the SDH. Given the impact of the SDH on health disparities, and Kingdon's theories on how problems gain the attention of policy makers, this chapter (1) identifies components of the Three Streams Approach, (2) applies the framework to a health disparity: diabetes, (3) includes select SDH that impact diabetes, and (4) provides examples of the type of health policies that can be developed that incorporate the SDH and applies Kingdon's theory (Exworthy, 2008). The goals are to provide a step-by-step process that would facilitate strategic thinking and appropriate planning for engaging in policy or advocacy-related activities.

CONCEPTUAL FRAMEWORKS: THREE STREAMS APPROACH

Kingdon (2011) proposed three variables in his Three Streams Approach to describe the policy process: the problem, policy, and political streams. This framework centers on how a social problem, such as health disparities, reaches the agenda-setting stage where policy makers are paying attention to the issue. According to Kingdon (2011), the *problem stream* consists of various social problems that unofficial actors want policy makers to consider and to formulate a solution to the problem. It is critical to increase awareness to the public and to policy makers on a particular issue, especially since one's perception of what is considered an issue for policy makers may not be shared by others (Kingdon, 2011; Theodoulou & Cahn, 1995). For instance, the need to pass a National Health Insurance Program has been the subject of debate throughout many Administrations (Blumenthal & Morone, 2010). Some perceive the uninsured problem as a matter of health and human rights that require government intervention, while others do not perceive it as a right, rather a social good that can be bought and sold in the health care market (Kingdon, 2011).

Policy communities consist of bureaucrats, academicians, researchers, or congressional staff, and they emerge in Kingdon's *policy stream*. These communities have a collective interest in a particular social problem, however, their positions on how to resolve the problem may differ. Hence, participants of policy communities compete against one another and develop persuasive policy proposals to have their solution to the problem gain the attention of policy makers (Kingdon, 2011; Smith, 2010). The policy proposals that have viable solutions and are perceived by policy makers as technically feasible are the ones that progress to policy enactment (Kingdon, 2011).

The *political stream* represents the national mood, which reflects how the nation as a whole perceives the significance of solving a particular social problem. The political mood also includes any changes in Administration that can influence the political agenda, mainly what issues are considered a higher priority to policy makers relative to others (Kingdon, 2011). A change in a political administration in Congress or the presidential office influences whether or not a problem advances on the policy makers' agenda (Kingdon, 2011). A newly elected Congress or administration may oppose the philosophies of a former administration. Under the new administration, new issues may be advanced and/or old issues may fall off the agenda (Kingdon, 2011; Theodoulou & Cahn, 1995). For instance, some administrations may consider investments in domestic programs a higher priority compared to other administrations. Take, again for example, the problem of the uninsured. By 2009, it became clearer to the nation and policy makers that the perceived issue of the uninsured was a problem and there was urgency from the Obama administration to formulate a remedy to this problem. The uninsured has been problematic for decades and expanding public insurance to solve this problem has gained the attention of many presidents prior to the Obama administration (Blumenthal & Morone, 2010). There were administrations that made the political decision not to do anything about this problem (Blumenthal & Morone, 2010). Ultimately, the politics were favorable, and the Affordable Care Act of 2010, passed under the Obama Administration, expanded access to health care for persons within a specific (low) income status (Kingdon, 2011).

The national mood may substantiate why policy makers would increase (or decrease) their attention to a social problem based on how the nation collectively perceives the problem. Public opinion surveys inform policy makers how the nation may collectively regard a particular problem (Sabatier, 2007). An example would be opinion polls that monitor the nation's perceptions on the practicality of the Health Care Reform Bill to solve the problem of the uninsured (Henry J. Kaiser Family Foundation, 2011).

According to Kingdon (2011), the three streams flow independently until they meet at a critical point, and this affords the opportunity for problems to be adopted into a policy. These opportunities are short lived and do not occur often. They may be stimulated by political events such

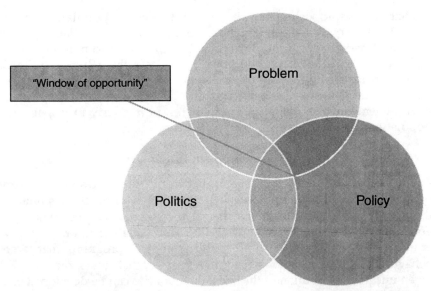

FIGURE 10.1   Venn diagram of Kingdon's Three Streams Approach that also reflects the small "window of opportunity" when a policy can be adopted.

as a change in administration or Congress or by a change in how insistent the public (national mood) is about the government responding to a particular problem. Figure 10.1 depicts a Venn diagram of the components in Kingdon's framework and a small "policy window" (2011, p. 165) available for policies to be enacted into law.

Case Study Exercises

Individually, or as a group, review the following case study and respond to the questions posed at the end of the study, as appropriate. Be sure to focus on the why, how, and what emphasized in each question. Your professor/instructor will provide you specific guidance on how you are to report your findings for the class.

Case Study 10.1: Diabetes: Three Streams Approach in Health Policymaking

Kingdon's framework can be used as a guide to assist stakeholders who plan to engage in the policymaking process to address a health disparity. The example below provides a step-by-step process on how Kingdon's theory can be used to block, enforce, or create policies that address the SDH for the elimination of disparities in diabetes prevalence. The steps described in this example are not prescriptive, such that they do not have to be performed sequentially and, to some degree, can be done simultaneously, depending on capacity. The SDH, access to resources, is used in this example.

Diabetes disproportionately impacts low-income populations (Rabi et al., 2006). Experts suggest that individual risk factors for diabetes, such as unhealthy diets, play a dominant role in morbidity and mortality rates, and interventions have been designed to address this (Ruggiero, 2000). Other experts attribute disparities associated with diabetes to the built environment. These experts believe that the social, economic, and physical environment impacts disparities in diabetes, particularly in low-income populations (Chen & Florax, 2010).

Step 1: Problem Stream

The first step is to frame the issue of diabetes in such a way as to justify why policy makers should intervene. If the problem of diabetes is built on the concept of individual behavior change, then there would be no need for government intervention. There would be a pressing desire only for governments and nonprofits to fund health-promotion programs that target behavior change strategies. However, if the issue of diabetes is framed based on an unequal distribution in the SDH, then policies can be developed centered on the concept of health equity. There are advocacy strategies that can be employed in the *problem stream* to convince both official and unofficial actors of the reasons why this problem persists in the context of the SDH. Quantitative statistics help to exemplify the magnitude of this problem— portraying morbidity and mortality rates in a given community framed around the scarcity in the SDH. The Composite Logic Model offers strategies on how to disseminate this information and includes: engaging the media (press releases), electronic outreach, grassroots organizing, educating policy makers, developing culturally sensitive brochures, public service announcements, or conducting presentations in key venues, such as community colleges, faith-based organizations, or nonprofit organizations (Figure 10.2).

Step 2: Conduct Your Research!

While this step is not a part of Kingdon's three streams, it is indeed a critical step that can inform your advocacy or policy approach. A policy assessment includes research on specific policies in a given locale, state, or nation. A policy assessment helps to determine if there are any policies associated with diabetes or select SDH that are on the policy makers' agenda, if any have been adopted as law or have been fully implemented into a program and accessible to its target population. Some examples of health policies that are associated with diabetes and the SDH may include, but are not limited to, the following:

- Zoning and planning policies that
  - Restrict fast-food outlets
  - Support incentivizing businesses to open grocers in low-income neighborhoods
  - Fund for police presence in unsafe neighborhoods

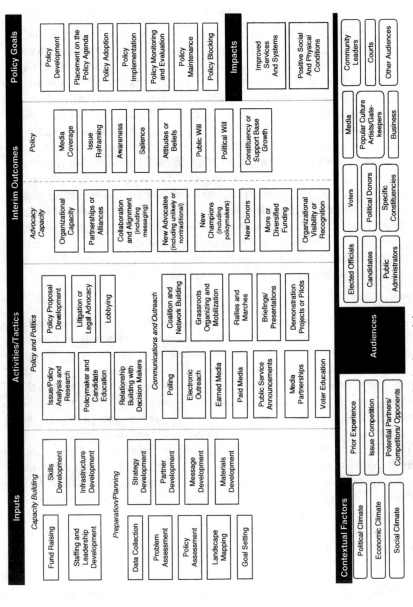

FIGURE 10.2   J. Coffman's composite logic model.
Source: Coffman, J. Advocacy and Policy Change Composite Logic Model. Reprinted with permission.

- Schools: regulations on balanced, nutritious meals
- Vending machine regulations in schools and workplaces
- Spaces for physical activity including bicycles and walking trails

Step 3: Policy Stream

After conducting the appropriate research, policy goals can be established for Kingdon's *policy stream*. Do you need to develop a new policy? Should you block an existing policy that would restrict access to the SDH? Will you aim to enforce an existing policy that supports the resources necessary to eliminate disparities in diabetes? Given the determined policy approach, proposals are developed to communicate with policy makers about a solution to the problem. The goal of policy proposals is to gain the attention of policy makers, such that the solution proposed advances on their agenda and is adopted into a law. Smith's (2010) book, *Writing Public Policy: A Practical Guide to Communicating in the Policy Making Process*, offers insight on how to write a policy proposal. Policy proposals should clearly and concisely state the issue for policy makers, an explanation of why a proposed solution to the problem is more feasible relative to other competing proposals, demonstrate the use of a political theory, and include credible resources. In the past, policy makers have responded to policy proposals that incorporated conceptual frameworks.

Politics Stream

How does the nation perceive the problem? Additional research on how the public and policy makers perceive the causes for diabetes is essential. Using public opinion polls or administrating surveys are ways to ascertain information. Key organizations associated with your cause state their position about causes for diabetes on their websites. Partnering with these organizations, including the populations most affected by the problem, to engage in policy action can strengthen your case to policy makers. Interviews with policy makers to understand their position is essential. This provides an opportunity to educate policy makers about the ways in which disparities in diabetes are associated with the SDH, with the intent to obtain their political support to champion your cause to their fellow constituents. It may be the case that the current administration does not support increasing resources for public programs to enhance the built environment due to the economic climate. Another alternative is perhaps to wait for a new administration that will soon take over and that would be more supportive of this issue.

Step 5: The GPS: Navigating the Policymaking Process

Using the Three Streams approach, select SDH and diabetes as an example, a plan of action can be constructed to serve as a guide (see Figures 10.3 and 10.4).

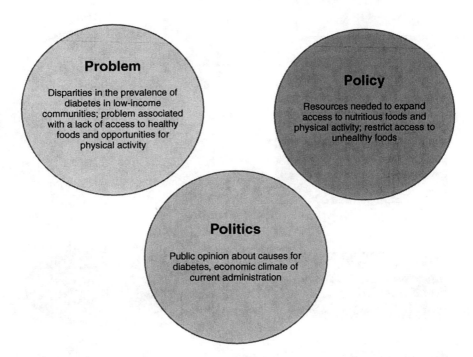

FIGURE 10.3   The utility of the Three Streams framework to address the issue of diabetes.

Study Questions

1. Consider Kingdon's problem stream and choose a health disparity.
2. How would you frame the problem of your selected health disparity?
3. What role does the SDH play in the problem of health disparities?
4. Does the problem warrant the attention of policy makers?
5. Does the issue need to be reframed in order to attain the attention of the public and policy makers?
6. What types of advocacy strategies would you consider to gain the attention of the general public, your target population, or policy makers?
7. Are there any policy proposals comparable to your policy goals?
8. What types of policies, systems, or environmental approaches currently exist that support or promote healthier environments?
9. What is your policy approach?
10. Will you need to develop new policies, block an existing policy, or enforce a policy?
11. Consider Kingdon's policy stream.
12. Describe the type of policy communities that would most likely support your cause.

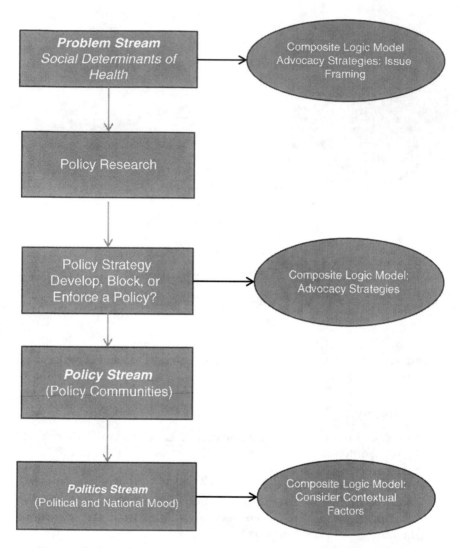

FIGURE 10.4   Framework (GPS) for integrating political theory (Kingdon), SDH, advocacy strategies, and policy research to promote policy change.

13. Are there any stakeholders that support your position, but oppose your solution to the problem?
14. What is the national mood's perception of health equity?
15. Is the national mood (your state or community) amenable to understanding how the SDH is associated with incidence, prevalence, morbidity, or mortality rates of the health disparity you selected?
16. What types of evidence can you ascertain to support this?

17. Does the current administration support environmental policies and programs that redistribute resources to create healthier
environments?

REFERENCES

American Nonsmokers' Rights Foundation. (2010). *Summary of 100% smokefree state laws and population protected by 100% U.S. smokefree laws.* Retrieved November 12, 2010, from www.no-smoke.org/pdf/SummaryUSPopList.pdf

Bell, J., & Standish, M. (2010). Building healthy communities through equitable food access. *Community Development Investment Review, 5*(3), 75–85.

Beltran, V. M., McDavid, H. K., Hall, H. I., & Dean, H. D. (2011). Collection of social determinant of health measures in U.S. national surveillance systems for HIV, viral hepatitis, STDs, and TB. *Public Health Reports, 126*(Suppl. 3), 41–53.

Bernstein, J., McNichol, E., & Lyons, S.K. (2006, January). *Pulling apart. A state by state analysis of income trends, State Fact Sheet.* Center for Budget and Public Priorities and Economic Policy Institute. Retrieved February 2007, from www.cbpp.org/1-26-06sfp-states.htm

Birkland, T. A. (2005). *An introduction to the policy process: Theories, concepts, and models of public policy making* (2nd Ed.). Armonk, NY: M.E. Sharpe.

Blumenthal, D., & Morone, J. (2010). *The heart of power: Health and politics in the Oval Office.* London, England: University of California Press.

Boushey, G. (2010). *Policy diffusion dynamics in America.* Cambridge: Cambridge University Press.

Braveman, P. (2011). Accumulating knowledge on the social determinants of health and infectious disease. *Public Health Reports, 3*(126), 28–30.

Chen, S., & Florax, R. (2010). Zoning for health: The obesity epidemic and opportunities for local policy intervention. *Journal of Nutrition, 140,* 1181–1184.

Cochran, C., & Malone, E. F. (1995). *Public policy: Perspectives and choices.* New York, NY: McGraw Hill.

Coffman, J., Hendricks, A., Masters, B., & Williams Kaye, J. (2009). The composite logic model. Retrieved on October 2009, from http://www.planning.continuousprogress.org

Commission on the Social Determinants of Health. (2008). *Closing the gap in a generation: Health equity through action on the social determinants of health.* Final Report of the Commission on Social Determinants of Health. Geneva: World Health Organization.

Daniels, N., Kennedy, B. P., & Kawachi, I. (1999). Why justice is good for our health: The social determinants of health inequalities. *Daedalus, 128*(4), 215–251.

Dery, D. (1984). *Problem definition in policy analysis.* Lawrence, KS: University Press of Kansas.

Dye, T. (2001). *Top down policymaking.* New York, NY: Seven Bridges Press.

Exworthy, M. (2008). Policy to tackle the social determinants of health: Using conceptual models to understand the policy process. *Health Policy and Planning, 23,* 318–327.

Henry J. Kaiser Family Foundation. (2011, January). *Kaiser public opinion. The public, health care reform and views on repeal.* Retrieved January 2012, from www.kff.org/healthreform/upload/8131.pdf

Hofrichter, R. (2003). The politics of health inequities. In R. Hofrichter (Ed.), *Health and social justice: Politics, ideology, and inequity in the distribution of disease* (pp. 59–88). San Francisco, CA: Josey Bass.

Hofrichter, R., & Bhatia, R. (2010). *Tackling health inequities through public health practice: Theory to action* (2nd Ed). New York, NY: Oxford University Press.

House, J. S., & Williams, D. R. (2003). Understanding and reducing socioeconomic and racial/ethnic disparities in health. In R. Hofrichter (Ed.), *Health and social justice: Politics, ideology, and inequity in the distribution of disease* (pp. 59–88). San Francisco, CA: Josey Bass.

Jann, W., & Wegrichand, K. (2007). Theories of the policy cycle. In F. Fischer (Ed.), *Handbook of public policy analysis: Theory, politics, and methods.* Boca Raton, FL: Taylor & Francis Group.

Kaiser Family Foundation. (2001). *Employer Health Benefits Survey Report.*

Kawachi, I., Daniels, N., & Robinson, D. E. (2005). Health disparities by race and class: Why both matter. *Health Affairs, 24*(2), 343–352.

Kim, J. Y., Millen, J. V., Irwin, A., & Gersham, J. (Eds.). (2000). Introduction. What is growing? Who is dying? In *Dying for growth: Global inequality and the health of the poor* (pp. 3–10). Monroe, ME: Common Courage Press.

Kingdon, J. (2011). *Agendas, alternatives and public policies* (2nd Ed). Glenview, IL: Addison-Wesley Educational Publishers.

Labonte, R., & Schrecker, T. (2006). *Globalization and social determinants of health: Analytic and strategic review paper.* Ottawa, ON: Globalization Knowledge Network.

Liburd, L. (2009). *Diabetes and health disparities: Community based approaches for racial and ethnic populations.* New York, NY: Springer Publishing.

Longest, B. (2010). *Health policymaking in the United States* (5th ed.). Chicago, IL: Foundation of the American Colleges of Healthcare Executives.

Malena, C. (2009). *From political will to political won't: Building support for participatory governance.* Sterling, VA: Kumarian Press.

Marmot, M. (2005). Social determinants of health inequalities. *Lancet, 365,* 1099–1104.

Marmot, M., Freil, S., Bell, R., Houweling, T., & Taylor, S. (2008). Closing the gap in a generation: Health equity through action on the social determinants of health. *The Lancet, 372*(9650), 1661–1669.

May, J., & Wildavsky, A. (1978). *The policy cycle.* Beverly Hills, CA: Sage Publications.

McGinnis, J. M., Williams-Russo, P., & Knickman, J. (2002). The case for more active policy attention to health promotion. *Health Affairs, 21*(2), 78–93.

Nakamura, R. (1987). The textbook policy process and implementation research. *Policy Studies Journal, 7*(1), 142–154.

Navarro, V. (2000). *The political economy of social inequalities: Consequences for health and quality of life.* Policy, Politics, Health, and Medicine Series. New York, NY: Baywood Publishing.

Navarro, V. (2009). What we mean by the social determinants of health. *International Journal of Health Services, 39*(3), 423–441.

Rampbell, C. (2009). U.S. Health Spending From the Pack. *The New York Times*. Retrieved January 2012, from http//:economix.blogs.nytimes.com/2009/07/08us-health-spending-breaks-from-the-pack

Raphael, D. (2003). A society in decline: The political, economic and social determinants of health inequalities in the United States. In R. Hofrichter (Ed.), *Health and social justice: Politics, ideology, and inequity in the distribution of disease* (pp. 59–88). San Francisco, CA: Josey Bass.

Raphael, D. (2008). Introduction to the social determinants of health. In D. Raphael (Ed.), *Social determinants of health: Canadian perspectives* (2nd ed., pp. 2–19). Toronto, ON: Canadian Scholars' Press.

Ruggiero, L. (2000). Helping people with diabetes change behavior: From theory to practice. *Diabetes Spectrum, 13*(3), 125.

Sabatier, J. A., & Jenkins-Smith, H. C. (1993). *Policy change and learning: An advocacy coalition approach.* Washington, DC: Westview Press.

Sabatier, P. (1991). Toward better theories of the policy process. *PS: Political Science and Politics, 24*(2), 147–156.

Sabatier, P. A. (2007). *Theories of the policy process* (2nd ed.). Boulder, CO: Westview Press.

Schlager, E., & Blomquist, W. (1996). A comparison of three emerging theories of the policy process. *Political Research Quarterly, 49*(3), 651–672.

Sharpe, T., Harrison, K., & Dean, H. (2010). Summary of CDC consultation to address social determinants of health for prevention of disparities in HIV/AIDS, viral hepatitis, sexually transmitted diseases, and tuberculosis. *Public Health Reports, 125*(4), 11–15.

Smith, C. (2010). *Writing public policy: A practical guide to communicating in the policy making process.* New York, NY: Oxford University Press.

Soldo, B. J., & Agree, E. M. (1988). America's elderly. *Population Bulletin, 43*(3), 1–53.

Stachowiak, S. (2007). *Pathways for change: Six theories about how policy change happens.* Seattle, WA: Organization Research Services.

Teitelbaum, J., & Wilensky, S. (2007). *Essentials of health policy and law.* Sadbury, MA: Jones and Bartlett Learning.

Theodoulou, S., & Cahn, M. (1995). *Public policy: The essential readings.* Upper Saddle River, NJ: Prentice Hall.

True, J. L., Jones, B. D., & Baumgartner, F. R. (2007). Punctuated-equilibrium theory: Explaining stability and change in public policymaking. In P. A. Sabatier (Ed.), *Theories of the policy process* (2nd ed., pp. 155–187). Boulder, CO: Westview Press.

United States Census Bureau. (2000). Retrieved from www.census.gov

Unites States Census Bureau. (2008). Retrieved from www.census.gov

Valente, T., & Pumpuang, P. (2007). Identifying opinion leaders to promote behavior change. *Health Education & Behavior, 34*(6), 881–896.

Van Meter, D., & Van Horn, C. (1975). The policy implementation process: A conceptual framework. *Administration and Society, 6*(4), 445–488.

Wilkinson, R., & Marmot, M. (2006). *Social determinants of health: The solid facts.* New York, NY: Oxford University Press.

Williams, D., & Sternthal, M. (2010). Understanding racial and ethnic disparities in health. *Journal of Health and Social Behavior, 51*(1), S15–S27.

11

Advancing Health Equity Through Public Health Policies

Noble Maseru

When Inequality is too great the idea of community cannot be realized.

Anonymous

LEARNING OBJECTIVES

What you can learn by studying this chapter:

- To identify broad social conditions (determinants)
- To identify effective primary prevention, addressing root causes
- How to define the meaning of formulating health disparity policy
- How decision makers influence resource allocation
- How public health practice is a discipline that requires recognition of the social context
- The use of Infant Vitality Surveillance Network (IVSN) as an effective application
- How to use a health equity lens in developing reproductive health policy
- How to involve policy formulation and evaluation
- To define health equity and structural social relations

Social justice is a core value of public health. One of public health's programmatic responsibilities is to provide preventive and primary health care services to poor, dependent, and high-risk populations. Local health agencies in urban settings are compelled to address variables such as income, occupational shifts, education, socioeconomic status, population heterogeneity, poverty, lack of access to transportation, safe affordable housing, nutritious foods, safe space, and other measures that affect population health. These variables have in some cases resulted in a disproportionate burden of disease and premature death for certain populations.

This chapter assesses the importance of health equity and how it can be achieved through public health policies and the practice of public health.

It recognizes the social determinants of health variables, which have an inordinate affect on poor and vulnerable populations such as children, pregnant women, infants, and the elderly. In addition to income, education, race, gender, sexual orientation, and ethnicity, geographic location is also a variable that should be considered, particularly for rural locations and some urban communities.

The policy examples we use in this chapter are taken from our experience with the Cincinnati Health Department (CHD). The City of CHD was established in 1826 and has been providing services as a public health agency chartered by the State of Ohio since 1871. The overall role of the CHD is to prevent disease and injury, promote health, and protect the environment. This is accomplished through partnerships with schools, hospitals, community health centers, health insurers, community action agencies, businesses, the faith community, health and human services stakeholder organizations, and other community-based groups to improve the Cincinnatians' quality of life and well-being.

In the chapter case studies, we examine policies related to infant vitality (maternal and reproductive health; Cook, Dickens, & Fathalla, 2003) and assessment. Evidence is offered demonstrating that improved infant survival and improved maternal and child health can be achieved through health policy that is prevention-oriented, and driven by interventions that are mostly outside the health care setting. Vitality is assessed by indicators of health, well-being, and mortality through the development and application of an IVSN data component that tracks inputs (deliveries) and birth outcomes (low birth weight, prematurity, and infant mortality). The IVSN and Maternal Health Improvement Initiative is a strategic partnership between the university hospital (UH) and the CHD. The UH is the nation's first teaching hospital; its mission includes providing care to the indigent. The UH is affiliated with the University of Cincinnati College of Medicine and Academic Health Center.

The results from our CHD program outcomes demonstrate that corrective public health policy that addresses *upstream* issues relevant to specific populations, using a health equity lens, and applying public health interventions can reduce the disparity that exists between advantaged and disadvantaged populations (Mays & Smith, 2011).

In this regard, consequent issues affecting the formulation of CHD public health policy and attendant utilization of health services by client populations, such as the rationale influencing health decisions, are incorporated in the discussion. Within that context, we will attempt to answer three questions regarding infant vitality and reproductive health policy in a public health setting (Sagar & Paul, 1983):

1. Are there differences in health outcomes by a CHD reproductive health subpopulation and the City of Cincinnati over all?

2. If yes, or conversely no, what type of action is needed by decision makers in a public health policy context to solve the dilemma?
3. What are the factors and rationales influencing health services delivery-intervention decisions that determine infant vitality and reproductive health policy affecting the public health and nonpublic health client populations?

Health inequity elimination strategies are cored around "systems change" and collaboration. The chapter concludes that equity in health is and/or can be achieved through the provision of public health policies that:

- Take into account the social context
- Offer core safety net services and multisector strategic collaboration
- Monitor and measure results with accountability
- Include clients in policy formulation and evaluation

BACKGROUND

Currently, largely due to Title XIX of the Social Security Act (Medicaid) and Title VI of the 1964 Civil Rights Act (PL 88–164 and PL 93–641), health services have become more available to the poor (Kane, Kasteler, & Gray, 1985). Nevertheless, the problem of infant mortality differentials remains formidable. There is considerable evidence that socioeconomic, racial, and ethnic factors are associated with gaps in reproductive health outcomes (low birth weight, prematurity, and infant survival). Studies also have shown that maternal and infant health services are less available to ethnic and low-income populations than to middle-income and upper-income communities; furthermore, the inequity is heightened by the underutilization of reproductive health services by the respective communities. Evidence also suggests that differential mortality rates have a singular statistically significant correlation with race and income (Kitagawa & Hauser, 1973).

DESCRIPTION OF THE PROBLEM

As stated above, this chapter examines the concomitant variables that impact reproductive health outcomes for infant vitality (infant mortality, prematurity, and low birth weight). It is generally accepted that infant mortality, the number of babies that die before their first birthday, is one of the most sensitive indicators of the overall health of a community.

With the lowering of financial and structural barriers to care through the institution of Medicaid Title VI, greater access to care was expected.

However, despite these measures, many of the poor still continue to experience barriers to care and, moreover, their utilization of services relative to actual need for care is still much less than middle- and upper-income communities (Aday, 1975). Unfortunately, much of the information and conclusions derived about the poor are made in contrast to economically advantaged populations. Hence, inferences do not genuinely reflect what is occurring in the populations that public health is mandated to serve.

The CHD has made inroads in the area of maternal health improvement and infant vitality. Historically (as will be described later in this chapter), infant mortality rates (IMRs) have been higher in certain racial and ethnic populations compared to the Caucasian population. There exists not only racial but also income disparity, particularly among those without health insurance or who live in poverty.

An analysis of birth outcomes to Cincinnati–Hamilton County Special Supplemental Nutrition Program for Women, Infants, and Children (WIC) clients from 2005 to 2007, revealed an IMR of 8.8 deaths/1,000 live births (Cincinnati is the largest city in the Hamilton County jurisdiction). Moreover, the county-wide intervention yielded a 9.6 IMR among African Americans in WIC compared to 21.0 for non-WIC users. The CHD-authored research published in the *American Journal of Public Health* (Khanani, Elam, Hearn, Jones, & Maseru, 2010), further demonstrates the effectiveness of public health intervention and innovative CHD health equity-oriented administered programs. The CHD/WIC program improved the birth outcomes of disadvantaged and low-income mothers.

In 2002 to 2004, there were 16,113 live births in Cincinnati. About 52.6% of these were to African American mothers. The Cincinnati IMR was 13.2 deaths per 1,000 live births for 2002 to 2004; the African American IMR of 15.6—nearly 2.5 times the White rate of 6.3—represented an unacceptable racial disparity in outcomes. The years of 2004 to 2007 saw the highest number of infant deaths annually in Hamilton County since data collection began by the Hamilton County Child Fatality Review Team (CFRT). The CFRT identified preterm birth as the major contributor to this high IMR. The second most common contributing factor identified was infant sleeping arrangements (March of Dimes, 2009).

THE ROLE OF PUBLIC HEALTH POLICY

The chapter is concerned not only with determining if there is inequity and disparity in use of public health care services by client subpopulations, but also what can be done with regard to policy to correct the dilemma—achieving health equity. Thus, the examination does not limit itself to determinations of disparities in health status and access to care that exists in a public health setting but, additionally, finds it equally important to identify problems in the decision-making equation responsible for health policy. Of course, it must be stated that not all program ineffectiveness is attributable to inappropriate policy. However, generally speaking, if there are sweeping and comprehensive patterns of disparity, then perhaps problem origin can be attributed to inappropriate policy.

Second, contrary to much of what the literature suggests, decision making and solutions to problems in public health are not simply managerial and technical. Not all problems can be reduced to managerial solutions unfettered by biased and special interest group persuasiveness. There is an increasing notion that decision making in public service at the managerial level is largely a neutral and valueless exercise. It is believed that because public service agencies are removed from the competitive arena, policy makers are not prone to competitive incentives and motivations that influence decision making in the private sector; instead the decisions are "un-ideological" (Goodnow, 1900). Epitomizing this value-neutral application in health are mathematical theorems that McNeil (1975) advocates, which "... can be applied to a wide range of clinical decisions involving individual patients to matters of public-health policy." Quite the contrary, as Kaufman (2007) states: "Public health is not passive observational... the focus of the field is on interventions and policy choices that improve the health of populations."

Third, there are some who subscribe to the notion that "... ours is a conflictive society with a daily battle of ideologies" (Amin, 1974). To arrive at conclusions in absence of examining the dynamics responsible for policy would be a partial examination of the total equation, limited to assessing the performance of health service areas and not that of the public health agency. Therefore, it is incumbent upon us to be cognizant of decision making among reproductive health policy makers and deliverers of prenatal care services. Succinctly stated, *public health practitioners' role in policy formulation is instrumental in affecting the distribution of resources that can diminish health inequities.* James Colgrove argues that a population's ability to benefit health improvement is shaped by resources allocated to society. Bruce Link and Jo Phelan's commentary on the influence social conditions have on population health states: "People who command more of these resources are able to gain a health advantage—that is, to benefit from the fruits of 'human agency for public health'; social conditions are not independent of the human agency" (Colgrove, 2002). The human agency is represented by policy makers, bureaucrats, and practitioners. The vital role that public health practitioners can play in eliminating health inequities is also recognized by Tony Iton. He writes: "Despite the apparently high priority that the elimination of health disparities receives in the public pronouncements of our nation's federal public health leaders, the public health strategies and practices that would operate to eliminate health disparities appear to be lacking" (Iton, 2008). Having a responsive public health practice possessing a health equity frame of reference is a corollary requirement to health policy. In the end, effective public health agencies *must* establish policies that eliminate health inequities.

HEALTH EQUITY

Eliminating Health Disparities Was One of Two Healthy People 2010 Goals

In the early 1980s, the then Health, Education and Welfare Secretary, Margaret Heckler commissioned the first U.S. government's report that comprehensively addressed the issue of racial and ethnic disparities, commonly referenced as the Heckler Report on Minority Health (U.S. DHHS, 2011). The report found that there were 60,000 excess deaths occurring annually because of health disparities, largely among African Americans. This finding became the impetus for the federal legislature establishing the Office of Minority Health. Subsequent developments included the establishment of minority health offices in other federal, state, and local branches of government. It should be noted that a 2005 study estimated African American excess deaths at 83,570 (Satcher et al., 2005).

In 1998, President Bill Clinton, through the U.S. Surgeon General, Dr. David Satcher, announced an initiative establishing a national goal of eliminating racial and ethnic disparities in health status by 2010. This goal ended the practice of past national health goal development that had separate benchmarks for different racial and ethnic groups. In this regard, in 1999, the Agency for Healthcare Research and Quality was directed by Congress to annually provide a report that monitors "prevailing dispari- ties" associated with raciality, ethnicity, and economy in "priority popu- lations." The first National Healthcare Disparities Report (NHDR) was released in 2004.

The most current and latest eighth NHDR was released in March 2010. The U.S. Department of Health and Human Services has initiated a National Stakeholder Strategy for Achieving Health Equity for Reducing Health Disparities.

The CHD is keenly attentive to the importance of recognizing social determinants' influence on health. Reducing health inequities is a CHD Board of Health ethical imperative; the department also has a center for health equity.

THE INFANT VITALITY SURVEILLANCE NETWORK

In October 2007, CHD, in concert with other agencies, began the process of documenting the public health burden of infant mortality in Cincinnati. Children of poverty largely reside in medically underserved areas and are less likely to access the health care system.

According to the CDC, "pockets of need" are areas or populations within each state or major city with low immunization coverage. Substantial numbers of women with inadequate prenatal care exist in pockets of urban areas with traditionally underserved populations. This description is applicable to CHD targeted zip codes where the "burden" of IMR is high (double digits).

As presented in Table 11.1, Cincinnati suffers from high IMR. Adverse birth outcomes are concentrated within the city. The Family and Children First Child Fatality Review Report reported in 2006 that 89 of 112 (79%) Hamilton County infant deaths occurred in the City of Cincinnati (Hamilton County Fatality Report, 2006).

But similarly within the city, as will be discussed below, the burden of infant death is inordinately greater in 14 of the city's 22 zip codes. The 14 targeted zip codes contain large ethnic and minority populations, are of low income, and have high rates of individuals without health insurance. Those 14 zip codes are the focus of the IVSN.

Figure 11.1 shows the zip code-specific IMR range from 0 to 27.1. The darker the area, the higher the IMR.

Table 11.1 shows CHD–UH favorable birth vitality outcomes in comparison to the city, county, state, and nation as a whole. The CHD–UH rate reflects women who complete their prenatal care at one of the five CHD health centers, are delivered by our partner UH, and receive perinatal and postnatal care by CHD home visitation program, using a CHD standardized tracking form. These women are typically considered to be a vulnerable population due to education levels, income, lack of insurance, and/or minority status. Thus, CHD–UH partnership patient's infant vitality outcomes reflect a strong public health and primary care system with accompanying public health interventions that have reduced IMR among its client population to below the national average. If the City of Cincinnati attained the 2006 5.3 IMR CHD–UH rate, *58 infant deaths would have been prevented.* The deaths saved in 2007 at the 7.1 IMR is 51.

In 2009, the reduction from the CHD–UH 12.3% prematurity to 8.1% (2010) was due to (among other aspects) improvement in the appropriateness of care. In 2008, there were 72 CHD preterm births. In 2009, there were 66 CHD preterm births. In 2010, there were 41 preterm births (31 fewer preterm births). The average first-year medical costs are 10 times greater for preterm babies ($50,000) than for full-term infants ($3,325) (March of Dimes Report, 2009).

TABLE 11.1   Infant Vitality

YEAR	CHD-UH	GOAL
LOW BIRTH WEIGHT (%)		
2008	10.9	11.0
2009	10.4	11.0
2010	9.0	11.0

YEAR	CHD-UH	CITY	COUNTY	STATE	USA
PRETERM BIRTH (%)					
2008	15.7	14.9			12.3
2009	15.6	14.9	13.1		
2010	8.1	16.8	14.7	12.6	

YEAR	CHD-UH	CITY	COUNTY	STATE	USA
INFANT MORTALITY RATE (%)					
2006	5.3	11.3	9.7	7.8	6.8
2007	7.1	13.5	10.9	7.7	6.7

City = Cincinnati; County = Hamilton; State = Ohio; CHD–UH-Cincinnati Health Department–University Hospital
Sources: Cincinnati Health Department and University Hospital Cincinnati (2011); Hamilton County Family and Children First Council Child Fatality Review Team Annual Report (2010); and National Center for Health Statistics State Profiles (2009).

The CHD–UH first-year medical cost saved from 41 fewer preterm births ($2,050,000–$136,325) equals $1,913,675.

The neonatal intensive care unit (NICU) cost of a preterm birth baby can range from $150,000 to $295,000 (National Academy of Sciences, 2007).[2] The CHD NICU cost savings range (41 fewer preterm births) equals $6,150,000 to $12,095,000.

We attribute the IMR and prematurity reduction success to the IVSN. The IVSN provides a "systemic change" framework that has the potential to eliminate health disparity in the select infant vitality measures and priority geographic areas. This UH Women's Health Center–CHD collaboration includes data sharing, home visitation, and a patient-centered medical home care coordination.

The data and tracking component will monitor 2,300 deliveries. The patient-centered medical home care dimension is in collaboration with

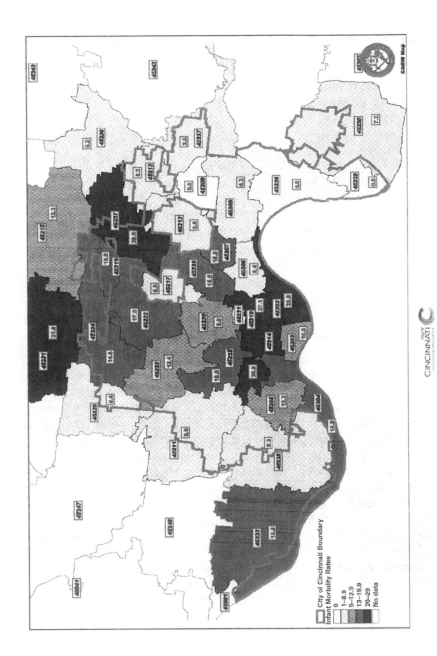

FIGURE 11.1 City of Cincinnati and contiguous area: infant mortality rates by zip code (2007–2008).
Source: Cincinnati Health Department Office of Vital Statistics and Records, 2010; Hamilton County Public Health
Division Of Epidemiology, 2010.

home-visitation agencies. Components (some in development) are listed below:

- Care coordination (home visitation)
- Case cross-match (home visitation)
- Case cross-match (WIC)
- Ensuring WIC
- Enrollment (WIC)
- Reports delivered and posted at CHD–UH clinic sites
- Monthly review with CHD–UH clinic team

The estimated number participating in the prenatal and postpartum field intervention for the targeted zip codes is approximately 2,000 mothers/expectant mothers.

SUMMARY

Social Policies Should Be Evaluated on Their Effect on Health Equity

This chapter presented a public health intervention surveillance and performance assessment model that expands on the *demonstrated* CHD–UH IMR improvement experience. It has attempted to advance the understanding of evidence-based strategies for improving the delivery of maternal and infant health to hard to reach target populations. Addressing the root causes of racial, ethnic, and geographic disparities, the model has included interventions, addressing environmental, economic, and social factors, and takes into account the community's values.

Furthermore, the chapter included in this effort recognition that decision makers' orientation and ideology are equally important in the calculus required to achieve equity in infant vitality and maternal health improvement. The principles that guide public health practice must be cored in (a) social justice, (b) evidence-based public health, (c) knowledge of the social determinants of health inequity, (d) recognize the socioecological framework of health equity, and lastly (e) adhere to the public health code of ethics (Public Health Leadership Society, 2002).

Health Equity in the IVSN Model

Public health practice strategies that are informed by core values of social justice and evidence-based social determinants research is the health equity lynchpin of the IVSN. The IVSN addresses the root causes of disparities in infant vitality by: (1) using data to make decisions, (2) assisting to empower, mobilize, and enfranchise communities, (3) monitoring, evaluating, and providing feedback that leads to ongoing adaptations and improvements, (4) facilitating a common understanding of the connection between health and development, and (5) identifying shared priorities and key obstacles to achieving health and equitable maternal and infant health improvement.

Using Data for Decisions: Developing Infant Mortality Data Sets for Cincinnati

The CHD–UH has utilized data on health status indicators to determine priorities and effectiveness of interventions. The UH delivery data provides birth outcome data by pay source, site, and provider. The collaboration demonstrates the value of a public health–clinical care services data-sharing partnership. The Institute of Medicine (IOM) study, *For the Public's Health: The Role of Measurement in Action and Accountability*, comments about the "... importance of population health statistics... and causal and interrelated pathways to health outcomes" (IOM Report, 2010).

Empowering and Mobilizing Communities to Engage and Lead

Cincinnati is composed of 52 distinct neighborhoods, which elect their own Community Councils. Each neighborhood functions as a unit of identity, with known names and boundaries, and leadership. Historically, Community Councils have focused on issues of housing and economic development. The city neighborhoods have historically been divided racially, politically, and economically, with class disparities and tensions existing even between neighborhoods of the same racial composition.

The CHD has worked to establish a positive relationship with the Community Councils. In 2008, CHD convened a town hall meeting entitled, "Building an Inclusive Cincinnati: Actions for Health and Equity through Neighborhood-Focused Decision Making." The meeting was in conjunction with the campaign by the National Association of City and County Health Officials to publicize the national public television series, "Unnatural Causes: Is Inequality Making Us Sick?" The CHD also held a series of "Local Conversations" that were neighborhood-based in African American, Hispanic, and Appalachian community settings. These were in support of the National Partnership for Action to End Health Disparities.

The CHD is poised to set up Health Impact Groups to address health concerns in their neighborhoods, assess health disparities, and develop health-related community action plans. Additionally, CHD health centers have Federally Qualified Look Alike designation requiring the Board of Governors be a 51% client majority.

In the field of public health, the model of "community-based participatory action" most closely relates to what the IVSN will achieve. The model proposes that agencies interested in developing knowledge about community health and promoting community action partner with communities. "Partners contribute their expertise and share responsibilities and ownership to increase understanding of a given phenomenon, and incorporate the knowledge gained with action to enhance the health and well-being of community members" (Israel et al., 2000).

Monitoring, Evaluating, and Providing Feedback That Leads to Ongoing Adaptations and Improvements

In addition to the performance measurement IVSN database, data about the health status of the community and how the quality of life is affected by the social determinants of health and risk factors in the community sectors are also maintained.

Facilitating a Common Understanding of the Connection Between Health and Development

This can be addressed in part by assessing the capacity of the local public health system to effectively address the root causes of health disparities; identifying the community's strengths, including cultural and psychosocial factors that can be used to shape the interventions and strategic themes to reduce the disparity in infant mortality. It is important to note that integral to this assessment is inclusion of other areas such as transportation, housing, and education. This was mentioned in the mobilizing communities' discussion.

Identifying Shared Priorities and Key Obstacles to Achieving Health and Equitable Maternal and Infant Health Improvement

Determining the forces of change that can reduce obstacles to the success of interventions and strategies is achieved by maintaining a feedback mechanism that enables evaluation, accountability, and transparency. Establishing performance benchmarks and "reporting" outcomes has proven to be effective in maintaining a constructive relationship between community stakeholders, the UH, and the CHD. Also, ascertaining the unique social, economic, and cultural circumstances of ethnic and racial populations in the respective target areas as well as the provider community will inform the development and sustainability of effective policy, system, and environmental strategies and interventions.

Case Study Exercises

Individually, or as a group, review the following case study and follow the exercises suggested at the end of the study, as appropriate. Be sure to focus on the why, how, and what emphasized in each exercise. Your professor/instructor will provide you with specific guidance on how you are to report your findings for the class.

Case Study 11.1

Eliminating health inequities in infant vitality is a daunting challenge, but one that must be confronted by local health departments, especially those situated in low socioeconomic urban communities. To respond to the Healthy People 2010 goal of eliminating racial and ethnic disparities, public health in a contemporary form must address the problem of inadequate clinical care services, exacerbated by poverty, income inequality, and social exclusion, as well as altering society's offending norms of behavior (Iton, 2008). The evidence presented in the IVSN model of the CHD in Table11.1 indicates that health equity can be impacted in infant vitality. Moreover, the model has the potential to impact maternal and infant populations on a large scale through systemic and structural change. It advances an intervention that reaches at-risk populations *but does not "let them go."* It uses a comprehensive strategic multisector approach that facilitates empowerment and establishes a social structure that promotes social justice (Braverman, 2004). The application of the IVSN model can indeed be pivotal in achieving health equity in infant vitality and maternal health improvement.

Study Exercises

1. Role play that you and your group are CHD public health practitioner. Describe how you would go about improving the maternal child health services in the community you serve.
2. Develop at least two strategies and methods for translating innovative ideas to reduce risk for mothers and infants in your target community.

REFERENCES

Aday, Lu Ann. (1975, June). Economic and non-economic barriers to the use of needed medical services. *Medical Care*, XIII(6), 447–456.

Amin, Samir. (1974). *Accumulation on a world scale: A critique of the theory of underdevelopment*. Vols. 1 & 2 Combined. New York, NY: Monthly Review Press, p. 10.

Braverman, P. (2004). An approach to studying social disparities in health and health care. *American Journal of Public Health*, 94(12), 2139–2148.

Colgrove, J. (2002). The McKeown thesis: A historical controversy and its enduring influence. *American Journal of Public Health*, 92(5), 725–729.

Cook, R. J., Dickens, B. M., & Fathalla, M. F. (2003). *Reproductive health and human rights: Integrating medicine, ethics, and law*. Oxford: Oxford University Press.

Goodnow, Frank. (1900). *Politics and administration* [especially Chapter 1]. New York, NY: The Macmillan.

Institute of Medicine (2010, December). *For the public's health: The role of measurement in action and accountability*.

Israel, B., Parker, E. A., Rowe, Z., Salvatore, A., Minkler, M., López, J., . . . Halstead, S. (2000, April 29). *The Detroit community – Academic Urban Research Center: Principles, rationale, challenges and lessons learned through a community based participatory research partnership.* Presented at the Community-Campus Partnerships for Health's 4th Annual Conference, Washington, DC.

Iton, T. (2008). The ethics of the medical model in addressing the root causes of health disparities in local public health practice. *Journal of Health Management Practice, 14*(4), 335–339.

Kane, R., Kasteler, J., & Gray, R. (1976). *The health gap: Medical services and the poor.* New York, NY: Springer Publishing, p. 140.

Kaufman, J. (2007). *Making causal inferences about macrosocial factors as a basis for public health policies.* New York, NY: Springer.

Khanani, I., Elam, J., Hearn, R., Jones, C., & Maseru, N. (2010, February 10). The impact of prenatal WIC participation on infant mortality and racial disparities. *American Journal of Public Health, 100*(Suppl. 1), S204–209.

Kitagawa, E. M., & Hauser, P. M. (1973). *Differential mortality in the United States: A study in socioeconomic epidemiology.* Cambridge, MA: Harvard University Press, pp. 11–32.

March of Dimes. (2009). *Study: Average preemie costs $49,000 in first year.* March of Dimes Report. White Plains, NY: Author.

Mays, G., & Smith, S. (2011). Evidence links increases in public health spending to declines in preventable deaths. *Health Affairs, 30,* 1585–1593.

McNeil, B. (1975). Primer on certain elements of medical decision making. *The New England Journal of Medicine, 293*(5), 215.

National Academy of Sciences. (2007). *Preterm birth: Causes, consequences, and prevention.* Washington, DC: The National Academies Press.

Ohio Department of Health Information Warehouse. *March of Dimes peristats system.* CFRT 2007 Report. Columbus, OH: Author.

Popper, Karl. (1957). *The poverty of historicism.* London: Routledge and Paul.

Public Health Leadership Society. (2002). *Principles of the ethical practice of public health.*

Sagar, John C., & Paul, John E. (1983). *Policy issues in personal health services: Current perspectives.* Rockville, MD: Aspen Publications, PL 93–641, pp. 109–133 and Chapter 4 regarding PL 88–352.

Satcher, D., Fryer, G. E., Jr., McCann, J., Troutman, A., Woolf, S. H., & Rust, G. (2005). What if we were equal? A comparison of the Black-White mortality gap in 1960 and 2000. *Health Affairs, 24*(2), 459–464.

U.S. DHHS. (2011). *Healthy People 2020 social determinants of health.* Washington, DC: U.S. Government Publications.

ADDITIONAL RESOURCES

Aday, Lu Ann, Economic and non-economic barriers to the use of needed medical services, *Medical Care* (Vol. XIII(6), June 1975).

Almond, G. (1966). Political theory and political science. *American Political Science Review, 60,* 869–879.

Amin, Samir, *Accumulation on a world scale: A critique of the theory of underdevelopment* (Vol. 1 and 2 combined; New York, NY: Monthly Review Press, 1974, p.

10); see also Navarro, Vicente, The underdevelopment of health of working America: Causes, consequences and possible solutions, *American Journal of Public Health* (Vol. 66(6), 1976, p. 544).

Appleby, P. H. (1965). *Policy and administration*. Birmingham: University of Alabama Press.

Bayles, Michael D. (1984). *Reproductive ethics*. Englewood Cliffs, NJ: Prentice-Hall.

Braverman, P., An approach to studying social disparities in health and health care, *AJPH* (Vol. 94(12), December 2004). Advancing health equity through public health policies.

Capron, A. M. (1984). The new reproductive possibilities: Seeking a moral basis for concerted action in a pluralistic society. *Law, Medicine and Health Care, 12*(5), 192–198.

Colgrove, J., The McKeown thesis: A historical controversy and its enduring influence. *American Journal of Public Health* (Vol. 92(5), 2002, pp. 725–729). See also Link, B. G. and Phelan, J. C., McKeown and the idea that social conditions are fundamental causes of disease, *The nation's health* edited by Phillip R. Lee (7th ed., Jones and Bartlett Publishers, 2003).

Easton, David. (1972). The new revolution in political science. *American Political Science Review, LXVI*, 796–817.

Elkington, J. (1986). *The poisoned womb: Human reproduction in a polluted world*. New York, NY: Pellican Press.

For the public's health: The role of measurement in action and accountability (Institute of Medicine Report Brief, December 2010).

Galea, S. (Ed.). (2007). *Macrosocial determinants of population health*. New York, NY: Springer.

Goldberg, R., & Koski, J. (1984). *The improved pregnancy outcome project: An analysis of the impact of a federal program on infant mortality*. Birmingham, AL: Division of Maternal Fetal Medicine, University of Alabama in Birmingham.

Golembiewski, R. (1977). *Public administration as a developing discipline*. New York, NY: Marcel Dekker.

Guendelman, S. and Pearl, M., Access to care for children of the working poor, *Archives Pediatric Medicine* (Vol. 155, June 2001).

Hamilton County Child Fatality Report 2006.

Israel, B., et al., *The Detroit community—Academic Urban Research Center: Principles, rationale, challenges and lessons learned through a community based participatory research partnership*, presented at the Community—Campus Partnerships for Health's 4th Annual Conference, Washington, DC, April 29, 2000.

Iton, Tony, The ethics of the medical model in addressing the root causes of health disparities in local public health practice, *Journal of Health Management Practice* (Vol. 14(4), 2008, pp. 335–339); see also *Tackling health inequities through public health practice: Theory to action* edited by Richard Hofrichter and Rajiv Bhatia (Oxford University Press, 2010).

Kane, et al., *The health gap*, p. 140. Also see Aday, Lu Ann, The impact of health policy on access to medical care, *Milbank Memorial Fund Quarterly* (Spring 1976). The Robert Wood Johnson Foundation, *Access to health care in the United States: Results of a 1986 survey*, Special Report Number 2 (1987). The Robert Wood Johnson study was a follow-up to the foundation's initial investigation. See

The Robert Wood Johnson Foundation, *A new survey on access to medical care,* Special Report Number 1 (1978).

Kaufman, Jay, *Making causal inferences about macrosocial factors as a basis for public health policies* (Springer, 2007); see also Galea, Sandro, *Macrosocial determinants of population health ed* (Springer, 2007).

Khanani, et al., The impact of prenatal WIC participation on infant mortality and racial disparities. *AJPH* (February 10, 2010).

Kirn, M. E. (1977). Behavioralism, post-behavioralism, and the philosophy of science: Two houses, one plague. *Review of Politics, 39,* 82–102;

Kitagawa and Hauser, *Differential mortality,* pp. 11–32. Also see Goldberg, Robert, and Koski, Judith, *The improved pregnancy outcome project: An analysis of the impact of a federal program on infant mortality* (Division of Maternal Fetal Medicine, University of Alabama in Birmingham). For a representative example of how infant mortality data is displayed see Figure 1 in Illustrations from, Georgia Center for Health Statistics, Division of Public Health, Department of Human Resources, Statistical Printout, 1987.

Kuhn, T. (1970). *The structure of scientific revolution.* Chicago, IL: University of Chicago Press.

Link, B. G., Phelan, G., & McKeown, J. C. (2003). Idea that social conditions are fundamental causes of disease. In Phillip R. Lee (Ed.), *The nation's health* (7th ed.). Boston, MA: Jones and Bartlett.

Marx, Fritz M. (1957). *The administrative state.* Chicago, IL: University of Chicago Press.

Max, W., Woodrow, W., Taylor, F., Guendelman, S., & Pearl, M. (2001). Access to care for children of the working poor. *Archives Pediatric Medicine, 155,* 651–658.

Mays, G. and Smith, S., Evidence links increases in public health spending to declines in preventable deaths, *Health Affairs* (July 2011). A study presented in the July 21, 2011, *Health Affairs Journal* affirms the hypothesis that increased investments in public health prevents deaths and improves population health over time. The authors show that mortality rates declined between 1.1% and 6.9% for each 10% increase in public health spending. Robert Wood Johnson Foundation funded the study.

McNeil, Barbara, Primer on certain elements of medical decision making, *The New England Journal of Medicine* (Vol. 293(5), July 31, 1975, p. 215).

Miller, E. (1972). Positivism, historicism, and political inquiry. *American Political Science Review, 66,* 796–817.

Musgrave, Alan (Eds.). (1970). *Criticism and the growth of knowledge.* Cambridge, MA: Cambridge University Press.

Navarro, V. (1976). The underdevelopment of health of working America: Causes, consequences and possible solutions. *American Journal of Public Health, 66*(6), 544.

Ohio Department of Health Information Warehouse, March of Dimes Peristats System, CFRT 2007 Report Columbus, Ohio.

Preterm birth: Causes, consequences, and prevention (National Academy of Sciences, 2007).

Principles of the ethical practice of public health (Public Health Leadership Society, 2002).

Richard, H., & Rajiv, B. (2010). *Tackling health inequities through public health practice: Theory to action.* New York, NY: Oxford University Press.

Satcher, D., et al., What if we were equal? A comparison of the Black-White mortality gap in 1960 and 2000, *Health Affairs* (Vol. 24(2), 2005, pp. 459–464). See also *Report of the Secretary's Task Force on Black and Minority Health* (Vol. I and IV; Vol. VI: Infant mortality and low birthweight; Vol. I: Executive summary (Washington, DC: U.S Department of Health and Human Services, August 1985).

See Sagar, John C. and Paul, John E., *Policy issues in personal health services: Current perspectives* (Rockville, MD: Aspen Publications, 1983); for both a discussion and description of PL 93–641 pp.109–133 and Chapter 4 regarding PL 88–352.

Stanworth, M. (Ed.). (1987). *Reproductive technologies: Gender, motherhood and medicine.* Minneapolis, MN: University of Minnesota Press.

Study: Average preemie costs $49,000 in first year (March of Dimes Report, 2009).

The definition we employ is that aspect of reproductive health pertaining to infant mortality, natality, and prenatal and postnatal care. Questions involving other important dimensions of reproductive health such as induced and spontaneous abortion, sterilization, contraception, maternal mortality, and sex education are notable but beyond the scope of this chapter's objective. For a discussion involving the comprehensiveness of the concept of reproductive health see Cook, R. J., et al., *Reproductive health and human rights: Integrating medicine, ethics, and Law* (Oxford University Press, 2003); Wilcox, Allen J., *Fertility and pregnancy: An epidemiologic perspective* (Oxford University Press, 2010); Capron, A. M., The new reproductive possibilities: Seeking a basis for concerted action in a pluralistic society, *Law, Medicine and Health Care* (October 1984); Bayles, Michael D., *Reproductive ethics* (Englewood Cliffs, NJ: Prentice-Hall, 1984); also Stanworth, Michelle. (Ed.), *Reproductive technologies: Gender, motherhood and medicine* (Minneapolis, MN: University of Minnesota Press, 1987) and Elkington, J., *The poisoned womb: Human reproduction in a polluted world* (New York, NY: Pelican Press, 1986).

The idea that decision making is apolitical and neutral fulfills the old notion of an administration–policy dichotomy that the administrator is to distance from politics; the adminstrator's function is to execute and carry out policy. The administration–policy dichotomy assumed a role of value neutrality for the administrator and nonpolicy-making bureaucracy. The dichotomy reflects the oversimplified view of the classical model of administration, comprising concepts of Max Weber, Woodrow Wilson, and Frederick Taylor. See Goodnow, Frank, *Politics and administration*, especially Chapter 1 (New York, NY: Macmillan, 1900) and Wilson, Woodrow, The study of administration, *Political Science Quarterly* (Vol. 2, June 1887, pp. 197–222); also Appleby, Paul H., *Policy and administration* (Birmingham, AL: University of Alabama Press, 1965) and White, L., *Introduction to the study of public administration* (New York, NY: Macmillan, 1934). An evolutionary perspective on the administrative state is provided by Van Ripper, Paul P., The American administrative state: Wilson and the Founders–An orthodox view, *Public Administration Review* (November/December 1983). See also Truman, David, Dillusion and regeneration: The quest for a discipline, *American Political Science Review* (Vol. 59(4), December 1965, pp. 865–873); Marx, Fritz M., *The administrative state* (Chicago, IL: University of Chicago Press, 1957); Golembiewski, R., *Public administration as a developing discipline* (New York, NY: Marcel Dekker). The behavioralist–postbehavioralist debate is also relevant in this regard. Where the behavioralists refer to themselves as "normal scientists," with postbehavioralists linking their views to a historicist or antipositivist position that relied to a large extent on Kuhn, Thomas, *The structure of scientific revolution* (University of Chicago Press, 1970). See also Miller, Eugene, Positivism, historicism, and political inquiry, *American Political Science Review* (Vol. 66, September 1972). For views of science according to behavioralists, see Popper, Karl, *The poverty of historicism* (London: Routledge and Paul, 1957); for a discussion of the debate between Popper and Kuhns views, see Lakatos, Imre, and Musgrave, Alan (Eds.), *Criticism and the growth of knowledge* (Cambridge, MA: Cambridge University Press, 1970). For a differentiation between the behavioralist and postbehavioralist approach, see Kirn, Michael E., Behavioralism, post-behavioralism, and the philosophy of science: Two houses, one plague, *Review of Politics* (Vol. XXIX, January, pp. 82–102);see also Easton, David, The new revolution in political science, *American Political Science Review* (Vol. LXVI, September 1972, pp. 796–817); Almond, Gabriel, Political theory and political science, *American Political Science Review* (December 1966, pp. 869–879). Amin, Samir, *Accumulation on a world scale: A critique of the theory of underdevelopment* (Vol. 1 and 2 combined; New York, NY: Monthly Review Press, 1974). See pp. 10–13 regarding Amins' remarks about reason, concepts of science, limits of methodology, and economic empiricism. The author castigates the notion of science being pure and immune to value. Having earlier stated that "The economic 'science' taught in the universities has died of impotence, as a social science, through rejecting the objective theory of value." Amin writes about social science and the art of management, commenting that "Insofar as the allegedly 'eternal' concepts of marginalist science are indeed immediately deduced from observation of the capitalist mode of production, they do enable development of an art of economic management, even though this art is far from perfect...." For insight on how the medical profession adopted the value-neutral outlook in its application, see also Brown, E. R., *Rockefeller medicine men*, pp. 60–97.

The Robert Wood Johnson Foundation. (1978). *A new survey on access to medical care"* Special Report Number 1. Princeton, NJ: Author.

The Robert Wood Johnson Foundation. (1987). *Access to health care in the United States: Results of A 1986 survey.* Special Report Number 2. Princeton, NJ: Author.

Truman, David. (1965). Dillusion and regeneration: The quest for a discipline. *American Political Science Review, 59*(4), 865–873.

U.S Department of Health and Human Services. (1985, August). *Report of the Secretary's Task Force on Black and Minority Health Volumes I & IV; Volume VI: Infant mortality and low birthweight; Volume I: Executive summary.* Washington, DC: Author.

U.S. DHHS 2011 U.S. Government Publications Healthy People 2020 has a social determinants of health content area, but objectives have not yet been developed for the measure.

Van Ripper, Paul P. (1983). The American administrative state: Wilson and the founders – An orthodox view. *Public Administration Review, 43,* 477–490.

White, L. (1934). *Introduction to the study of public administration.* New York, NY: The Macmillan.

Wilcox, Allen J. (2010). *Fertility and pregnancy: An epidemiologic.* New York, NY: Perspective Oxford University Press.

Wilson, Woodrow. (1887). *The study of administration. Political Science Quarterly, 2,* 197–222.

12

Using the Power of Media to Influence Health Policy and Politics in CEOD

Jessie Daniels, Barbara Glickstein, and Diana J. Mason

Whoever controls the media—the images—controls the culture.

Allen Ginsberg

LEARNING OBJECTIVES

What you can learn by studying this chapter:

- To differentiate the traditional model of media versus new media
- To identify the power of media in influencing electoral campaigns and health policy
- How to describe the shift in who controls the media in a Web 2.0 world
- To define a "distributed campaign"
- What the role of documentaries and entertainment media is in influencing public policy
- How to define media advocacy
- How to develop a frame for accessing and using media to get a health policy issue on the public's agenda
- How to evaluate the credibility and reliability of a health story reported in the public media
- To identify three strategies for positioning oneself in the media as an expert in policy matters
- To identify three strategies for using media to distribute a message about a health policy matter

In February 2007, United States Senator Barack Obama (D-IL) had a conversation with Marc Andreessen, a founder of Netscape (one of the original browsers, predating Google) and member of the board of directors of Facebook. The conversation was about using social media to build a political campaign that could upset frontrunner Hillary Rodham Clinton in the Democratic primary election for the U.S. presidency. In 2004, presidential candidate Howard Dean had used a viral web strategy to build a campaign war chest through small donations from large numbers of people.

Obama had a vision for building upon Dean's success, and he hired Chris Hughes, another founder of Facebook, to manage his presidential campaign's social media effort. David Axelrod, Obama's top adviser, was formerly a partner in ASK Public Strategies, a public relations firm. Together, Hughes and Axelrod built a team that marshaled every tool in the social media and marketing tool box to create and sustain the Obama campaign and brand.

They launched an expert viral marketing campaign including Obama ringtones, product placement (Obama ads in sports video games), and a 30-minute infomercial that was played on YouTube. The campaign's effort spawned additional digital videos as well, including the "I Got a Crush...on Obama" video and the celebrity-filled video called "Yes We Can" featuring Black-Eyed Peas front man, Wil.I.Am, both of which went viral, spreading to millions of viewers in just days of being posted online. The Obama campaign led competitors in using social media to connect with a growing audience of followers on Facebook, Twitter, MySpace, and blogs. In the general election, he had 118,107 followers on Twitter, outpacing his opponent John McCain's 2,865 followers by a factor of 40 to 1 (Lardinois, 2008). Obama used social media to build a grassroots movement that resulted in his historic election (Talbot, 2008).

But, he knew that the use of social media is not simply a campaign technique—it is a way of interacting, building an activist community, and engaging people in ways that matter to them. As president, he quickly launched www.change.gov for people to share their ideas for reforming the country, sending the message that he had no intention of regressing to a traditional media operation as president. Rather, he was going to continue to engage people in supporting his agenda for the nation. When health care reform was teetering from a growing army of discontents blocking its passage, he continued using social media to mobilize supporters to pressure Congress to act before the April 2010 recess. President Obama also took to the road and held town meetings in key communities because he knew that these town meetings would garner reports on primetime television, get radio coverage, and have a front-page position in newspapers. He could count on the primetime news including a sound bite and visual image of him speaking before a crowd of enthusiastic Ohioans, cheering for passing some form of health care reform legislation. The personal appearances were a way to get his message to those who were not yet social media mavens and to reinforce it with those who were already his followers on Twitter and Facebook.

The web has dramatically changed how we think about communicating with others, whether to connect with family or build a grassroots political movement to push policy makers to pass new laws. Even traditional media outlets are now augmenting their work with all sorts of social media to extend their reach and impact. Legislators are launching blogs, using Facebook, and "Tweeting" to make their voices heard and to connect with their constituents. In fact, engaging citizens in government is reshaping the way government works. This chapter looks at the integration of traditional and social media as powerful tools for health professionals and community health leaders to harness shaping health policy and politics.

SEISMIC SHIFT IN MEDIA: ONE-TO-MANY AND MANY-TO-MANY

There has been a seismic shift in the way media is created and distributed. For many years, the dominant paradigm in media was a model in which one broadcaster sent a message out to a mass audience. This broadcast model is referred to as "one-to-many." Today, this model is being challenged by the advent of the Internet and user-generated content in which many people create media and distribute it to their networks. This new model is sometimes referred to as "many-to-many."

MASS MEDIA: THE ONE-TO-MANY MODEL

Traditional media in radio, television, film, and newspapers was based on the idea that one broadcaster would try to reach as many audience members as possible. But, for those interested in influencing health policy and politics through the media, there were many advantages and some significant disadvantages to the one-to-many model of broadcast media (Abramson, 2003).

Radio, film, and television have all been used to communicate messages about health to consumers and policy makers alike. What all these media share is the ability to broadcast a message to a mass audience, sometimes in the millions or tens of millions. When there were very few media outlets, it was possible to broadcast a consistent message to a wide audience. The use of mass media has been a major tool in health-promotion campaigns because it reaches a large audience. Media is a powerful tool that is capable of promoting healthy social change (Whitney & Viswanath, 2004).

There are also disadvantages to mass media communications. Large corporations own media outlets and control what goes out through their channels. The expense of buying time or space in major media outlets can be prohibitive, especially for nonprofit organizations. Mass media campaigns, by definition, are intended to reach a wide audience but are not as effective at reaching specific, target populations. For example, a mass media campaign about HIV prevention may reach a wide audience but may fail to reach the specific population that is most vulnerable to infection. However, political operatives have developed increasingly sophisticated approaches to segmenting and targeting specific electoral districts with mass media when they want to pressure a policy maker who may hold a deciding vote on an important bill. They buy commercial time on the dominant television station in that policy maker's district. But what no form of mass media does very well (or at all) is to allow users to create and distribute their own content with messages they find most important.

MANY-TO-MANY: USER-GENERATED CONTENT AND THE RISE OF THE "PROSUMER"

The rise of the Internet, and specifically websites, that rely on users to generate content are part of a new landscape of media creation and distribution. The early Internet featured "brochure" websites that were one-way flows of information. The paradigm-shifting quality of the Internet began to emerge with the rise of Web 2.0 (pronounced: "web two point oh"), a term coined by O'Reilly (2005) at a conference in 2004. Web 2.0 refers to a range of web-based Internet practices based on information sharing, social networks, and collaboration rather than the one-way communication style of the early era of the Internet. The key idea with the concept of Web 2.0 is that people are using the Internet to connect with other people, through their old face-to-face networks and through newly formed online networks. "Prosumption" is another way that some people talk about this shift. Prosumption is the idea that "producing" and "consuming" are combined in this new many-to-many paradigm. Rather than an elite few who "produce" media for a mass audience to "consume," now we are all both "producers" and "consumers," or prosumers of media. The many-to-many paradigm does not refer to a new form of technology but rather a new way that everyday people make use of that technology (Ritzer & Jurgenson, 2010).

The collaborative, information-sharing Internet practices have broad implications for health media, policy, and politics, but they do not mean the end of mass media.

THE POWER OF MEDIA

Mobile phone initiatives are revolutionizing the way that health care is delivered in developing countries. Mobile health, or mHealth, is a term used for the practice of health care delivery and public health supported by mobile devices. In the developing world, lack of infrastructure prevents health workers from delivering efficient health care to rural areas. As health workers travel from clinics to reach isolated patients, they are often as disconnected from central clinics as the patients they are trying to serve. In 2010, mobile phones represented more than 90% of all telephone lines in Africa. Today, close to 50% of people on the African continent own a mobile phone and it is projected that the number will reach 100% in a few years (Schwartz, 2010).

Medic Mobile (http://medicmobile.org) is a nonprofit company and early innovator in open-source mobile health technology. The company is working on 20 projects in 10 countries throughout Africa, Asia, and Latin America. In 2011, it developed the first SIM application for health care that can operate on 80% of the world's phones. This SMS-based platform allows patients to get home-based care, even if they can't be physically visited by a caregiver. This new technology provides the ability to monitor data and design evaluation tools to validate the impact of the mobile health programs. Medic Mobile launched a pilot program in Malawi and was able to report through research finding that in 6 months it saved the clinical staff an estimated 1,200 hours follow-up time and more than $3,000 in fuel and transportation costs. In addition, more than 100 patients received treatment for tuberculosis (TB) after their symptoms were noticed by the community and reported by text message.

Mobile health in the hands of health workers and people in communities is one way to strengthen the capacity and capability of health workers to improve the health of people globally. But it is increasingly being harnessed to shape the political and policy landscape globally.

A classic example of the power of traditional media in shaping health policy arose during the first months of William Jefferson Clinton's presidency, when he tried but failed to enact health care reform legislation despite campaigning on a policy platform that sought to guarantee comprehensive health care coverage for every American. In September 1993, he proposed the Health Security Act to Congress and the public with the hope and anticipation that this would become landmark legislation. Clinton's proposal initially had substantial public support, because many believed the country had a moral imperative to extend health care coverage to all who live here. However, according to an analysis by the Annenberg Public Policy Center of the University of Pennsylvania (1995), one of the top factors that unraveled the legislation's progress was the "Harry and Louise" campaign (a series of television advertisements about two curious characters, Harry and Louise), which was sponsored by the Health Insurance Association of America (HIAA), an ardent opponent to the president's plan.

Actors portrayed this couple voicing grave concerns about the bill. They said, "Under the President's bill, we'll lose our right to choose our own physician," and "What happens if the plan runs out of money?" Although the advertisements were not the only reason for the demise of the Health Security Act, the Harry and Louise television spots effectively planted fear and negativity in the hearts and minds of many citizens within the span of 60 seconds. Suddenly, many of the Americans who had been concerned about the growing numbers of uninsured became more concerned about how the bill would affect their own health care options and withdrew their support from the Act.

What many do not realize about the Harry and Louise ads is that the target audience was not the public directly. Rather, it was policy makers and those who could influence how the public perceived the issue: journalists. The ads originally aired in the country's major media centers: Washington, DC; Los Angeles; New York City; and Atlanta. They were seen and reported on by journalists. In fact, the ads got more airtime by becoming part of the journalists' news stories. Many people who saw the ads did so through viewing them as part of the evening news, not as a paid advertisement.

The Harry and Louise commercials are an example of a deliberate media strategy to reframe a public policy issue and mobilize a public constituency around it. It is one illustration of the power of the media in policy and politics. The media saturate this nation and much of the world with images that change people's opinions, shape their attitudes and beliefs, and transform their behavior (McAlister, 1991). In today's media landscape, the Harry and Louise television ads would also be posted on YouTube for millions more to view. Bloggers would include links to the video, as would people who write about it on their Facebook or Twitter pages. Yet, the current media landscape would also spawn critical analyses of the ads by bloggers and unmasking of the HIAA and their motives, potentially limiting the impact of the ads.

Media campaigns such as these often rely on cloaked websites to enhance the effectiveness of their deception. Cloaked websites are published by individuals or groups who conceal authorship in order to deliberately disguise a hidden political agenda (Daniels, 2009). Consider an ad from the more recent, successful effort to pass the Affordable Care Act of 2010. During this political battle, an unknown political group with no clear affiliation to a political party created a video opposing the reform. In the ad, a variety of attractive-looking people declare, "I guess I'm racist" because they oppose health care reform. The central message of the video, although not immediately obvious, was a signal that a growing number of people opposed Obama's policy on health care reform but that opposition was not rooted in any individual racism. The video had fairly high-quality production values, meaning it looked professionally produced and good enough to appear on broadcast television; yet, it was released exclusively on YouTube. The provocative video quickly went viral (meaning it was very popular and links to it spread via e-mail and blogs from person to person, much like a biological virus). Within 24 hours, it was one of the most viewed videos on YouTube—no small accomplishment among the millions of videos on the site. Once again, the political operatives behind this video did not have to buy airtime on television to get their message out. After the video became the top video on YouTube, several mainstream broadcast news media outlets re-aired it on television. Some of these were critical of the video, such as the Rachel Maddow Show on MSNBC, but the fact is that what started as a YouTube video was featured on several broadcast television shows within 24 hours. Health care reform legislation did eventually pass despite these types of campaigns. Yet, this instance of converging media (Geary, Mahler, Finger, & Shears, 2005) illustrates just how sophisticated the use of multiple forms of media has become.

WHO CONTROLS THE MEDIA?

The traditional media industry has been owned by six major corporations that, prior to the growth of social media, controlled 90% of the news Americans read, saw, or heard (Harris, 2005). In 2003, the Federal Communications Commission (made up of political appointees reflecting the then dominant Republican Party's values) voted to ease the restrictions on cross-ownership between different news entities, permitting one corporation to own the primary television, radio, and newspaper outlets in a community, thus enabling one corporation to control messages and put forth a particular perspective. CNN founder Ted Turner objected to this consolidation of corporate media power, arguing that allowing this cross-ownership "will extend the market dominance of the media corporations that control most of what Americans read, see, or hear" and "give them more power to cut important ideas out of the public debate" (Harris, 2005, p. 83).

Today, social media can actually drive traditional media to cover issues that major newsrooms may not deem worthy of their limited space and time. On June 12, 2009, Iran held its presidential elections between incumbent Mahmoud Ahmadinejad and rival Hossein Mousavi. The result was a landslide victory for Ahmadinejad, yet there was strong suspicion of voting fraud. This led to violent riots across Iran and protests worldwide. As protests erupted in the streets of numerous cities in Iran and, in some cases, turned violent, major broadcast media in the United States had almost no news on these events at all. Americans and others around the world and in Iran used the Twitter hash tag (e.g., a # symbol used to group messages on a specific topic) "#CNNfail" to track and share updates on what was happening in Iran that were pouring in from around the world. Twitter was the best source of information for second-by-second updates and breaking news on what was happening in Iran. People on the ground and across the globe chatted about the news out of Iran fed by social media more than mainstream news divisions. YouTube was a central distribution medium for the Iran riots with videos shot by people on the ground using their cell phones and small handheld cameras. The blogosphere was far quicker with news and multimedia from Iran then traditional news, illustrated by the spectacle of highly paid cable news anchors reading Twitter and blog updates on the air as part of their "reporting" a story. The social media photo site Flickr was quickly filled with gut-wrenching imagery from the ground showing photos of beatings, protests, and military action. This groundswell of news from and about Iran spread globally and, nearly instantly through social media, turned into a news item itself and was reported on by all traditional media outlets. Eventually, the focus shifted and CNN and other news outlets started covering stories about Iran. This example illustrates the power of social media to offset the corporate take-over of traditional media. This bodes well for health professionals and community health leaders who have not always been able to garner media attention for their issues.

Organizations of health professionals are particularly well positioned to mount focused social media campaigns because they already have a list of people who can begin the viral spreading of messages. But the social network lines are getting crowded and establishing a reputation for reliable, important information that others want to regularly take note of requires a thoughtful strategy. Distributed campaigns are increasingly a part of the political strategy, whether for winning an election, getting an issue on policymakers' or the public's agenda, or garnering support for a new policy initiative.

DISTRIBUTED CAMPAIGNS

Obama's social media campaign strategy is called a distributed campaign—a bottom-up rather than a top-down approach to political campaigns that depends upon viral spreading from the grassroots rather than message broadcasting and control by the campaign staff (Ozimek, 2005). These campaigns are designed to involve more than core supporters. They seek to engage swing voters, provide opportunities for core supporters to craft messages that may appeal to these swing voters more effectively than messages created by central campaign staff, and thereby strengthen the commitment of core supporters to the campaign. E-mail, blogs, and various other social media venues are used by campaign staff to begin a dialogue that is subsequently taken over and developed by a broad community of supporters.

Whether people are reached by e-mails, Facebook or Twitter updates, or other means, distributed campaigns provide people with tools for activism, such as petitions to sign, e-mail scripts to send, or letters to sign and send to legislators. Organizations such as Democracy In Action (http://salsalabs.com/democracyinaction) are available to help build the capacity of groups that want to develop action tools that reach diverse audiences in distributive campaigns. Living in a media-saturated world can sometimes feel like being in a cacophony of conflicting voices. The challenge is how to use these powerful tools most effectively as the media model changes.

GETTING ON THE PUBLIC'S AGENDA

One of the most important roles that the media plays is getting issues on the agendas of the public and policy makers. What the mainstream media do or do not cover is equally powerful in determining what issues are considered by policy makers.

The news media are instrumental in getting issues onto the agenda of policy makers, but non-news entertainment television programs can mobilize public constituencies around an issue. Television continues to be the dominant form of media in most people's lives, despite the rise of new forms of media online. The television is on more than 8 hours a day in the average American household (Nielsen Reports, 2007). Teenagers still spend more time watching TV than they do online (Kaiser Family Foundation, 2010). The Internet may be where people go to find out about a health issue, but they often first become aware of the issue through television.

Turow (1996) points out that non-news television entertainment is particularly loaded with rhetoric that often stereotypes power relationships and may be more successful than the news in shaping people's images of the world. Highly viewed TV presentations of health care hold political significance that should be assessed alongside news. Medical and nursing dramas on broadcast and cable television, such as *Grey's Anatomy*, *ER*, and *Nurse Jackie*, are often important sources of information about health and health policy for a wide audience. Researchers Turow and Gans (2002) systematically evaluated one television season of 4 hour-long medical dramas and found that health care policy issues appeared regularly in the programs. Evidence from a national telephone survey indicates that the percentage of regular viewers of the show *ER* who were aware that HPV is a sexually transmitted disease was higher (28%) 1 week after viewing an episode of the show about HPV than before seeing the show (9%). Even 6 weeks after viewing the episode, 16% had retained this knowledge. This capacity to quickly get a message out to millions of people through an hour-long drama is part of the reason that many health advocates work to get their particular issue included in a storyline of a major network drama. For many working in public health, storyline placement is considered the "gold standard" for achieving advocacy goals.

Perhaps not surprisingly then, when National Institutes of Health (NIH) wanted to get out a message that "drug addiction is a brain disease," they turned to HBO. In a landmark collaboration between HBO, the NIH, and the Robert Wood Johnson Foundation, the cable network launched *The Addiction Series* (2007), an award-winning collection of documentary films about substance use, each by a leading director. Of course, *The Addiction Series* also included a website with more information about treatment options and a lively discussion board (Bauder, 2007).

Documentary films, in conjunction with online campaigns, are influencing health policy and politics, while achieving mainstream commercial success. For example, Morgan Spurlock's *Super Size Me* (2004) explored the health impact of fast food on childhood obesity, fueling changes in local school and community policies, requiring posting of calories in fast-food stores, changing the foods and beverages available in schools, and ramping up exercise options in schools. Michael Moore's documentary *SiCKO* (2005) examined health care policy in the United States, helping to raise the public's awareness of how bad the U.S. health care system had become at a time when health care reform was on the nation's agenda. Many of those who were uncertain about whether or not health care reform was needed became converts after watching *SiCKO*.

For some media activists concerned with health policy, Internet technologies have transformed documentary films into just one element in a multimodal social action campaign. Perhaps the archetypal example of how media is converging across multiple platforms and creating change in awareness about health and galvanizing movement for policy change around an important health issue is the development of Food, Inc. (2008). In 2001, journalist and filmmaker Robert Kenner read *Fast Food Nation*, a book by Eric Schlosser about the rise of agribusiness, and Kenner was appalled. He wanted to do something about the industrialization of the food supply, so he started work on the documentary that would eventually become *Food, Inc.* Kenner collaborated with Schlosser on the film (Schlosser is listed as coproducer). The online presence for *Food, Inc.* (http://www.foodincthemovie.com) is a vast repository of further information about the issues surrounding the industrialization of food. It includes opportunities to participate in activism, such as signing the online petition to reauthorize the Child Nutrition Act, which would support healthy food choices in schools. The film also inspired another book (*Food, Inc.*), an e-version that can be downloaded at the website, or a hard copy that can be ordered from online booksellers. The social action campaign around *Food, Inc.* started with a heavily researched book and became a documentary film, a website, another book, and links for people to take action. This exemplifies how people are converging media to shape health and health policy.

MEDIA AS A HEALTH-PROMOTION TOOL

Media can promote health in three ways: public education, social marketing, and media advocacy. The first two are often used to help people change their health behaviors by acquiring important information that they lacked (public education) or through visual or verbal messaging that can shift the individual's thinking, attitudes, and values (social marketing). Both of these can also be used to shape public policy and political campaigns, but media advocacy specifically targets public policy.

MEDIA ADVOCACY

Media advocacy is the strategic use of media to apply pressure to advance a social or public policy initiative (Dorfman, Wallack, & Woodruff, 2005; Jernigan & Wright, 1996; Wallack & Dorfman, 1996). It is a tool for policy change—a way of mobilizing constituencies and stakeholders to support or oppose specific policy changes. It differs from social marketing and is a means of political action (DeJong, 1996).

The success of Mothers Against Drunk Driving (MADD) is illustrative of the power of media advocacy. MADD was formed in 1980 at a time when a drunk driver could kill a child and it would not be treated as a crime. MADD developed a policy agenda aimed at preventing drunk driving. It developed a "Rating the States" program to bring public attention to what state governments were and were not doing to fight alcohol-impaired driving. Then, just after Thanksgiving (the beginning of a period of high numbers of alcohol-related traffic accidents), MADD representatives held local press conferences with their state's officials and members of other advocacy groups to announce the state's rating. Local and national broadcast and print press brought the story to an estimated 62.5 million people. Subsequently, lawmakers in at least eight states took action to address drunken driving (Russell, Voas, DeJong, & Chaloupka, 1995). Today, MADD's website (www.madd.org) advocates a number of policy changes that people can sign onto, a walk to raise funds to support the organization's work, a link to its Twitter page, and news about drunk driving initiatives.

Getting on the news media's agenda is one of the functions of media advocacy (Wallack, 1994). With numerous competing potential stories, media advocacy employs strategies to frame an issue in a way that will attract media coverage. For example, MADD often created media events by putting a wrecked car in front of a local high school a few days prior to a prom. Journalists flocked to these events. The visual of the wrecked car got people's attention, particularly reporters. The news accounts and parental outrage that resulted from these media events eventually led to wide social support for the concept of "designated driver" and harsher penalties for "driving under the influence."

How a message is presented is as important as simply getting the attention of the news media. The demise of Clinton's Health Security Act demonstrates this point. It got on the media's agenda, but the important messages were lost in the strategic use of the Harry and Louise commercials.

FRAMING

Getting an issue on the agenda of the public and policy makers and shaping the message require framing (Dorfman et al., 2005). Framing "defines the boundaries of public discussion about an issue" (Wallack & Dorfman, 1996,

p. 299). Reframing involves breaking out of the dominant perspective (or frame) on an issue to define a new way of thinking about it that can lead to very different ideas about potentially effective policy responses. Reframing requires working hard to understand the dominant frame, the values that undergird it, and its limitations, and then exploring new frames.

Framing applies to all messaging and policy work, whether changing staffing policies in a hospital or promoting legislation that will remove soft drinks from school vending machines. From a media perspective, framing for access entails shaping the issue in a way that will attract media attention. It helps to attach the issue to a local concern or event, anniversaries, or celebrities, or to "make news" by holding events that will attract the press, such as releasing new research at a press conference (Jernigan & Wright, 1996). Most importantly, it requires some element of controversy (albeit not over the accuracy of advocates' facts), conflict, injustice, or irony. The targeted medium or media will shape how the story is presented. For example, television requires compelling visual images. If a broad audience is to be reached, a powerful, brief message on television can provide a quick frame for an issue and narrow how people will view it. But the interactive nature of social media provides the opportunity for others to continue to reframe a message, helping people to break out of a dominant frame.

Framing for content is more difficult than for access. A compelling individual story may gain visibility in some media, but there is no guarantee that the reporter or social media activists will focus on the public policy changes that you want. Wallack and Dorfman (1996) suggest that this reframing can be accomplished by the following:

- Emphasizing the social dimensions of the problem and translating an individual's personal story into a public issue
- Shifting the responsibility for the problem from the individual to the corporate executive or public official whose decisions can address the problem
- Presenting solutions as policy alternatives
- Making a practical appeal to support the solution
- Using compelling images
- Using authentic voices—people who have experience with the problem
- Using symbols that "resonate with the basic values of the audience" (Wallack & Dorfman, 1996, p. 300)
- Anticipating the opposition and knowing all sides of the issue

Framing is not just about verbal messages. Jacob Riis was a social reformer who used visual imagery and the latest technology to frame issues in ways that would influence policy makers. Riis emigrated to the United States from Copenhagen in 1871 and found work as a reporter in New York City. As a reporter, his beat was writing about the Lower East Side of New York where, in the 1880s, 334,000 people were crammed into a single square mile, making it the most densely populated place on earth. The people there were living in disease-ridden tenements, often with 10 or 15 to a room (Burrows & Wallace, 2000). Riis wrote often about their plight for his newspaper; he identified with the people on the Lower East Side, mostly immigrants like himself. Moved as he was, he grew frustrated by the lack of response from his readers. Riis had considered using photography to tell the stories of these New Yorkers, but the photographic technology of the day required a lot of light—which was scarce in a dark, airless tenement. Then, Riis read about a new technology from Germany called "flash photography." Riis started using flash technology to photograph some of the poorest New Yorkers and the deplorable conditions in which they lived and worked. In 1899, Scribner's Magazine published an 18-page article by Riis that included 19 of his photographs. Based on that article, a publisher invited Riis to publish an entire book, and his *How the Other Half Lives* became influential in shaping the early progressive movement working on behalf of immigrants' rights. Riis's photographs also influenced a young New York politician by the name of Theodore Roosevelt to implement public health laws that improved the city's health and are still in place today.

Today, many bloggers include a photo or image with each post to draw attention to an entry. The images help to convey the frame that the bloggers want.

FOCUS ON REPORTING

One can argue that individual journalists are equally responsible for their choice of issues to cover and how they cover them. Journalists rarely have the same depth of knowledge about a topic as insiders. In fact, prior to the rise of social media, journalists and traditional media contributed to a public cynicism of politics and policy makers that resulted in a largely uninvolved citizenry (Fallows, 1996). This is due partially to journalists' having limited expertise on particular issues; as a result, they often cover only the political dimensions of an issue rather than the details of the policy options. This, in combination with the growth in polarized television "news" programs and politicized talk radio shows, requires careful analysis of "news." But, social media also provides myriad opportunities for false, biased, and inflammatory messaging.

Getting to know the nature and quality of a particular journalist's or cyberactivist's work can help you to decide how much trust to place in it. Ask the following questions:

- Do they frequently misrepresent issues?
- Are their stories sensationalized, overplayed, or exaggerated?
- Do they present all sides of an issue with accuracy, fairness, and depth?

■ Can you substantiate wild claims through sites such as www.snopes. com, www.urbanlegends.about.com, and www.truthorfiction.com?

In reality, few journalists have the time and the editorial support or the breadth and depth of knowledge about science to provide thorough reporting on health issues that have policy implications. This often results in less-than-adequate reporting on important issues, such as the reporting on how communities should respond to the West Nile virus. Roche (2002) examined print media coverage of the approaches for reducing the mosquito population to reduce the incidence of and mortality from West Nile encephalitis. None of the newspapers or magazines examined gave any information about risk of mortality from pesticide exposure or a cost analysis of this approach. Roche concluded that the public is "operating 'in the dark' in evaluating the question of whether pesticides should be deployed."

Health professionals and community health leaders can assist journalists and cyberactivists by both reframing health policy issues and providing the depth of detail that others may lack. For example, a journalist covering a story on obesity in poor neighborhoods has focused on individual health behaviors like lack of vegetable consumption and low rates of exercise. Health advocates could assist the journalist by reframing the story as a structural issue by focusing attention on the lack of fresh produce and park space in low-income neighborhoods, as well as the subsidizing of foods with corn-syrup additives, which are disproportionately sold and consumed in low-income neighborhoods. While talking with this journalist does not ensure that your frame will be incorporated into the journalist's story, you can push out the frame you believe is important through your blog, Facebook page, or Twitter account.

One strategy is to facilitate information exchange in the public arena by becoming news makers, aggregators, or curators of health news. Posting links to news articles and research on critical policy issues on social media sites such as Facebook makes the news easy to find. Health professionals and community health leaders are positioned to explain complex health policy issues by breaking them down, not just for information sharing but for civil engagement, so people will act, whether by having a conversation with a coworker about the issue or contacting government representatives. Facebook friends, including other health professional colleagues or community members, can click "share" on Facebook, which reposts these articles to their personal networks to widen the community in infinite ways. Social networking can generate a buzz and create conversations about an issue or policy. It is "digital activism" and has enormous potential to build networks, propagate power, and frame issues.

EFFECTIVE USE OF MEDIA

Formal training for health professionals and community leaders rarely includes information about how to use traditional media or new forms of social media. The following recommendations provide readers with a starting point for effectively using traditional and social media.

POSITIONING YOURSELF AS AN EXPERT

Whereas health policy was once the domain of a limited field of experts setting the agenda for the rest of us, the rise of user-generated content signals a radical departure from this approach. The emergence of user-generated content means a profound transformation in what it means to be an expert and opens the possibility of a wider range of types of expertise. New media provides health professionals with platforms to reach the public as media makers and aggregators of reliable health research information.

Gain Credentials. There are many types of credentials, although they are typically thought of as degrees from educational institutions, work titles, and affiliations. Some institutions require that their employees notify them of any interaction with media, but this may be unnecessary if you don't name the institution in your interview or other communication. For example, you could be a "health professional at women's clinic."

Become an Expert in Your Field. Becoming the "go to" person who is the expert on a topic or particular field is another way to establish yourself as an expert. You can establish this by launching your own professional website, blog, and Twitter and Facebook pages, as well as by meeting with local journalists who cover health.

Use Personal Experience. Part of why the MADD campaign has been compelling is their strategic use of stories from women whose children have been killed as a result of drunk driving. These bereaved mothers involved with MADD have transformed themselves into experts on the policy of driving while intoxicated and used their experience to make this point with policy makers. Similarly, people who were infected with HIV/AIDS in the 1980s and believed that the federal government was acting too slowly to move treatment through clinical trials made themselves experts on the science of the disease and, using a variety of tactics, forced policy makers to speed up the time for drugs to market. The Internet facilitates the rise of this kind of expertise.

Create Your Own Brand of Expertise. You can also become an expert in your field through some unique-to-you combination of all of these. Individual policy makers weigh these differently. For example, after the death of her two-and-half-year-old son from *Escherichia coli*, Barbara Kowalcyk became an expert in food-borne illness. Eventually, she started a nonprofit organization called Center for Foodborne Illness & Prevention (CFI) (www.foodborneillness.org) and lobbied Congress to adopt laws for better food safety.

GETTING YOUR MESSAGE ACROSS

Getting your message to the appropriate target audience requires careful analysis and planning. For example, you might want to target a message to local homeowners, many of whom watch a particular TV station's evening news. To get television coverage, you must have a visual story. Health advocates in California staged a media event on a senior health issue with a "rock around the clock" marathon, with seniors in rocking chairs outside an insurance company. They received press coverage of the event, which elicited some supportive letters to the editor, as well as some negative press from seniors who said that they were stereotyping older adults.

Reaching ethnically and linguistically diverse populations requires a familiarity with their preferred media and tapping into the growing use of social media. According to a 2009 study by the Pew Internet and American Life Project, African Americans were the most active users of the mobile Internet through frequent use of smart phones—at a rate that was twice the national average (Horrigan, 2009). While social media technology and its use are moving targets, the expectation is that smart phones and ordinary cell phones will continue to transform how we distribute messages, including to provide health care and to influence health policy. The Connecticut Health Foundation (www.cthealth.org) realized that online and offline conversations about ethnic disparities in health and health care were not occurring outside of academia. With the aim of creating "public will to decrease racial and ethnic health disparities in access and treatment," the foundation launched a social media project that included training of nonprofits in the use of social media (http://tinyurl.com/6kuak4d).

BLOGGING AND MICROBLOGGING

A 2006 random sample telephone survey conducted by the Pew Internet and American Life Project found that the American blogosphere was dominated by those who use their blogs as personal journals. When asked to choose just one topic that they blog about, 37% of bloggers responded that "my life and experiences" as their primary focus. Politics and government ran a very distant second with 11% of bloggers citing issues of public life as the main subject of their blog. Entertainment-themed topics were the next most popular category of blog (7%); followed by sports (6%); general news and current events (5%); business technology (4%); religion, spirituality, or faith (2%); and a specific health problem or illness (2%). Of interest here is the 2% that blog about a specific health problem or illness. While this is a comparatively small percentage of the total blogosphere, this 2% still constitutes a vast universe of health blogs. A conservative estimate would place the number of health blogs in the hundreds of thousands, and a less conservative estimate would be upwards of five million; and these blogs are consulted by an estimated 60 million users in the United States, according to research conducted in 2008 (Manhattan Research, 2008). While most blogs are maintained by individuals who are affected by a particular health condition, some health-related blogs are sponsored by traditional newspapers or by community activist organizations.

Theresa Brown is an oncology nurse living and working in Pittsburgh. Her first career was as a doctorally prepared English professor before deciding that she wanted to work more closely with people. She wrote a narrative about a dying patient that was published on the first page of the *New York Times* Science section, which until then had been dominated by physicians' narratives. She was then invited to contribute to the *Times's* health blog, *Well*, and now does so on a regular basis. As a result, issues of concern to practicing nurses and patients get regular visibility through her posts. Her expertise as a nurse in cancer care is clearly valued by those who post responses to her blog entries.

Twitter, an example of microblogging, is a great way for health professionals to listen as well as talk to others on a very direct level. Twitter allows users to post short, 140-character, messages. For longer conversations, people use hash tags (# symbols) to track topics. People are very creative in the way they use Twitter, and it holds a great deal of potential for health professionals. For example, you can use it to convey your position on legislation that is up for a vote on the local, state, or national level to inform public debate on how this policy will impact the health and well-being of individuals and communities. You can also use Twitter—and other social media such as Facebook—to link to relevant data supporting your position and to see what others are saying about this policy: Is it positive? Negative? Misinformed? Journalists frequently use Twitter to find sources and information on stories they're covering, or to simply uncover new stories. Following key health journalists can provide opportunities for recommending yourself or other health professionals as experts on specific topics or to help them to reframe their stories.

FACEBOOK AND MYSPACE: USING SOCIAL NETWORKING SITES

The development of Web 2.0 has meant increased participation and media attention on virtual communities, most frequently in social networking sites (SNS) such as Facebook and MySpace. The impact that SNS will have on health policy is still emerging, but there are some intriguing early examples of the advantage they may hold for advocacy. For instance, Facebook has emerged as an important venue for debate about health policy, and not just among people typically thought of as policy makers. The health care reform battle sparked a large number of for- and against-themed pages, such as Ohio Against Health Care Reform (81 fans), Wyoming for Health Care Reform (247 fans), and the perennial Facebook meme, "I bet we can find 1,000,000 people who support/ oppose" health care reform. While measuring the effectiveness of such Facebook campaigns remains elusive, we should expect to see more of this type of activity as health care reform continues to be implemented over the coming years.

The promise of online communities and social networking sites (SNS) for community health advocacy has captured the attention of major funders in health policy, including the Robert Wood Johnson Foundation (www.rwjf. org) and the Benton Foundation (www.benton.org). In a unique joint venture between Robert Wood Johnson and Benton in 2007, the two foundations launched New Routes to Community Health (www.newroutes.org/). New Routes, a Madison, Wisconsin-based initiative, is an attempt to bring the power of a SNS to bear on improving the health of immigrants. It does this through immigrant-created media and by funding other immigrant-led collaborations across the United States. In each of these efforts, immigrants have worked to create locally focused media and outreach campaigns that speak directly to immigrants' health concerns in their area.

BUILDING COMMUNITY AND WORKING WITH PARTNERS

In the pre-Internet era, activists made use of existing technology to mobilize supporters through the use of "phone trees." One person would call 10 others, and each of those 10 would call 10 others, and so on. In the digital era, cyberactivists use Web 2.0 to accomplish a number of different goals, including public representation of their cause through an online presence, information distribution to and solidarity with other cyberactivists, outreach to potential new supporters, fund-raising, and direct action (Costanza-Chock, 2003). With Web 2.0 technologies, social networks can be built, accessed, and amplified, particularly with features such as always-on connectivity. Taken together, these features allow tremendous potential to leverage Web 2.0 to advocate for change with cybertools that are constantly evolving.

ANALYZING MEDIA

The first obligation that all health professionals and community leaders have is to be knowledgeable consumers of media. They must seek out factual unbiased information from many sources before taking positions on policy issues and be able to critically evaluate media messages, assess who controls the media, and identify whose vested interests are being protected or promoted. Those working in the health fields should add www.

mediachannel.org and www.mediareform.net to their Internet favorites and evaluate their sources.

WHAT IS THE MEDIUM?

The first step is to ask yourself where you get your information and news.

- What TV and radio news programming do you regularly tune in to? Do you read a daily newspaper or go online to a trusted news website every morning?
- What is the station's, program's, paper's, or website's reputation? Is it known for balanced coverage of health-related issues? Is it partisan?
- Does it cover national as well as state and local issues?
- Is it a credible source of information about health issues and policies?

These questions provide a basis for you to judge whether or not the information and news you are getting are credible and representative of a broad sector of public opinion. For any particular issue of concern, you will want to sample various media presentations of the issue and evaluate their messages and effectiveness.

WHO IS SENDING THE MESSAGE?

Part of understanding what the real message is about comes from knowing who is behind the message and why. You could interpret the real message behind the Harry and Louise commercials against President Clinton's health care reform legislation once you knew they were sponsored by the HIAA. If the legislation had passed, the majority of insurance companies would have been locked out of the health care market. Instead, their media success left them in control of health care in the United States until 2010.

For news media, ask the following questions: Who owns this medium? Who sponsors the website? What are the owner's biases? In addition, more and more newspapers and online venues are using the Associated Press (AP), or other major national papers, as their source for stories. The AP does not investigate; they attend events, accept news releases, and file reports. If newspapers are using abridged stories from other papers, the news slant or bias of the other paper reflects the bias or slant of the paper you are analyzing. As newspaper and television newsroom budgets get slashed, few news outlets are able to afford investigative journalism. To preserve this important aspect of journalism, nonprofit investigative news organizations have arisen to fill the void, such as the online Kaiser Health News (www.kaiserhealthnews.org) founded and supported by Kaiser Family Foundation (KFF), and ProPublica, supported by a major multiyear commitment of funding by the Sandler Foundation. While Kaiser Health News is specific to health, ProPublica is not. Nonetheless, the latter does cover health issues. For example, ProPublica conducted an investigation in the influence drug companies exert over regulators (www.propublica.org/blog/item/e-mails-show-drug-company-used-third-party-medical-groups-to-influence-regu). Pharmaceutical company Sanofi-Aventis launched an advocacy campaign to influence the U.S. Food and Drug Administration and protect their brand-name blood thinner "Lovenox." Sanofi-Aventis wanted to delay generic competitors and did so by contacting medical societies and researchers, urging them to write in to the FDA—or in one case, to write an "advertorial" for the *Wall Street Journal*—to raise safety concerns about generics.

WHAT IS THE MESSAGE AND WHAT RHETORIC IS USED?

What is the ostensible message that is being delivered, and what is the real message? What rhetoric is used to get the real message across? In a protracted debate on social security during the administration of George W. Bush, his administration attempted to create a "crisis" of solvency that needed immediate reform.

Economists and organizations such as the AARP were successful in pointing out that the government's own actuaries demonstrate that the Social Security Trust is solvent through 2042 and that the fund will begin to spend more than it is receiving only in 2018, so there is no immediate crisis. But Bush's messages also appealed to individual self-interest in talking about an "ownership society" and "private accounts," which are contrary to the purpose of the social security system, which was set up in 1935 to protect all of society—especially older adults, the widowed, and the disabled. Bush's message avoided talking about the trust's solvency because his proposals actually contributed to insolvency earlier than what had been projected without any changes.

In 2005, pollster Luntz of the Luntz Research Companies provided an analysis of the rhetoric used in the 2004 presidential campaign and outlined rhetoric that Republicans would use to win legislative battles and political campaigns in 2006. Luntz's analysis also provides insight into the language used to frame some of the major issues that would confront the federal Republican policy makers. For example: "Sometimes it is not what you say that matters but what you don't say. Other times a single word or phrase can undermine or destroy the credibility of a paragraph or entire presentation...[E]ffectively communicating the New American Lexicon requires you to stop saying words and phrases that undermine your ability to educate the American people. So from today forward YOU are the language police. From today forward these are the words never to say again" (Luntz, 2005, Appendix, p. 1).

BANISH PRIVATIZATION FROM YOUR LEXICON

One of the words "never to say" was "privatization/private accounts." Rather, the document advocated the phrase "personalization/personal accounts." The report noted that "Many more Americans would 'personalize' Social Security than 'privatize' it. Personalizing Social Security suggests ownership and control over your retirement savings, while privatizing it suggests a profit motive and winners and losers" (Luntz, Appendix, p. 1).

Democrats were well aware of this difference in language and consistently framed the issue as "privatization." On health care, the document admonished never to say "healthcare choice" but rather to say "the right to choose," noting: This is an important nuance so often lost on political officials. Almost all Americans want "the right to choose the healthcare plan, hospital, doctor and prescription drug plan that is best for them," but far fewer Americans actually want to make that choice. In fact, the older you get, the less eager you are to have a wide range of choices (Luntz, 2005, Appendix, p. 4)

Every issue has "spin doctors" who develop believable messages based on focus groups and polling. As messages are repeated in the media, they become normalized and believable. It is essential to be attentive to the language used in media messages—whether delivered directly by policy makers, pundits, or advocates—and evaluate the credibility, bias, and intentions of sources.

WHAT AND WHOM SHOULD WE BELIEVE?

Images also convey important messages. As the Luntz document notes, "Language is your base. Symbols knock it out of the park. The American people cannot always be expected to directly grasp the connection between your policies and your principles. Symbols bridge this gap, so use them" (Section 2, p. 2). The document promotes the obvious symbols of the American flag and Statue of Liberty. But consider the symbols used by health insurance companies to advertise to employed individuals and families. These ads use pictures of healthy active adults and bright-eyed children. Health insurers have never used images of obese individuals or people disabled by arthritis to attract new members to their insurance products. These are examples of targeted media messages in which images are symbols to augment carefully crafted rhetoric to sway a target audience to believe or act in a particular way.

IS THE MESSAGE EFFECTIVE?

Does the message attract your attention? Does it appeal to your logic and to your emotions? Does it undermine the opposition's position?

IS THE MESSAGE ACCURATE?

Who is the reporter or cyberactivist, and what reputation do they have? Are they credible, with a reputation for accuracy and balanced coverage of an issue? What viewpoints are missing? Whose voice is represented in the message or article?

RESPONDING TO THE MEDIA

One of the most important ways to influence public opinion is to respond to what is read, seen, or heard in the media. Letters to the editor or call-ins to talk radio programs can be powerful ways to reframe an issue or put it on the public's agenda. Opinion editorials ("op eds") allow more in-depth response to current issues and provide a way to get an issue on the public's agenda. Although they are often solicited by a newspaper or magazine, particularly in large cities, local community papers are often eager to receive editorials that describe an important issue or problem, include a story that illustrates the local impact of the problem, and suggest possible solutions.

Tips for successful op eds include the following:

- Keep it short and within the word limit specified by the publication.
- Hook it to a national event if the publication or website has a national focus, or to a local event for local publications.
- Have a timely topic, concisely and clearly written in a conversational style, and with an unexpected or provocative slant.
- Include details or examples to bring the commentary alive.
- Define the problem and the solution(s).

Similarly, letters to the editor should be written immediately after the original story is published and follow the publication's guidelines for letters. They should be concise and make a specific point relevant to the article. Calling in to talk radio provides another opportunity for sharing your perspectives. Remember to identify yourself as a health professional and to stay on the line while the host or program guest responds to your point or question. You may need to correct a misunderstanding or offer additional clarifying information.

Finally, it's always a good idea to contact a journalist to thank him or her for a good story. If you have a blog, be sure to link to the story in a post. If you see a Tweet you like, you can "re-Tweet" it to others who follow you. If you're on Facebook and like someone's posting, you can click on the "Like" button to register your approval and continue the viral spread of the posting.

CONCLUSION

Health professionals and community health leaders have not always been taught how to use the media as a health-promotion tool. But sometimes we have to teach ourselves how to navigate in this rapidly changing world. Certainly, harnessing the new social media will provide myriad opportunities for health professionals and community health leaders to shape healthy public policies and engage in political activism. But use of traditional media can also help to spread a message.

Case Study Exercises

Individually, or as a group, review the following case Studies and respond to the questions posed at the end of the study, as appropriate. Be sure to focus on the why, how, and what emphasized in each question. Your professor/instructor will provide you with specific guidance on how you are to report your findings for the class.

Case Study 12.1. "Staying Alive"—HIV Programming From MTV and KFF Partnership

The partnership between MTV and the KFF has been a remarkably successful one for raising awareness about HIV and AIDS.

In the late 1990s and early 2000s, MTV produced several stand-alone HIV/AIDS documentaries for the annual World AIDS Day. Then, the television network decided to develop a more comprehensive media response to the global HIV epidemic. To realize this vision, MTV partnered with the KFF.

In 2002, MTV and KFF launched Staying Alive, a series of programs intended to heighten awareness about HIV prevention. The programs aired on TV stations serving nearly 500 million households. When China's CCTV aired the *Staying Alive* documentary in March 2003 that number rose to nearly 800 million households. This amounted to 64% of all television households worldwide at that time.

The degree of exposure to the campaign was measured at three global locations: Kathmandu, Nepal; Sao Paolo, Brazil; and Dakar, Senegal. Among youth ages 16 to 25, 12% in Nepal had seen the campaign, compared to 23% in Brazil and 82% in Senegal. Evaluation of the Staying Alive campaign suggests that media messages about HIV/AIDS increase interpersonal communication about the disease, which may lead to positive changes in policies about HIV/AIDS (Geary, Burke, et al., 2007; Geary, Mahler, et al., 2005).

Study Questions

1. In what way does the partnership between MTV and KFF illustrate the "one-to-many" media paradigm?
2. What are the advantages of such a partnership, especially in terms of "reach"?
3. Are there any disadvantages to a global media campaign such as Staying Alive?

Case Study 12.2: "Mobileactivistas" in Argentina

In regions of the world without a well-developed infrastructure for landline telephones, as in many parts of South American and Africa, mobile phones are much more prevalent. In addition, the pricing structure for mobile phone service in the rest of the world and the United States is completely different, such that sending a text message (or SMS) is much cheaper, even free, compared to making a voice call. Taken together, these have resulted in some interesting uses of mobile phones by activists concerned about issues that affect health.

For example, Greenpeace Argentina successfully used an SMS campaign to stop the destruction of the Pizarro Reserve (a nature reserve) from being sold and subsequently destroyed. First, Greenpeace Argentina introduced legislation to parliament that would prevent future destruction of the Pizarro Reserve. Next, they launched a communication strategy rooted in SMS technology. The group placed print-ads in public bathrooms and in their (print) magazine asking people to join them as "mobileactivistas" (mobile activists) by sending a specific word to their mobile number. The sender's number was then stored in an SMS database used primarily for real-time communication and action. Through this extremely inexpensive strategy more than 4,500 *mobileactivistas* participated in this campaign so far. Mobile-activists sent text messages to legislators and key players involved in the bill's various hearings. SMS was also used to arrange spontaneous meeting points and public demonstrations.

The SMS campaign allowed *mobileactivistas* to stay informed and act quickly during the bill's journey through the legislative process. When Greenpeace Argentina learned that the bill was at risk due to a strong waste industry, they immediately sent text messages to all the mobile-activists on the database. The *mobileactivistas* responded by pressuring specialists and members of the commission to approve the bill and move it on to the next round of discussions. Throughout the campaign to save the Pizarro Reserve, SMS was the primary means of communication between movement organizers and *mobileactivistas* (Greenpeace Argentina).

Study Questions

1. In what way do the "mobileactivistas" illustrate the "many-to-many" media paradigm? How did Greenpeace Argentina incorporate "old" forms of media to get the word out about the SMS campaign?
2. What are the advantages of such a partnership, especially in terms of speed? What else?

REFERENCES

Abramson, A. (2003). *The history of television, 1942 to 2000.* New York, NY: McFarland.

Annenberg Public Policy Center of the University of Pennsylvania. (1995). *Media in the middle: Fairness and accuracy in the 1994 health care reform debate.* Philadelphia, PA: Annenberg Public Policy Center.

Bauder, D. (2007, March 14). *For HBO executive, series on "addiction" is personal.* Boston Globe. Retrieved from www.boston.com/ae/tv/articles/2007/03/14/for_hbo_executive_series_on_addiction_is_personal

Burrows, E., & Wallace, M. (2000). *Gotham: A history of New York City to 1898.* New York, NY: Oxford University Press.

Costanza-Chock, S. (2003). Mapping the repertoire of electronic contention. In A. Opel & D. Pompper (Eds.), *Representing resistance: Media, civil disobedience and the global justice movement* (pp. 173–191). New York, NY: Greenwood Press.

Daniels, J. (2009). Cloaked websites: Propaganda, cyber-racism and epistemology in the digital era. *New Media & Society, 11*(5), 659–683.

DeJong, W. (1996). MADD Massachusetts versus Senator Burke: A media advocacy case study. *Health Education Quarterly, 23*(3), 318–329.

Dorfman, L., Wallack, L., & Woodruff, K. (2005). More than a message: Framing public health advocacy to change corporate practices. *Health Education and Behavior, 323,* 320–336.

Fallows, J. (1996). *Breaking the news: How the media undermine American society.* New York, NY: Vintage Books.

Geary, C. W., Burke, H. M., Castelnau, L., Neupane, S., Sall, Y. B., & Wong, E. (2007). Exposure to MTV's global HIV prevention campaign in Kathmandu, Nepal; São Paulo, Brazil; and Dakar, Senegal. *AIDS Education and Prevention, 19*(1), 36–50.

Geary, C. W., Mahler, H., Finger, W., & Shears K. H. (2005). *Using global media to reach youth: The 2002 MTV Staying Alive campaign.* Arlington, VA: Family Health International, YouthNet Program.

Greenpeace Argentina. Retrieved from www.greenpeace.org/argentina/es/

Harris, J. (2005). To be our own governors: The independent press and the battle for "popular information". In E. D. Cohen (Ed.), *News incorporated* (pp. 79–95). Amherst, MA: Prometheus Books.

Horrigan, J. (2009). *Wireless Internet use.* Pew Internet and American Life Project. Retrieved from www.pewinternet.org/Reports/2009/12-Wireless-Internet-Use/1-Summary-of-Findings.aspx

Jernigan, D. H., & Wright, P. A. (1996). Media advocacy: Lessons from community experiences. *Journal of Public Health Policy, 18,* 306–329.

Kaiser Family Foundation. (2010). *Generation M2: Media in the lives of 8- to 18-year-olds.* Menlo Park, CA: Author.

Lardinois, R. (2008, November 5). *Obama's social media advantage.* ReadWriteWeb. Retrieved from www.readwriteweb.com/archives/social_media_obama_mccain_comparison.php

Luntz, F. (2005). *The new American lexicon.* Alexandria, VA: The Luntz Research Companies. Retrieved from www.dailykos.com/story/2005/2/23/3244/72156

Manhattan Research. (2008). *Cybercitizen Health™, v 8.0.* Retrieved from www.manhattanresearch.com/cch

McAlister, A. L. (1991). Population behavior change: A theory-based approach. *Journal of Public Health Policy, 12*(3), 345–361.

Nielsen reports television tuning remains at record levels. (2007, October 17). Retrieved from http://en-us.nielsen.com/content/nielsen/en_us/news/news_releases/2007/october/Nielsen_Reports_Television_Tuning_Remains_at_Record_Levels.html

O'Reilly, T. (2005, September 30). *What is Web 2.0: Design patterns and business models for the next generation of software.* Retrieved from www.oreillynet.com/pub/a/oreilly/tim/news/2005/09/30/ what-isweb-20.html?page=1

Ozimek, T. (2005). Distributed campaigns: Using the Internet to empower action. In D. Mason, J. Leavitt, & M. Chaffee (Eds.), *Policy and politics in nursing and health care* (5th ed., pp. 171–176). St. Louis, MO: WB Saunders/Elsevier.

Ritzer, G., & Jurgenson, N. (2010). Production, consumption, prosumption: The nature of capitalism in the age of the digital "prosumer". *Journal of Consumer Culture, 10*(1), 13–36.

Roche, J. P. (2002). Print media coverage of risk-risk tradeoffs associated with West Nile encephalitis and pesticide spraying. *Journal of Urban Health, 79*(4), 482–490.

Russell, A., Voas, R. B., DeJong, W., & Chaloupka, M. (1995). MADD rates the states: Advocacy event to advance the agenda against alcohol-impaired driving. *Public Health Reports, 110*(3), 240–245.

Schwartz, M. (2010, April 9). *Research and markets: 50% mobile penetration in Africa this year.* Developing Telecoms. Retrieved from www.developingtelecoms.com/research-and-markets-50-mobile-penetration-in-africa-this-year.html

Talbot, D. (2008, September/October). *How Obama really did it: The social-networking strategy that took an obscure senator to the doors of the White House.* Technology Review. Retrieved from www.technologyreview.com/web/21222

Turow, J. (1996). Television entertainment and the U.S. health-care debate. *Lancet, 347*(9010), 1240–1243.

Turow, J., & Gans, R. (2002). *As seen on TV: Health policy issues in TV's medical dramas.* Menlo Park, CA: The Henry J. Kaiser Family Foundation.

Wallack, L. (1994). Media advocacy: A strategy for empowering people and communities. *Journal of Public Health Policy, 15,* 420–436.

Wallack, L., & Dorfman, L. (1996). Media advocacy: A strategy for advancing policy and promoting health. *Health Education Quarterly, 23*(3), 293–317.

Whitney, R., & Viswanath, K. (2004). Lessons learned from public health mass media campaigns: Marketing health in a crowded media world. *Annual Review of Public Health, 25,* 419–437.

13

Community Resilience, Disasters, and the Public's Health

Rose L. Pfefferbaum and Richard W. Klomp

LEARNING OBJECTIVES

What you can learn from studying chapter:

- To identify and list public health's main roles and responsibilities with respect to disasters
- How to define resilience
- How to describe resilience as an emergent process as distinct from an attribute
- How to distinguish community resilience from personal resilience
- What the role of human agency is in community resilience
- How to describe attributes, properties, and adaptive capacities associated with community resilience
- How to describe strategies for developing community resilience to disasters

With the ubiquitous threat of disasters, it is incumbent upon government, business, nonprofit organizations, and the general public to create a culture that fosters disaster readiness, response, and recovery. Everyone has a role, everyone has responsibilities. This is emphasized by the call for resilient communities, a "proactive and positive expression of community engagement" (Cutter et al., 2008b, p. 598) that can help "break the cycle of destruction and recovery" associated with major disasters (Subcommittee on Disaster Reduction, 2005, p. 1). Public health and the health care sector constitute essential components of disaster management that can help rally and direct multiple, sometimes disparate, players toward a common goal, while establishing systems to foster effective prevention and mitigation, preparedness, response, and recovery.

The role of public health is "to assure the conditions necessary for people to live healthy lives, through community-wide prevention and protection programs" (Centers for Disease Control and Prevention [CDC], n.d., p. 1). Public health's obligation to respond to disasters and assist with recovery is both explicit and implied by other obligations such as preventing epidemics and the spread of disease, protecting against environmental hazards, preventing injuries, promoting and encouraging healthy behaviors and mental health, and ensuring the quality and accessibility of health services. Public health meets these obligations—within the context of disasters and otherwise—by providing an array of essential services, including (1) monitoring health status to identify and address community health problems, (2) diagnosing and investigating health problems and community health hazards that may preexist and lead to public health crises or that may result from disasters, (3) informing, educating, and empowering the public about health issues, (4) mobilizing community stakeholders and stimulating action to identify and address health problems, (5) developing policies and plans to support individual and community health efforts, (6) enforcing laws and regulations to protect health and safety, (7) connecting individuals with needed personal health services and ensuring the provision of care when otherwise unavailable, (8) ensuring a competent health care workforce, (9) evaluating the effectiveness, accessibility, and quality of personal and public health services, and (10) conducting research to solve health problems (CDC, n.d.).

Homeland Security Presidential Directive 21 (HSPD 21) establishes a National Strategy for Public Health and Medical Preparedness, which will "transform our national approach to protecting the health of the American people against all disasters" (U.S. Department of Homeland Security [USDHS], 2007, p. 2). Identifying community resilience as one of the four most critical components of public health and medical preparedness, HSPD 21 describes community resilience and directs the federal government to assist states and local authorities to build community resilience to health catastrophes:

> *Where local civic leaders, citizens, and families are educated regarding threats and are empowered to mitigate their own risk, where they are practiced in responding to events, where they have social networks to fall back upon, and where they have familiarity with local public health and medical systems, there will be community resilience that will significantly attenuate the requirement for additional assistance. The Federal Government must formulate a comprehensive plan for promoting community public health and medical preparedness to assist State and local authorities in building resilient communities in the face of potential catastrophic health events. (USDHS, 2007)*

Not always consistently defined, community resilience has emerged recently as a construct that is viewed sometimes as a goal and sometimes as a mechanism for achieving disaster readiness, response, and recovery. Community resilience both supports and requires effective disaster management. This chapter addresses community resilience and its relationship to disaster readiness, response, and recovery in the context of the public's health. After providing definitions, characteristics of community resilience and attributes, properties, and adaptive capacities of resilient communities are described. Seven strategies for building community resilience are offered for consideration. The chapter concludes with two case studies that explore approaches to developing community resilience.

DEFINITIONS

Community resilience is the foundation for the *National Health Security Strategy of the United States of America* (National Health Security Strategy) (U.S. Department of Health and Human Services [USDHHS], 2009), which envisions that the nation and its people be prepared for, be protected from, respond effectively to, and be able to recover from, incidents with potentially large-scale, negative health consequences such as disease outbreaks, natural disasters, and terrorist attacks. Appreciating community resilience and its role in mitigating the adverse effects of disasters requires an understanding of basic terminology, specifically the meaning of *disasters* and *resilience*.

Disasters

Disasters are extreme events that overwhelm the resources of a community or region, causing excess morbidity and mortality. They may result from internal or external forces, of natural and/or human origin, over which a community has no effective control. Disasters include, for example, hurricanes, tornados, and earthquakes; airplane crashes, industrial accidents, and major power outages; terrorist attacks, suicide bombings, and biological warfare; and epidemics and other mass-casualty events.

Often sudden and unexpected, disasters have both ecological and psychosocial effects. They erode the conditions necessary for people to live healthy lives by maiming and killing, destroying property, damaging built infrastructures, disrupting government and commerce, creating chaos and confusion, generating immeasurable emotional devastation, and unraveling the social fabric of communities. Disasters are collectively experienced (McFarlane & Norris, 2006), affecting the structure and functioning of communities by changing, at least temporarily, how individuals relate, the roles and the rules governing behavior, social networks and processes, and the allocation and use of resources. The ensuing physical, emotional, and socioeconomic destruction associated with disasters threatens the public's health and impedes productive interactions that could revive communal existence. Social support may deteriorate or be mobilized after a disaster depending, in part, on characteristics of the disaster and of the community and its membership (Jerusalem, Kaniasty, Lehman, Ritter, & Turnbull, 1995).

Resilience

As part of the lexicon of various disciplines (e.g., computer science, ecology, economics, engineering, geography, health, physical science, psychology, sociology), resilience is defined differently depending on context and purpose. The term may be used in reference to individuals, materials, networks, ecosystems, or communities, any of which is potentially relevant in relationship to disasters. For purposes of this chapter, resilience is defined as *the process of successfully adapting to, and recovering from, adversity*. This simple definition conceals differences among researchers, practitioners, and policy makers that may be important, especially for assessing resilience and generating evidence-based strategies for improving it. Several issues related to the meaning of resilience deserve exploration for a better understanding of community resilience.

UNDERSTANDING COMMUNITY RESILIENCE

Resilience can be best appreciated within the context of the adversity from which it emerges. While both involve human agency, community resilience must be distinguished from personal resilience. Some attributes, properties, and adaptive capacities of resilient communities are described below.

Resilience as an Emergent Process

Resilience is defined herein as a *process* of adaptation and recovery rather than as an *attribute* or an *outcome*. R. L. Pfefferbaum and colleagues (2008, p. 52) adopt a similar definition in describing community resilience as "a process evident in adaptation to threat or attack, stress, disruption, and security concerns." From this perspective, adaptation (rather than resilience) is the *outcome*. Norris, Stevens, Pfefferbaum, Wyche, and Pfefferbaum (2008, p. 130) also define resilience as a process, one "linking a set of adaptive capacities to a positive trajectory of functioning and adaptation" following a disturbance to a system. Resilience emerges from the adaptive capacities and leads to adaptation, an outcome characterized by wellness.

Plodinec (2009, p. 2) refers to the distinction between resilience as an *attribute* and resilience as a *process* as one of "Being vs. Becoming." Many authors define resilience as an attribute, commonly either as the *ability* or *capacity* of a system to resist, absorb, respond, adapt, and/or recover from adversity (see, e.g., Bruneau et al., 2003; Cutter et al., 2008a, 2008b; Federal Emergency Management Agency [FEMA], 2011; Longstaff, 2005; Plodinec, 2009; Subcommittee on Disaster Reduction, 2005; USDHS, 2010a). For example, resilience is defined in *The National Disaster Recovery Framework* as the "ability to adapt to changing conditions and withstand and rapidly recover from disruption due to emergencies" (FEMA, 2011, p. 81).

Butler, Morland, and Leskin (2007) define resilience by a set of *outcomes* associated with recovery following challenge. They also recognize that there are aspects of the recovery *process* that exemplify or signal elements of resilience. For them, resilience refers to recovery and the means and mechanisms of that recovery. They thereby link process with outcomes. Masten and Obradovic (2008, p. 2) complete the link between process, attributes, and outcomes, defining resilience as "the processes of, capacity for, or patterns of positive adaptation" during, or in the aftermath of, adversity.

The emphasis herein is on resilience as a process that emerges in response to adversity as opposed to being an inherent characteristic of a system. Resilience is not the absence of distress and adversity, but successful progress in spite of, in the midst of, and in response to distress and adversity (B. Pfefferbaum, Pfefferbaum, & Norris, 2009). A system may respond differently to different stressors and may respond differently to a given stressor at different points in time. Thus, a system may be resilient with respect to some adversities and not others. Those who define resilience as an attribute are likely to recognize that it can be affected by circumstances, thus lending a dynamic quality to it (see, e.g., Cutter et al., 2008a). In such characterizations, as with process definitions, resilience can be influenced by a variety of determinants, which is important for those who seek to build, as well as understand, resilience.

Differences Between Personal Resilience and Community Resilience

While similar definitions may apply, community resilience is not simply a collection of personally resilient individuals. The distinction between the two, which is enormous and often missed, may be understood, in part, by recognizing that the whole is more than the sum of its parts (Aristotle, translated in Ross, 2007). Thus, a community consisting of personally resilient individuals is not necessarily resilient (Brown & Kulig, 1996/1997; B. Pfefferbaum, Reissman, Pfefferbaum, Klomp, & Gurwitch, 2007; R. L. Pfefferbaum et al., 2008). Brown and Kulig (1996/1997, p. 43) describe relational aspects of communities in which members "are resilient together, not merely in similar ways." Community resilience emerges from collective activity in which individuals join together in efforts that foster response and recovery for the whole. Moreover, in resilient communities, individual and collective actions are buttressed by physical and social conditions and structures that enable resilience to manifest itself in the face of adversity (Brown & Kulig, 1996/1997; B. Pfefferbaum et al., 2007; R. L. Pfefferbaum et al., 2008). The health and public health infrastructures provide examples of systems that help create resilient communities by their roles in identifying, studying, preventing, and resolving threats and potential threats to healthy lifestyles.

Just as a collection of personally resilient individuals does not guarantee resilience of the community, a resilient community does not guarantee the resilience of individual members. While community resilience may strengthen the personal resilience of some, perhaps many, members by addressing functional and behavioral problems at the individual level (B. Pfefferbaum et al., 2007), some members of resilient communities tend not to adapt well to various adversities. Indeed, communities may rebound successfully from disasters even when some individual members do not.

The Role of Human Agency

Community resilience generally reflects an ability to adapt and change (Cutter et al., 2008a; Longstaff, 2005; Norris et al., 2008) and, according to some authors, the potential to grow from a crisis (Brown & Kulig, 1996/1997; B. Pfefferbaum et al., 2007; R. L. Pfefferbaum et al., 2008). Brown and Kulig (1996/1997) ground the concept of community resilience in human agency, that is, the capacity for deliberate, meaningful action. As such, community resilience consists of both proactive and reactive elements that link recovery with choices and efforts by individuals and groups to transform their physical and social environments to mitigate future adversities. Community members must be able to communicate effectively to interpret their environment and act collectively to remedy the effects of a crisis (Brown & Kulig, 1996/1997; Norris et al., 2008; B. Pfefferbaum et al., 2007; R. L. Pfefferbaum et al., 2008).

Attributes of Resilient Communities

R. L. Pfefferbaum and colleagues (2008) describe eight attributes of community resilience, which they identified through a review of the community competence and capacity literatures (Cottrell, 1976; Gibbon, Labonte, & Laverack, 2002; Goeppinger & Baglioni, 1985; Goodman et al., 1998; Labonte & Laverack, 2001a, 2001b), key informant interviews, and community surveys. The eight attributes are (1) connectedness, commitment, and shared values; (2) participation; (3) support and nurturance; (4) structure, roles, and responsibilities; (5) resources; (6) critical reflection and skill building; (7) communication; and (8) disaster management. These attributes are described below with examples.

Connectedness, Commitment, and Shared Values

A strong mutual interest; connection to a place; and a group of people with shared history, laws, values, interests, and customs are common ways to describe a community. The perception that community members are treated fairly and that one's personal well-being is improved by membership in the community can enhance one's sense of belonging and commitment to a community and may foster cooperation and consensus building. When diversity among members is supported, communities should be better able to address the needs of its members before, during, and after disasters. An example of this would be celebrating a city's birthday by having a fair at which the fire department gives away fire-prevention coloring books and the police department provides interested parents with instruction on basic principles of first aid.

Participation

A sense of belonging and feelings of ownership and identification can be strengthened by participation in community activities and organizations. This can lead to increased personal contribution and a commitment to safeguarding community life. Communities that encourage participation may find their members more actively engaged and invested in civic roles. When opportunities for involvement are extended to diverse members of the community in ways that are respectful and sensitive to the interests and demographics of those members, community leaders should be better able to identify and address concerns that arise in the absence of, as well as during and after, disasters. An example of this would be enlisting support of local service organizations (e.g., the Rotary Club, Kiwanis Club, Boy Scouts) to participate in service projects on Martin Luther King Day to clean up a local senior citizens center or paint over graffiti in a city park.

Support and Nurturance

Communities can bolster personal and collective resilience by attending to the needs of their members regardless of socioeconomic status, ethnicity, or level of education. Caring communities meet basic human needs, listen to members, help members to overcome challenges and achieve goals, promote well-being, empower individuals and groups, and instill hope. Communities that become adept at acquiring and equitably allocating resources should be better able to provide support and nurturance. In resilient communities, support mechanisms provide assessment of, and assistance to, vulnerable members before, during, and after disasters. Support must be sustained through crises if it is to buffer the personal, social, and economic losses that accompany these events. An example of this would be reaching out to the faith-based community, which often has commercial kitchens and buses, to invite their participation in preparedness, planning, and response efforts focused on providing emergency food services for vulnerable populations (e.g., individuals with limited mobility, non-native English speakers, individuals with vision impairment) within the community.

Structure, Roles, and Responsibilities

Resilient communities tend to reflect an appreciation for equity in establishing and applying community standards, rules, and procedures that foster social interaction and governance. Members learn and teach others to navigate the complex reciprocal links and overlapping networks among entities (e.g., individuals, groups, organizations, agencies) that comprise their community. Interactions tend to be relatively frequent and supportive, with individuals and groups identifying and addressing, rather than ignoring, common concerns. Solutions may emerge from formal or informal associations focused on establishing priorities and resolving issues. Strong and responsive leadership, teamwork, transparent organizational structures, and well-defined roles, responsibilities, and lines of authority facilitate collaboration. Reducing adverse secondary consequences of disasters requires structure, roles, and responsibilities that create the capacity for prevention, mitigation, and preparedness, as well as decisive and timely response to crises. In an all-hazards approach, structural elements must be flexible to address unforeseen vulnerabilities and threats. An example of this would be an elected official building a reputation as a good listener and consensus builder by regularly meeting with, sharing information with, and seeking input from a local advisory council comprised of representatives from the business, education, health care, mental and behavioral health, faith-based, media, and service sectors of the community.

Resources

In addition to land and other raw materials, resources include financial, human, and social assets belonging to members of the community and the community itself along with the built infrastructure and machinery and tools used in production. Money and credit constitute financial resources that facilitate the acquisition of other resources, the production and distribution of goods and services, and exchange within the community and across communities. Human resources include the workforce, expertise, and leadership, as well as member qualities such as hope, work ethic, and the will to improve community well-being. Social resources include relationships and support systems within a community and characteristics such as cohesion and collaboration. In resilient communities, redundancy in some resources is beneficial to maintain essential functions. Resilient communities generally acquire, mobilize, allocate, invest in, and use their resources effectively to serve members and meet community goals. Ongoing investment in physical, human, and social capital may be necessary to create infrastructures and systems that can endure and respond to a wide variety of potential disasters and threats. One example of this would be investing in improvements in schools, local health facilities, job-training programs, and neighborhood development. Another example would be establishing mutual aid agreements with neighboring communities that might facilitate access to scarce resources in an emergency.

Critical Reflection and Skill Building

Establishing structures to collect, analyze, and use information; identifying and addressing local issues, needs, and problems; recognizing and framing collective experiences; and planning, managing, and evaluating programs are activities at which resilient communities tend to excel. Critical reflection about values, their history and experiences, and the experiences of others, should permit formal and informal community leaders to establish worthwhile goals and objectives, make decisions, and develop and implement strategies for the benefit of the community and its members. Resilient communities assess their performance, study their successes and failures, learn from adversity, and support skill building at individual and systemic levels. Learning, accommodation, and growth may lead to enhanced capacity and improved disaster resilience. An example of this would be establishing a confidential and anonymous method of accessing feedback to generate a lessons-learned report from participants in a table-top exercise of an emergency response effort.

Communication

Clear, timely, accurate two-way communication among members, between authorities and community residents, and with other communities and the larger society is essential to community resilience. Productive communication requires shared meanings and understandings and the perception of honesty and openness. Diverse community members and groups should have opportunities to express their views and their needs, and they should be encouraged to participate in community problem solving. This can foster trust in leadership and, in the face of disasters, it can enhance preparedness, compliance with directives, effective response, and successful recovery. Effective communication also can identify and facilitate the resolution of existing and emerging unmet needs, as well as those that accompany disaster. Resilience to disasters depends on sufficient redundancy in communication channels to ensure timely resource mobilization and deployment. One example of this would be broadcasting public health reminders on popular local radio shows or including them in city water bills. Another example would be taking steps to generate dialogue with individuals from different sectors of the community through formal channels (e.g., citizen advisory groups, town hall meetings) and informal mechanisms (e.g., through conversations at barber shops, beauty parlors, sporting events).

Disaster Management

Implementing measures to prevent and mitigate, prepare for, and respond to disasters, thereby limiting adverse consequences and setting the stage for reconstruction and recovery, is required to achieve community resilience. Prevention and mitigation include activities to avoid or control an incident, to decrease risks to people and property, and to reduce potential or actual adverse effects. Mitigation measures, implemented prior to, during, or after an incident, should decrease the likelihood of hazardous incidents and limit exposure to, or potential loss from, such events. Preparedness is an ongoing process that assesses threats and vulnerabilities and identifies resource requirements. Preparedness also involves efforts to prevent and mitigate adverse consequences and to stockpile resources for response and recovery. Response addresses the direct, short-term effects of a disaster. In addition to emergency assistance, disaster response includes efforts to decrease further damage during or immediately after a disaster; to support basic human needs; and to maintain the social, economic, and political structure of an affected community. Survivors begin to rebuild their lives and their community as the relatively short-term response phase transitions into a longer period of recovery. An example of this would be establishing local Community Emergency Response Team (CERT) programs or immersing community leaders in disaster response training (e.g., free, online, training through the Federal Emergency Management Agency or the Red Cross) related to successfully implementing basic emergency response processes and systems.

Community Resilience Properties

Defining community resilience in the context of earthquakes, Bruneau and colleagues (2003) describe four properties of resilience for physical and social systems: (1) *robustness,* referring to strength or the ability to withstand stress without degradation or loss of function; (2) *redundancy,* referring to the functional substitutability of elements and systems; (3) *resourcefulness,* referring to the ability to identify problems, determine priorities, and mobilize resources in response to threats and disruptions; and (4) *rapidity,* referring to the ability to meet priorities and reach goals in a timely manner to limit losses and prevent future disruption. Robustness and rapidity are reflected in the description of resilience in the 2010 *Quadrennial Homeland Security Review Report* (QHSR Report) (USDHS, 2010b), which identifies resilience at the individual, community, and system levels as one of three key concepts essential to, and part of the foundation for, a comprehensive approach to homeland security. In describing resilience, the QHSR Report calls for "individual, community, and system robustness, adaptability, and capacity for rapid recovery" (USDHS, 2010b, p. 15).

Adaptive Capacities

Norris and colleagues (2008) describe four adaptive capacities from which community resilience emerges: economic development, social capital, information and communication, and community competence. These resilience resources have one or more dynamic attributes described by three of the properties identified by Bruneau and colleagues (2003): robustness, redundancy, and rapidity. Resilience depends on the resources themselves, as well as these dynamic properties. Health and public health systems contribute to the adaptive capacities of communities to the extent that they establish conditions necessary for the health and wellness of community members through personal and community prevention, preparedness, protection, response, and recovery programs and services.

Economic Development

As a capacity, economic development involves the level and diversity of economic resources (such as raw materials; machinery, tools, and equipment; the built environment; and a workforce), equity of resource distribution, and fairness of risk and vulnerability to hazards. Unfortunately, poor communities are not only at greater risk for destruction, they are frequently less successful in mobilizing support postdisaster. Community resilience is directly influenced by the capacity to distribute resources to those most in need (Norris et al., 2008).

Social Capital

Social capital can be defined as the aggregate of resources, both actual and potential, linked to possession of a durable network of relationships (Bourdieu, 1986; Norris et al., 2008). As an adaptive capacity associated with community resilience, social capital involves network structures and linkages; social support; and community bonds, roots, and commitments. Network structures and linkages include overlapping, interorganizational systems characterized by reciprocal links, frequent supportive interactions, and processes for cooperative decision making (Goodman et al., 1998; Norris et al., 2008). Social support includes social interactions that provide assistance (received or enacted social support) and those that are expected to provide assistance when the need for it arises (perceived or expected social support). Community bonds, roots, and commitment involve a sense of community, place attachment (i.e., an emotional connection to one's community), and citizen participation and grassroots leadership (Norris et al., 2008).

Information and Communication

A communication infrastructure, including responsible media, is an important aspect of this adaptive capacity since information and communication are essential for effective emergency management. A trusted source of accurate information is, according to Longstaff (2005), the most important resilience asset an individual or group can have. Communal narratives that give shared meaning and purpose to a traumatic experience also are a valuable part of the information and communication resource (Norris et al., 2008).

Community Competence

This adaptive capacity entails collective action and decision making, which may stem from collective efficacy and empowerment. Collective efficacy derives from mutual trust and willingness to work toward the common good (Norris et al., 2008). According to Cottrell (1976, p. 197), a competent community—one which "will be competent to cope with the problems of its collective life"—is one in which various components of the community collaborate effectively in identifying community problems and needs; come to a working consensus on goals and priorities; agree on ways and means for implementing agreed-upon goals; and take effective, collaborative action.

COMMUNITY RESILIENCE STRATEGIES

Community resilience is seen both as part of the vision for, and as a mechanism to accomplish, disaster readiness, response, and recovery. The construct is now imbedded in public health and homeland security policies and is becoming part of the discourse of emergency management. If the process of community resilience is to be supported, community leaders, professionals, and policy makers will have to generate and implement strategies for improving disaster resilience in the great variety of communities that populate the landscape. Norris and colleagues (2008) identify five resilience strategies for disaster preparedness based on their four adaptive capacities: (1) decrease risk and resource inequities, (2) engage members in mitigation, (3) create organizational links, (4) enhance and protect social supports, and (5) plan for the unexpected. R. L. Pfefferbaum and colleagues (2008) identify similar strategies with two notable additions: use a holistic wellness approach and promote a consciousness of community resilience. Seven strategies based on these recommendations are described below; they are explored in greater detail elsewhere with respect to Hurricane Katrina and its impact on children (see B. Pfefferbaum et al., 2009): (1) develop economic resources and address risk and resource inequities, (2) foster community engagement and participation, (3) create and strengthen organizational links, (4) enhance social supports, (5) undertake effective disaster planning and management, (6) adopt a holistic wellness approach, and (7) create a conscious awareness of community resilience.

Develop Economic Resources and Address Risk and Resource Inequities

The local resource base of a community becomes particularly important when there is a dearth of resources prior to, and/or as a result of, a disaster. When confronting similar environmental vulnerabilities and threats, poor communities that lack a solid economic base, individual and collective resources, and competent transformational leadership will be less able to mount an effective emergency management program than communities that are better endowed (R. L. Pfefferbaum et al., 2008). Communities that rely on a single business sector also are likely to be more vulnerable than those with a more diversified economic base (Cutter et al., 2008a). Some demographic and social characteristics increase a community's social vulnerability including, for example, inequities in income and wealth; limited access to information and resources; and marginalization due to ethnicity, language, or citizenship (Cutter et al., 2008a). Impoverished populations that routinely live with danger and insecurity often are less able to anticipate and respond effectively to external threats without assistance (Morrow, 2008). Thus, resources essential to community resilience, disaster response, and public health must be made available to them (Norris et al., 2008; B. Pfefferbaum et al., 2009). But, the creation of disaster-resilient communities within a disaster-resilient nation will require more than that. It will require economic development and public policies and programs that address resource inequities across and within communities (Morrow, 2008). It also will require the provision of functional infrastructure and essential public health services in all communities, rich and poor, so that equitable conditions exist to enable people to live truly healthy lives.

Foster Community Engagement and Participation

Social capital and community competence, two of the adaptive capacities associated with community resilience, can be enhanced through the engagement and participation of community residents. Informing, educating, and empowering community members about health issues is one of the major obligations of public health (CDC, n.d.), essential to the creation of communities more resilient to disasters. Kretzmann and McKnight (1993) maintain that when residents come together to address problems and when local organizations collaborate, communities are enriched and become more self-reliant. Community members will have increased capacity for self-direction when they believe in their ability to solve problems. Kretzmann and McKnight (1993) argue for engaging community members who are marginalized by age or label. Such individuals are likely to (1) perceive roles, responsibilities, and circumstances differently from the majority; (2) ask unanticipated questions; and (3) bring new energy and insight to the development process. Fullilove and Saul (2006) recognize the importance of the social and psychological investment of community members for the sustainability of community development programs.

Glass and Schoch-Spana (2002) make the case for public engagement in planning for bioterrorism response. They recommend that public and civic organizations be involved in practical public health activities, that communities invest in public outreach and communication, and that planning and intervention reflect the values and priorities of affected populations.

Community members also should assess and address their vulnerability to hazards, develop problem-solving abilities and specific strategies, and identify and access networks that provide information and assistance (Norris et al., 2008; B. Pfefferbaum et al., 2009).

Create and Strengthen Organizational Links

Relationships and connections among the entities that comprise a community, along with those that cross community boundaries, are essential for effective disaster management and public health. While many of these relationships will exist before a disaster, some may be established as part of prevention, preparedness, and planning, and others will emerge as part of response and recovery. Improved communication, information sharing, and collaboration among various sectors of a community (e.g., health care, business, education, social services, faith-based organizations, the media, and the public sector) can increase the efficiency and effectiveness of disaster management and public health by helping a community to (1) become aware of local needs and assets, (2) identify and address health hazards and service gaps, (3) reduce unnecessary duplication, (4) curtail interagency conflict, (5) build mutual respect and trust, and (6) create a sense of shared ownership and responsibility. Organizational links and networks can be built around shared concerns and specific issues such as disaster readiness, response, and recovery. Relationships can be strengthened through cross-representation on boards and committees; cosponsorship of community activities; support for professional, practitioner, and provider organizations; and the creation of coalitions to address common concerns (B. Pfefferbaum et al., 2009). Networks also extend beyond the community as illustrated by the federal system for disaster management that establishes a hierarchy of responsibility based on an understanding that disasters are local, requiring the involvement of individuals who are familiar with the affected community and who will remain in the community after response and recovery activities are complete. State and, if necessary, federal assistance is available if local resources are insufficient in response (FEMA, 2011).

Enhance Social Supports

Disaster interventions should protect and enhance existing social supports to help ensure that communities and families maintain the capacity to give and receive support throughout and beyond response and recovery. Unfortunately, altruism and cohesion, which are often abundant in the initial aftermath of a disaster, tend not to endure across all disaster phases. Thus, deliberate efforts may be necessary to create and build social support in the aftermath of a disaster. Ideally, such efforts will provide participants with attitudes, knowledge, and skills they can use to develop their own supports (Norris et al., 2008).

Undertake Effective Disaster Planning and Management

Disaster resilience requires comprehensive emergency management involving four traditional elements: prevention and mitigation, preparedness, response, and recovery. The QHSR Report (USDHS, 2010b) identifies ensuring resilience to disasters as one of five missions, which it grounds in these four traditional elements. According to the QHSR Report, resilience will require a shift from a primary focus on response and recovery to one that balances response and recovery with mitigation and preparedness in a process that engages all stakeholders. Thus, communities must create a culture of preparedness. They must develop flexible, all-hazards, community emergency plans that include effective risk communication based on trusted sources of information and that recognize the potential for unforeseen and unknown events (Longstaff, 2005; Norris et al., 2008; B. Pfefferbaum et al., 2009; R. L. Pfefferbaum et al., 2008). Stakeholders must be trained and must practice plans.

Adopt a Holistic Wellness Approach

Community resilience is buttressed by "the promotion of healthy lifestyles; disease prevention; access to culturally informed, timely and high-quality health care; and a robust public health system" (USDHHS, 2009, p. 6). This suggests a holistic wellness approach in which formal and informal services and systems reinforce and inform health-seeking behaviors, promote effective coping, provide for the maintenance and restoration of healthy physical and mental functioning, attend to those who suffer serious physical and psychological illnesses, defend from adverse physical and psychological consequences of disasters, and care for the injured (Friedman, 2005; R. L. Pfefferbaum et al., 2008). These are all elements of essential public health services.

Create a Conscious Awareness of Community Resilience

Community resilience relies on intentional, collective action to prepare for and remedy the impact of a problem, including the ability to interpret the environment, diagnose the community's health status, intervene, and move on. Community resilience requires a diverse collection of resources that can be acquired and developed, and it relies on skills that can be taught and practiced at personal (American Psychological Association, n.d.) and community levels (McGee et al., 2009). When community members and organizations have a conscious awareness of community resilience, they are more likely to recognize the importance of engagement, surveillance, collaboration, skill development, critical analysis, and strategic planning that underlie it. Awareness alone, of course, does not create healthy communities. Awareness alone does not mobilize resources, train individuals, establish plans, or ensure that plans are practiced, but it may be a first step. In creating a consciousness of and appreciation for community resilience, it is important to reinforce the concept of resilience as a process that must be sustained over time and across adversity lest people begin to feel either complacent or discouraged and defeated.

SUMMARY

The National Health Security Strategy was developed by the U.S. Department of Health and Human Services to address many threats with potential large-scale health consequences such as, for example, disease outbreaks, natural disasters, technological accidents, and terrorist attacks (USDHHS, 2009). It recognizes that managing these threats requires commitment and cooperation across all segments of society including all levels of government; private commerce; academic, civic, faith-based, fraternal, nonprofit, and professional organizations; households; local communities; the media; and international partners. The vision of the National Health Security Strategy—that the nation and its people be prepared for, be protected from, respond effectively to, and be able to recover from incidents with potentially negative health consequences—reflects, at its core, an appreciation for community resilience (USDHHS, 2009).

Defined simply as the process of successfully adapting to, and recovering from, adversity, community resilience involves deliberate, meaningful, collective action to transform social and physical environments. Connectedness, commitment, and shared values; participation; support and nurturance; structure, roles, and responsibilities; resources; critical reflection and skill building; communication; and disaster management are attributes associated with resilient communities. These attributes contribute to four adaptive capacities from which resilience emerges: economic development, social capital, information and communication, and community competence. Four properties characterize resilient systems: robustness, redundancy, resourcefulness, and rapidity.

The attention to community resilience in health and homeland security policy makes it increasingly likely that health and public health professionals will be called upon to develop strategies, programs, services, and interventions for building community resilience to disasters. It is recommended that these include (1) developing economic resources and addressing risk and resource inequities, (2) fostering community engagement and participation, (3) creating and strengthening organizational links, (4) enhancing social supports, (5) undertaking effective disaster planning and management, (6) adopting a holistic wellness approach, and (7) creating a conscious awareness of community resilience. Ideally, programs and interventions will engage individual community members and organizations in activities with common purpose, creating synergies that permit fulfillment of communal goals, promote health and wellness, instill hope, and engender trust.

Case Study Exercises

Individually, or as a group, review the following case studies and follow the exercises at the end of the study, as appropriate. Be sure to focus on the why, how, and what emphasized in each exercise. Your professor/instructor will provide you specific guidance on how you are to report your findings for the class.

Case Study 13.1: The Communities Advancing Resilience Toolkit (CART)©

The Communities Advancing Resilience Toolkit (CART) (R. L. Pfefferbaum, Pfefferbaum, & Van Horn, 2011) is an evidence-informed community intervention designed to enhance community resilience to disasters and other adversities through assessment, group processes, planning, and action. Created by the Terrorism and Disaster Center, a partner in the National Child Traumatic Stress Network, CART uses community assessment to prompt and facilitate strengths-based community development, engages community members and organizations, initiates and reinforces community connections, promotes disaster management, and creates a consciousness of community resilience.

TABLE 13.1   Description of the Four Domains and Their Relationship to the Eight Attributes

THE FOUR DOMAINS	ATTRIBUTES THAT MAP TO EACH DOMAIN
Connection and caring: Community members feel connected to a place or group of people with shared history, customs, laws, and values. They feel like they belong and are committed to the community; have hope; and believe the community treats people fairly.	• Connectedness, commitment, and shared values • Participation • Support and nurturance • Communication
Resources: The community effectively acquires, mobilizes, allocates, invests in, and utilizes natural, financial, physical, human, and social resources to meet community goals and serve the community.	• Structure, roles, and responsibilities • Resources • Communication
Transformative potential: Community members recognize and frame collective experiences. They engage in intentional, meaningful, collective action involving critical analysis, planning, intervention, and resolution related to community issues.	• Structure, roles, and responsibilities • Resources • Critical reflection and skill building • Communication
Disaster management: The community acts effectively to prevent and mitigate, prepare for, respond to, and recover from disasters.	• Disaster management • Communication

Source: Pfefferbaum, R. L., Pfefferbaum, B., & Van Horn, R. L. (2011). Communities Advancing Resilience Toolkit (CART)©. Oklahoma City, OK: Terrorism and Disaster Center, University of Oklahoma Health Sciences Center.

Originally based on attributes associated with community competence and capacity, CART research has identified four domains that are the foundation for CART: (1) connection and caring, (2) resources, (3) transformative potential, and (4) disaster management. Table 13.1 displays the four domains and their relationship to the eight community resilience attributes.

The CART process engages community stakeholders in collecting and using assessment data to develop and implement strategies for building community resilience. Participants may include a homogeneous or heterogeneous mix of community leaders, neighborhood members, selected professionals, and/or representatives of community organizations convened by local partners that sponsor a CART application. The CART survey and other assessment information are used to generate a community profile reflecting the perspective of the participants. The profile provides information useful in developing strategies for building community resilience. The CART process is displayed in Figure 13.1.

The CART survey instrument, which has evolved through key informant input and field testing, includes 21 community resilience items that assess resilience across the four domains. Standard demographic

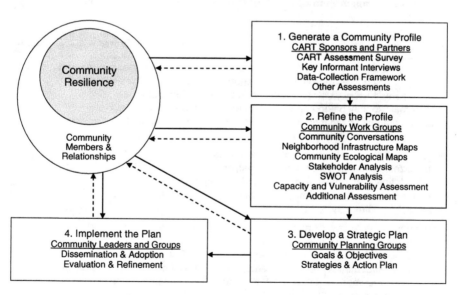

FIGURE 13.1 The CART process. The solid lines show data and information flows. The dotted lines show potential changes in, or effects of, the CART intervention on community resilience characteristics.
Source: Pfefferbaum, R. L., Pfefferbaum, B., & Van Horn, R. L. (2011). Communities Advancing Resilience Toolkit (CART)®. Oklahoma City, OK: Terrorism and Disaster Center, University of Oklahoma Health Sciences Center.

questions are included along with items assessing the personal relationship of respondents to their community. Additional, customized, community- and organization-specific questions are developed in conjunction with community partners. The survey can be administered via interview (in person or over the telephone), in written form (distributed at meetings or through postal mail), or online.

Questions available for interviews and community conversations explore the perceived meaning of community and the four community resilience domains within the context of the participating community. Key informant interviews and community conversations also provide opportunities for participants to review and interpret survey findings. Interpretation of findings is important because the meaning of survey results may differ across communities and across CART participants.

CART is designed to strengthen and empower communities, not to compare or rank them. It provides a structure and avenues to information to guide analysis of community concerns from a resilience perspective. CART stimulates communication, critical reflection, analysis, and action. Community member participation in the CART process, while time- and labor-intensive, contributes to the development of human and social capital, both of which are essential to community resilience. The collaboration, skill building, resource sharing, and purposeful action that are part of a successful CART application contribute to the transformative potential of a community.

More information about CART is available at the website: http://www.oumedicine.com/tdc.

Study Exercises

1. CART was originally built on the eight community resilience attributes (B. Pfefferbaum et al., 2007; R. L. Pfefferbaum et al., 2008). Discuss how implementing the CART process also can contribute to the expansion of the eight attributes within a specific community.
2. Note that communication is an attribute associated with each of the four CART domains. Information and communication is also one of the four adaptive capacities from which resilience emerges (Norris et al., 2008). Explain what the role of communication is in each of the four CART domains.
3. CART employs a community-based participatory approach to community resilience assessment and intervention, which fosters collaboration between investigators and those being studied. Community-based participatory action research builds on the strengths of a community, using relationships to generate mutual understanding, enhance interactions, and stimulate collective problem solving (Norris, Sherrieb, & Pfefferbaum, 2011). Discuss why this would be a suitable approach for building community resilience.

4. The CART survey can be administered by interview (over the telephone or in person), online, or in written format (delivered in person or via postal mail). Consider the costs and benefits of each approach. What factors or characteristics should be considered to determine which method is most likely to engage local community members? Why are those factors relevant?

Case Study 13.2: Community Emergency Response Teams (CERTs)

CERTs are part of disaster preparedness and response in many communities across the country. The CERT Program, one of five Citizen Corps partner programs, is administered by the Federal Emergency Management Agency (FEMA). CERT members are trained to care for themselves, their families, and their neighbors and coworkers in the event of a major disaster. Training consists of 21 clock hours of a FEMA-approved curriculum in which CERT members learn about a variety of hazards that may impact their local area and through which they acquire disaster response skills associated with fire safety, light search and rescue, disaster medical operations, disaster psychology, and team work (Citizen Corps, n.d.).

Individuals who are on-site when a disaster strikes are often inclined to, and do, assist others until professional responders arrive. Their ability to do so is enhanced when they are trained for this role and are organized into teams. Standardized training and teamwork facilitate the integration of CERTs into formal response and recovery activities and in mitigation and preparedness efforts before new disasters strike (Citizen Corps, n.d.). CERT training encourages people to assume personal responsibility for preparedness, response, and recovery. CERT training also empowers individuals and communities at a time when local resources may be overwhelmed by circumstances.

Ideally, CERT members continue to learn and work together over time, with teams providing a basis of support integrated within a community. CERT members often complete supplemental training and perform service projects in communities and workplaces. For example, some CERT members receive training and participate in Points of Dispensing (POD) exercises under the direction of their public health department. These exercises help prepare a volunteer workforce to assist in the distribution of mass amounts of vaccine or antibiotics in response to public health crises.

CERTs are about people helping people, making a difference, and doing the greatest good for the greatest number. CERTs are about readiness. They are a positive and proactive component of disaster preparedness. CERTs can save lives and property, help communities remain intact, and hasten recovery for areas hit by disaster. CERTs can transform a potentially dangerous, anxiety-ridden environment into one characterized by capacity and a realistic sense of control.

More information about CERTs is available at the website: www.citizencorps.gov/cert.

Study Questions

1. Local CERT programs can contribute to the personal and family resilience of team members, as well as to the resilience of the community in which teams operate. Distinguish between personal and community resilience and explain what the role of CERTs would be in fostering each.
2. How do CERTs contribute to the four properties of resilient systems described by Bruneau and colleagues (2003): robustness, redundancy, resourcefulness, and rapidity?
3. Which of the four adaptive capacities described by Norris and colleagues (2008) are addressed by CERTs: economic development, social capital, information and communication, and community competence? In what ways might CERTs build these capacities in a major metropolitan area? In a rural community? In an impoverished neighborhood?

REFERENCES

American Psychological Association Task Force. (n.d.). *Fact sheet: Fostering resilience in response to terrorism: A fact sheet for psychologists working with adults.* Retrieved from www.deep.med.miami.edu/media/FostResilRspTerAdltsAPA.pdf

Bourdieu, P. (1986). The forms of capital. In J. Richardson (Ed.), *Handbook of theory and research for the sociology of education* (pp. 241–258). New York, NY: Greenwood. doi: 10.1002/9780470755679.ch15. Retrieved from www.marxists.org/reference/subject/philosophy/works/fr/bourdieu-forms-capital.htm

Brown, D. D., & Kulig, J. C. (1996/1997). The concept of resiliency. Theoretical lessons from community research. *Health and Canadian Society, 4*(3), 29–50.

Bruneau, M., Chang, S. E., Eguchi, R. T., Lee, G. C., O'Rourke, T. D., Reinhorn, A. M.,...von Winterfeldt, D. (2003). A framework to quantitatively assess and enhance the seismic resilience of communities. *Earthquake Spectra, 19*(4), 733–752. doi: 10.1193/1.1623497

Butler, L., Morland, L., & Leskin, G. (2007). Psychological resilience in the face of terrorism. In B. Bongar, L. Brown, L. Beutler, J. Breckenridge, & P. Zimbardo (Eds.), *Psychology of terrorism* (pp. 400–417). New York, NY: Oxford University Press.

Centers for Disease Control and Prevention. (n.d.). *Ten essential services.* Atlanta, GA: Centers for Disease Control and Prevention, U.S. Department of Health and Human Services. Retrieved from http://www.cdc.gov/stltpublichealth/hop/pdfs/Ten_Essential_Public_Health_Services_2011-09_508.pdf

Citizen Corps. (n.d.). *Community Emergency Response Teams*. Retrieved from www. citizencorps.gov/cert/

Cottrell, L. S., Jr. (1976). The competent community. In B. H. Kaplan, R. N. Wilson, & A. H. Leighton (Eds.), *Further explorations in social psychiatry* (pp. 195–209). New York, NY: Basic Books.

Cutter, S. L., Barnes, L., Berry, M., Burton, C., Evans, E., Tate, E., & Webb, J. (2008a). *Community and regional resilience: Perspectives from hazards, disasters, and emergency management*. Community and Regional Resilience Initiative (CARRI) Research Report No. 1. Oak Ridge, TN: Community and Regional Resilience Institute. Retrieved from www.resilientus.org/library/FINAL_CUTTER_9–25-08_1223482309.pdf

Cutter, S. L., Barnes, L., Berry, M., Burton, C., Evans, E., Tate, E., & Webb, J. (2008b). A place-based model for understanding community resilience to natural disasters. *Global Environmental Change, 18*, 598–606.

Federal Emergency Management Agency. (2011, September). *National disaster recovery framework*. Washington, DC: Author. Retrieved from www.fema.gov/pdf/recoveryframework/ndrf.pdf

Friedman, M. J. (2005). Every crisis is an opportunity. *CNS Spectrums, 10*(2), 96–98.

Fullilove, M. T., & Saul, J. (2006). Rebuilding communities post-disaster in New York. In Y. Neria, R. Gross, & R. D. Marshall (Eds.), *9/11: Mental health in the wake of terrorist attacks* (pp. 164–177). Cambridge, England: Cambridge University Press.

Gibbon, M., Labonte, R., & Laverack, G. (2002). Evaluating community capacity. *Health and Social Care in the Community, 10*(6), 485–491. doi: 10.1046/j.1365-2524.2002.00388

Glass, T. A., & Schoch-Spana, M. (2002). Bioterrorism and the people: How to vaccinate a city against panic. *Clinical Infectious Diseases, 34*, 217–223. doi: 10.1086/338711

Goeppinger, J., & Baglioni, A. J., Jr. (1985). Community competence: A positive approach to needs assessment. *American Journal of Community Psychology, 13*(5), 507–523. doi: 10.1007/BF00923264

Goodman, R. M., Speers, M. A., McLeroy, K., Fawcett, S., Kegler, M., Parker, E., . . . Wallerstein, N. (1998). Identifying and defining the dimensions of community capacity to provide a basis for measurement. *Health Education & Behavior, 25*(5), 258–278. doi: 10.1177/109019819802500303

Jerusalem, M., Kaniasty, K., Lehman, D. R., Ritter, C., & Turnbull, G. J. (1995). Individual and community stress: Integration of approaches at different levels. In S. E. Hobfoll & M. W. de Vries (Eds.), *Extreme stress and communities: Impact and intervention* (pp. 105–129). Dordrecht, The Netherlands: Kluwer Academic.

Kretzmann, J. P., & McKnight, J. L. (1993). *Building communities from the inside out: A path toward finding and mobilizing a community's assets*. Chicago, IL: Acta Publications.

Labonte, R., & Laverack, G. (2001a). Capacity building in health promotion, Part 1: for whom? And for what purpose? *Critical Public Health, 11*(2), 111–127.

Labonte, R., & Laverack, G. (2001b). Capacity building in health promotion, Part 2: whose use? And with what measurement? *Critical Public Health, 11*(2), 29–138.

Longstaff, P. H. (2005, November). *Security, resilience, and communication in unpredictable environments such as terrorism, natural disasters, and complex technology.* Cambridge, MA: Center for Information Policy Research, Harvard University.

Masten, A. D., & Obradovic, J. (2008). Disaster preparation and recovery: Lessons from research on resilience in human development [online]. *Ecology and Sociology, 13*(1), 9. Retrieved from www.ecologyandsociety.org/vol13/iss1/art9/

McFarlane, A. C., & Norris, F. H. (2006). Definitions and concepts in disaster research. In F. H. Norris, S. Galea, M. J. Friedman, & P. J. Watson (Eds.), *Methods for disaster mental health research* (pp. 3–19). New York, NY: The Guilford Press.

McGee, S., Bott, C., Gupta, V., Jones, K., & Karr, A. (2009). *Public role and engagement in counterterrorism efforts: Implications of Israeli practices.* Arlington, VA: Homeland Security Institute. Retrieved from www.hstoday.us/images/public_role_in_ct_israeli_practices_task_08-22.pdf

Morrow, B. H. (2008). *Community resilience: A social justice perspective.* Community and Regional Resilience Initiative (CARRI) Research Report No. 4. Oak Ridge, TN: Community Regional Resilience Institute. Retrieved from www.resilientus.org/library/FINAL_MORROW_9-25-08_1223482348.pdf

Norris, F. H., Sherrieb, K., & Pfefferbaum, B. (2011). Community resilience: Concepts, assessment, and implications for intervention. In S. M. Southwick, B. T. Litz, D. Charney, & M. J. Friedman (Eds.), *Resilience and mental health: Challenges across the lifespan* (pp. 149–161). Cambridge, UK: Cambridge University Press.

Norris, F. H., Stevens, S. P., Pfefferbaum, B., Wyche, K. F., & Pfefferbaum, R. L. (2008). Community resilience as a metaphor, theory, set of capacities, and strategy for disaster readiness. *American Journal of Community Psychology, 41,* 127–150. doi: 10.1007/s10464-007-9156-6

Pfefferbaum, B., Pfefferbaum, R. L., & Norris, F. (2009). Community resilience and wellness for the children exposed to Hurricane Katrina. In R. P. Kilmer, V. Gil-Rivas, R. G. Tedeschi, & L. G. Calhoun (Eds.), *Helping families and communities recover from disaster: Lessons learned from Hurricane Katrina and its aftermath* (pp. 265–288). Washington, DC: American Psychological Association. doi: 10.1037/12054-011

Pfefferbaum, B., Reissman, D. B., Pfefferbaum, R. L., Klomp, R. W., & Gurwitch, R. H. (2007). Building resilience to mass trauma events. In L. S. Doll, S. E. Bonzo, J. A. Mercy, D. A. Sleet, & E. N. Haas (Eds.), *Handbook of injury and violence prevention* (pp. 347–358). New York, NY: Springer. doi: 10.1007/978-0-387-29457-5_19

Pfefferbaum, R. L., Pfefferbaum, B., & Van Horn, R. L. (2011). Communities Advancing Resilience Toolkit (CART)©. Oklahoma City, OK: Terrorism and Disaster Center, University of Oklahoma Health Sciences Center.

Pfefferbaum, R. L., Reissman, D. B., Pfefferbaum, B., Wyche, K. F., Norris, F. H., & Klomp, R. W. (2008). Factors in the development of community resilience to disasters. In M. Blumenfield & R. J. Ursano (Eds.), *Intervention and resilience after mass trauma* (pp. 49–68). Cambridge, UK: Cambridge University Press. doi: 10.1017/CBO9780511585975.004

Plodinec, M. J. (2009, November). *Definitions of resilience: An analysis*. Oak Ridge, TN: Community and Regional Resilience Institute. Retrieved from www.resilientus.org/library/CARRI_Definitions_Dec_2009_1262802355.pdf

Ross, W. D. (2007). *Metaphysics by Aristotle*. eBooks@Adelaide. South Australia: University of Adelaide Library. Retrieved from http://ebooks.adelaide.edu.au/a/aristotle/metaphysics/

Subcommittee on Disaster Reduction. (2005). *Grand challenges for disaster reduction*. Washington, DC: National Science and Technology Council. Retrieved from http://www.sdr.gov/docs/GrandChallengesSecondPrinting.pdf

Terrorism and Disaster Center. (n.d.). *Information about TDC*. Retrieved from http://www.oumedicine.com/tdc

U.S. Department of Health and Human Services, Office of the Assistant Secretary for Preparedness and Response. (2009, December). *National health security strategy of the United States of America*. Washington, DC: Author. Retrieved from www.hhs.gov/aspr/opsp/nhss/nhss0912.pdf

U.S. Department of Homeland Security. (2010a). *DHS risk lexicon*. Retrieved from www.dhs.gov/xlibrary/assets/dhs-risk-lexicon-2010.pdf

U.S. Department of Homeland Security. (2010b). *Quadrennial Homeland Security review report: A strategic framework for a secure homeland*. Washington, DC: The White House. Retrieved from www.dhs.gov/xlibrary/assets/qhsr_report.pdf

U.S. Department of Homeland Security Presidential Directive-21. (2007, October 18). *Public health and medical preparedness*. Washington, DC: The Whitehouse. Retrieved from http://www.fas.org/irp/offdocs/nspd/hspd-21.htm

14

Evaluating the Community-Engaged Organization

*Roland Bernard Welmaker, Sr., Arletta T. Brinson, and
Adrienne C. Smith*

LEARNING OBJECTIVES

What you can learn by studying this chapter:

- Why an organization should be evaluated
- How to establish an evaluation framework
- How to construct an evaluation Logic Model
- How to prepare an evaluation report and why
- How to fit the evaluation into the planning process

This chapter will introduce the reader to evaluation as a component of the planning process. It will provide a definition of evaluation and answer the question, why we evaluate. Further, this chapter will address the following areas: how to design an evaluation framework; the use of Logic Models; steps in the evaluation plan; preparing the evaluation report; and fitting the evaluation into the planning process.

DEFINITION

Organizational evaluation is an assessment of an orgranization based upon data, its structure, activities, and/or interactions that provide a foundation upon which to measure performance, outcomes, and impact within the purview of intended and unintended results. In the evolving community-engaged organization (CEO), evaluation is a crucial part of the planning process because it is used to provide the information necessary for informed decisions to shape future decisions and directions.

WHY EVALUATE

CEOs are very often nonprofit entities established to provide needed local programs and/or services. Like any effective organization, CEOs should be guided by a vision; have a structure conducive to their vision, mission, goals, and objectives; and develop a plan that provides for their sustainability and continuing development. Activities centered around the development of community organizations are viewed as attempts to increase organizational capacity and effectiveness, whereas assessment and evaluation activities are necessary components to maintain the organization's fidelity to vision and purpose.

Organizations are assessed and evaluated to become more effective, efficient, and attractive to funders, and to provide increased accountability. Fully and competently executed evaluations build a case for future investments in the organization or in a particular program of the organization. A well-executed evaluation can be summarized as "a means to help organizations get the information they need to develop and execute effective strategies as evaluation is essential to improving and maintaining the quality of all programs, services, and organizations" (Rasing, 2010).

Broadly speaking, evaluations are also undertaken to determine:

1. Where opportunities and challenges have occurred
2. What accounted for successes and failures
3. What lessons were learned
4. How past lessons learned were applied

Specifically, organizational evaluations can be used to:

1. Provide information about organizational effectiveness for current and future funders regarding the institution's benefits to the community and participants
2. Strengthen organizational operations
3. Provide pathways to strengthen staff capabilities and performance
4. Determine baselines and/or historical trends in organizational efficiency and provide a rationale for improving or maintaining those efficiencies
5. Strengthen strategies that will improve participant outcomes

Evaluation for the CEO is just as crucial as it is for any type of organization that wishes to increase its effectiveness and efficiency. Evaluation is used to assess organizational strengths and weaknesses as they relate to the organization's ability to implement its strategies and to assess the discrete activities performed to meet organizational missions, goals, and objectives.

FRAMING THE EVALUATION

Dedicating time to frame the evaluation—its scope, the questions to be answered, how to fit the evaluation into the organization's planning process and into program activities—is non-negotiable. The framework for the evaluation is crucial to its success.

The framework, or at least the rudimentary beginning of one, must be established before an external evaluator is determined or an internal evaluator is identified. Without the framework, you will not know what qualifications you need in an evaluator or have a basis for opting for an internal or an external evaluator.

Critical to any project is the scope, that is, what is going to be covered and what is going to be omitted, what is in-bounds and what is out-of-bounds. By placing boundaries, the evaluation does not attempt to assess everything that may arise during the measurement phase of the evaluation. Otherwise, without boundaries the evaluation could never reach a conclusion. The scope is used to align administration, stakeholders, staff, and participants as to what to expect (the breadth and depth) in the evaluation reports.

Evaluations that are designed to answer research questions are the easiest for stakeholders, administration, and staff to understand and utilize. The framing of the research questions at the start of the evaluation is again a means of communicating all the parameters for which the organization will be held accountable.

The evaluation framework should be viewed as the foundation that makes an evaluation a "living" document, in other words used and referred to when making operational and/or programming decisions and not stored on a shelf until the next time an update is due to a funding agency. The Centers for Disease Control and Prevention (CDC) has an excellent website (www.cdc.gov/eval/framework/index.htm) devoted to program evaluation framework. The WF Kellogg Foundation also has a popular evaluation handbook that may be downloaded from www.wkkf. org/knowledge-center/resources/2010/W-K-Kellogg-Foundation-Evaluation-Handbook.aspx.

THE EVALUATOR

Evaluations are time consuming, deal with sensitive questions, and requires the evaluator to make unbiased assessments of data/information provided organizationally. It is best if the evaluator is a skilled and impartial outside entity. However, often that person (or group of persons) for economic reasons has to be an existing member of the organization's staff. There are inherent advantages and disadvantages, regardless whether the evaluator is external or internal.

The advantages of an outside evaluator reside in that person's independence and degree of freedom from normal organizational influences and pressures. That person also brings a fresh perspective to the activities, interactions, and personalities of the organization. A disadvantage of an outside evaluator can be the cost, especially during tight budget times. Also, the outside evaluator may not be as well versed in the organization's climate—its needs, purposes, issues, desires, and so on. The advantage of the inside evaluator may be the cost factor and intimate knowledge of organizational nuances and operations. However, the inside evaluator may be hampered by previously drawn conclusions, established biases, or real and/or perceived needs to provide certain conclusions. Lastly, many times internal evaluators feel the pressures of being *an employee* and, thus, potentially anyone in their up-line/chain of supervision can unduly influence or outright dictate the evaluation findings. The amount of time and internal resources that may be required to do a credible job may also be formidable.

With either option, internal or external evaluator, the cooperation or support of staff will be required to conduct the evaluation. It is incumbent that evaluation procedures be established to provide the most bias-free process and to meet, within the budget available, the established scope of the evaluation. Evaluation elements are as follows:

1. Type of evaluation (i.e., formative or summative, or both; participatory or not)
2. Research questions evaluation will answer
3. Questions to ask
4. Data-collection instruments to use (i.e., surveys, interviews, and/or focus groups)
5. Assumptions, limitations, and constraints
6. Data sources, numbers required, and selection methods (all or subset of organization members; community key informers, program participants, etc.)
7. Data to collect (qualitative or quantitative)
8. Data-collection techniques (phone, person-to-person, mail, and/or electronic; individual and/or group settings; etc.)
9. Methods of data analyses (descriptive and/or inferential techniques)

Evaluations, whether for the review of the entire community organization or for its individual initiatives or programs, may be used to assess such processes or results as organizational performance, program delivery methods, desired program outcomes, financial practices and per capita costs, community or participant perceptions and/or satisfaction, fidelity to organizational ideals, and adherence to standards or expectations.

The evaluator should develop a plan that organizes the evaluation within the scope and intent of the evaluation framework provided by the organization. The plan will indicate how resources will be allocated, the relationship of evaluation tools to specific goals, objectives, outcomes, and/or questions that are to be answered, sources of information, tools, and activities to be undertaken, and plan for analyses. The evaluation plan calls for the identification of evaluation goals, resources and capacity, required evaluation activities, type of evaluation to be implemented, and data-collection and handling methods (CDC, 2007).

INFRASTRUCTURE OF THE ORGANIZATION

Evaluation of an organization differs from the evaluation of one or more of the organization's programs or initiatives, first and foremost, in that it asks the question "Is the current organizational structure conducive to efficiently and effectively meeting the organization's stated mission?" Thus, an organizational evaluation includes the assessment of the board, the staffing, and potentially even interactions with any other stakeholders.

In addition to mandates from grantors or other funders, the nature of the evaluation should be determined by the organization's members from the board to the line personnel and/or volunteers, as each will have a role to play in the process and should have some type of positive buy-in into the process. The evaluation, whether with an internal or external evaluator, will usually involve the participation of the organization's staff members, who often are responsible for collecting data for the evaluator, and are often either observed in the delivery of programmatic services and/or in interaction with other staff and program recipients.

Board members may also be called upon to provide personal insight into board activities, assessments of the organization in relation to their roles, responsibilities, and the achievement of goals and objectives. Frequently, organizational charters outline profiles of desired board members, statements of vision and mission, types of activities to be accomplished by the organization, and community problems to be addressed. This part of the evaluation will delve into how the organization and the board are organized as well as the board's internal relationships juxtaposed to its purpose. It can assess the composition and performance of the board in fulfilling its responsibilities. It is incumbent upon the organization to decide whether the evaluation is to include the infrastructure, and if so, to what extent.

NEEDS ASSESSMENT

The evaluation may need to reassess the impetus for the very formation of the organization. Usually, there is a needs assessment made of the community to be served. The needs assessment, whether formal or informal, would form the rationale, the foundation of the organization's very existence.

The needs assessment is a composite of a series of analyses—that is, windshield surveys of the community, interviews of key stakeholders, individual interviews of community members, focus group sessions of stakeholders, and/or surveys of community members and concerned stakeholders—used by the organization to establish its vision, mission, goals, objectives, and strategies. Analysis of the needs assessment would have included a SWOT analysis—Strengths, Weaknesses, Opportunities, and Threats—present at the time.

Evaluations of organizations should revisit this foundation by answering the following questions:

- How have the community's needs changed? Are those needs still within the purview of the organization's mission?
- What is the organization's capacity to meet the current needs? What changes are required in organizational capacity to meet identified needs?

Communities are always evolving; members move in and members move on. Remember, an organization that is 100% successful at addressing a community need will ultimately eliminate that specific need within that community.

Organizational capacity is measured in such terms as financial requirements, funding sources, board expertise, board roles, board structure, staff expertise, and so on. One aspect of capacity may include the types of expertise and backgrounds desired of board members. Such expertise may include finance, fund raising, marketing, governmental department, local politician, clergy, community liaison, education, health care, and so on, to provide ready insight into community issues and contacts within the given greater community/profession represented.

PROGRAMS AND STRATEGIES

The second thrust of evaluation should be to assess the organization's strategies—its efforts and methods to provide services to its community. Strategies are the assumptions and approaches an organization believes will lead to successful outcomes for the target population. Strategy dictates the course of action to be taken if a program derails. In a CEO evaluation, the evaluator should assess the "goodness of fit" of the selected strategies with respect to both the intended outcome and to the implementation of program activities. This assessment uses the "body of knowledge" for the selected outcome, the lessons learned, and other such collective intelligences to assess "fit." A real-life example of a strategy is the current educational trend to include the parents in the education process. This strategy is actualized by having the parents, students (of a certain age), and the school administration sign an agreement. As part of an organizational evaluation, the evaluator would investigate if the strategy is sound given the desired outcome, and then assess whether or not the activities follow logically from the strategy. Program evaluation would then assess whether or not the activities effectively impacted the short or long-term outcomes.

Regardless of purpose, a well-crafted and well-implemented evaluation will provide continuous and timely feedback, which can be used to enhance organizational performance and the probability of maximizing desired attributes and attaining stated goals and objectives. It can also lead to an external evaluator gaining a more comprehensive understanding of the community organization, the community, and the context in which the evaluation is occurring. The evaluation should be such that it addresses all aspects of the organization's mission, functions, methods, and structure. It investigates the operational and program objectives/outcomes, answers any questions posed, and provides insight into any hypotheses that may have been offered or suggested.

Evaluations of organizational programs and strategies should answer the following questions:

- How was success measured? Were the strategies used appropriate? Were the measures used appropriate given the stated strategy?
- How successful have organizational strategies been in meeting past needs?
- What changes are required in the strategies to meet identified needs?
- Were objectives met?
- What were the outcomes—short term, intermediate, and long term?

LOGIC MODEL

Often, the evaluation plan is assisted through the use of a Logic Model (Table 14.1).

A Logic Model typically is a single-page document with columns reading from left to right displaying the chain of logic moving from the planned work through to the intended results. Resources or inputs typically are the left-most column; however, a Logic Model may go deeper and include

TABLE 14.1   Logic Model Defined

DEFINITION: A logic model is a planning tool to clarify and graphically display what your project intends to do and what it hopes to accomplish and impact.

A logic model:
- Summarizes key program elements
- Explains rationale behind program activities
- Clarifies intended outcomes
- Provides a communication tool

Think of a logic model as a map that you develop to clarify and communicate what your project intends to do and its presumed impact.

Source: National Network of Libraries of Medicine (2006).

TABLE 14.2   Logic Model Example

RESOURCES	ACTIVITIES	OUTPUTS	OUTCOMES	GOAL
Resources dedicated to or consumed by the program	What the program does with the inputs to fulfill its mission	The direct products of program activities	Benefits for participants during and after program activities	Desired long-term result of the program

Source: **National Network of Libraries of Medicine (2006).**

the underlying assumptions. The next column lists the programming activities and from each activity flows its related outputs, outcomes, and impacts. The difference between outputs and outcomes is that outputs are basically counts, such as the number of community education seminars offered. Outcomes might be that community members are more knowledgeable about home buying as measured by a facts-based pre-/posttest comparison. The impact is the long-term result of the activity such as a more stable neighborhood as the result of an increase in the proportion of home owners to renters.

There is latitude in the rows of the Logic Model depending upon the model's viewpoint (high-level view vs. detailed view). In one version, each row represents a "need" to be addressed by the organization's programming. Another version centers on the activities and connects each to their "logical" outputs, outcomes, and impacts (Table 14.2).

An Evaluation Logic Model, an alternative version, has as column headers the logical sequence resulting from following the research questions through data collection to analysis (Table 14.3).

EVALUATION PLAN

Evaluations occur for many purposes, including to answer questions or address issues related to governance, finances, operational and/or program effectiveness, and so on. Therefore, it is important for the community organization to identify its intended purposes for any evaluation to provide focus and appropriate oversight. The organization and the evaluator, as appropriate, establish the questions that need to be answered, objectives that need to be measured, outcomes needing assessment, grantor requirements, and so on. For whatever reason an evaluation is undertaken, it can be summarized in a Logic Model that may contain the following:

1. The questions to be answered and the goals and objectives to be assessed
2. The concomitant processes and activities related to the questions and objectives

TABLE 14.3   An Evaluation Logic Model Example

Goal:				
Objective/Research Question	Information Source	Evaluation Activity	Tool	Analysis
What are board members' perceptions of community needs?	Board members	Interviews	Interview protocol	Qualitative assessments
How successful has the organization been in meeting its objectives?	1. Program reports 2. Annual reports 3. Program data files 4. Community 5. Board	Review program objectives and data analyses; focus groups interviews	Activity counts, inferential stats, as appropriate; focus group and interview protocols	Qualitative assessments and statistical testing as appropriate
Was the program successful?	Program objectives/desired outcomes; participants; community	Review of program surveys; focus groups	Program data and activity information; focus group protocols	Qualitative assessments and statistical testing as appropriate

3. Instruments and standards upon which to measure success
4. Appropriate analytical techniques to be used
5. Timelines for each phase
6. Persons responsible for implementation

From the Logic Model, an evaluation plan is easily developed. Together, they become the roadmap for the evaluator to follow and upon which needed changes may be made and documented.

The evaluation plan should contain not only the elements of the Logic Model, but the specifics needed to implement the evaluation. The operative term here is *plan*. More time spent in developing a quality plan will result in an evaluation implementation process less fraught with problems that should or could have been foreseen. Such a plan will have specifics that will, in the context of the community organization and its community, speak to information/data needed, information sources, data-gathering methods, data-gathering instruments, data analyses, and reporting.

INFORMATION SOURCES

Data gathering will be dictated by the evaluation questions and objectives. For questions concerning perceptions related to organization operations, a combination of interviews and surveys may be desired. Questions that may be answered from documents should not be included in either interviews or surveys, but gathered from the actual files. Community organizations' program evaluations may find data in enrollment/application forms, attendance sheets, activity worksheets and summaries and pretests and posttests from program staff, participants, participant family members, community members, and the community at large. It is best to collect raw rather than previously summarized data. The evaluation plan should address, for each evaluation question, the anticipated source of information.

Choosing who to include in interviews/focus groups and surveys or what pieces from organization records will allow for the greatest possibility of securing an unbiased look at the organization. Selection bias is introduced when participants are chosen by the organization, the evaluator, or even by self-selection by participants. The best evaluation is performed when the sampling that does occur results in a subgroup that mirrors the population studied as much as possible. If the evaluation cannot include all persons or records, then the best methodology is to develop a randomized process that eliminates any possibility of organization or evaluator bias in the selection process. One may wish to assign unique numbers to persons or records and use tables of random numbers, with an arbitrary beginning point, but a planned route through the table to identify a previously agreed upon number of participants or records.

All participants requested to participate should be provided informed consent forms. Minors, as well as their parents, should also be provided with informed consent forms. The informed consent provides an overview of the evaluation, guaranteed confidentiality and anonymity, risk factors, and assurances of nonparticipation or withdrawal without penalty or threat of retaliation.

DATA COLLECTION

Data collection is guided by the evaluation questions and/or outcomes that are to be asked and/or measured. Since evaluations are time consuming, and even sometimes viewed suspiciously by those staff and community members who do not have a buy-in into the process, information gathering should be limited to only facts and perceptions that relate directly to the evaluation questions and/or outcomes.

Information comes in two formats—quantitative (numerical) and qualitative (nonnumerical). Evaluations for organizational development most often include both types and may require the use of such qualitative data as can be found in stakeholder (staff, program participants, community members, board members, and funders) interviews or focus group sessions, surveys with open-ended questions, and organizational records (i.e., meeting minutes, charters, past plans, contracts, funded grants, intake forms, etc.). Each process is best when a protocol is developed for its administration. Numeric data may also be obtained from the same sources, but are less often sought through interviews or focus groups.

Additional considerations may be made to use not only paper surveys or personal interviews, but also web-based tools such as Survey Monkey or even handheld personal digital assistant devices to collect data.

DATA-GATHERING METHODS AND INSTRUMENTS

Data-gathering protocols should be developed to ensure consistent treatment of subjects and records and the elimination of possible interviewer or survey administrator biases from occurring. The established protocols provide for scripts so that all interviewers and survey administrators say the same thing, in the same order, and hopefully in the same manner.

A basic warning about interviews and focus groups: The interviewers, session leaders, and survey administrators should follow their protocols (scripts) and not dominate the conversations. Interview questions should not seek responses in a predetermined favorable or unfavorable vein. They should not assume prior knowledge and should only include one thought or idea upon which to respond. Keep questions clear and simple and make sure they relate to the evaluation questions you wish to have answered. Focus groups should last for 1 hour or less, include no more than 10 persons and no more than six questions. The first (key) question should lead into your topic, while the middle four speak directly to your objectives for conducting the focus group, and the last question is your summary of what you heard.

Survey administrators should also make sure their instruments are easy to code for data entry. Data-gathering instruments should only ask those questions or elicit information from records that relate to the evaluation purpose. Data are also gathered from other sources. Organizational records and files, reports, case management records, and so on may need to be accessed for the evaluation. If needed information can be found in files, which is a preferable source rather than putting the question in a survey or protocol for an interview or focus group.

Data handling is important to ensure that confidential information is protected. Although data are collected from individuals, whether in groups or singly, they are reported as composite or group information to encourage continued sharing of personal perceptions and assessments. Further, data are seen by only those who must do so in order to enter it into the computer. Afterward, the data are kept in locked desk or cabinet drawers, separate from respondent names. Electronic data should be appropriately secured.

DATA ANALYSES

The plan for data analyses should include a descriptive section that draws a picture of the organization—including its history, composition, place in the community, achievements, future plans, and so on—and the

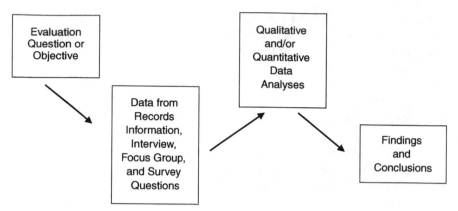

FIGURE 14.1   Relationship of evaluation question to analyses.

nature of the evaluation (why, how it is to be used, etc.). Data drawn from asking questions that relate to the purpose of the evaluation will result in information that can be successfully used to draw conclusions (Figure 14.1).

Initial analyses should be the descriptive analyses that relate pertinent basic information about the community organization—how many in the organization, how many programs, how much money in the budget, percentage of persons in the evaluation, groups, and so on. General descriptive information gathered from participants should also be presented here.

Evaluation questions and the accompanying data should be presented next. Quantitative data and any statistical analyses or qualitative data and their findings are then presented. However, only after the findings are presented should the evaluator attempt to present interpretations of the data. This would be followed by the implications of the findings and recommendations.

Results of the evaluation are due to the person responsible for commissioning the evaluation.

THE EVALUATION REPORT

The evaluation report of the developing organization is first and foremost for the organization. Generally, the organization wishes to have the evaluation done to assess its performance, to make sure it is not only on the correct path for solving problems, but is also doing a good job. Primarily, organizations wish to determine how to improve their efforts for their communities, how to be more successful in their programs, and how to become better advocates. It is most likely that the evaluator's report will provide the framework that may be used to adjust strategies to accomplish goals and objectives.

A suggested outline for the evaluation report follows.

- Executive summary: A brief description of the organization and the evaluation framework, the evaluation plan, major findings, and interpretations (1 page).
- Introduction
- Evaluation framework
- Evaluation plan
- Findings regarding infrastructure and strategies
- Conclusions, implications, and recommendations regarding infrastructure and strategies

PLANNING PROCESS

The traditional planning process is cyclical in that it may begin at a certain point, but it never really ends—at least not in the continuing organization. Beginning with the organization's SWOT analysis or needs assessment, the organization develops its vision, goals, and objectives. Then strategies are developed and implemented for accomplishing the objectives. The implemented strategies are *evaluated* to provide feedback to the organization. The feedback is used to reassess the organization's performance in relation to previously identified information found in the SWOT analysis or needs assessment and the cycle begins again. The evaluation leads to the restart of the planning cycle, and the evaluation has an impact on the process.

Case Study Exercises

Individually, or as a group, review the following case study and respond to the questions posed at the end of the study, as appropriate. Be sure to focus on the why, how, and what emphasized in each question. Your professor/instructor will provide you specific guidance on how you are to report your findings for the class.

Case Study 14.1: Westside Community

The Westside Settlers has existed in this neighborhood for 42 years. Originally, most of its members lived in this historic community, but now the organization draws members from throughout the metropolitan area. Membership is open to community members at a reduced rate.

To implement its community service-related initiatives, a CEO, Westside Cares, was formed over 20 years ago. Its purpose was to encourage the revitalization of the community through the provision of daycare services, after-school tutorials and homework help, health literacy and awareness programs, parenting support groups, a teen center, career development seminars, and financial literacy programming.

Westside Cares' structure calls for a board of 11 directors led by the executive board and the chairpersons of each of the continuing committees. The majority of the executive board members must be from the leadership of the Westside Settlers. Westside Cares' bylaws have been established to detail membership, officers, terms of office, standing and ad hoc committees, programmatic concerns, and other structural and directions of service guides. Westside Cares has an operating budget of about $200,000 and a program budget, developed through grants and donations, that has been as low as $25,000 and as high as $300,000.

There has *never* been an evaluation of the organization and you, the evaluator, have been called upon to assess Westside Cares' effectiveness.

Study Questions

1. Given that there has never been an evaluation and that you are dealing with two organizations, what would you recommend to be the direction of the evaluation? What are the major areas you would want your evaluation to cover? Justify your decisions.

   What do you need to do to establish your evaluation framework—in terms of understandings, directions, data/information, and so on. Describe the roles you will assign to whom to assist you in completing this evaluation. Estimate the resources needed to complete this evaluation.

   What criteria are you going to use to measure *Westside Cares'* effectiveness? What types of data might you examine, and from what sources might you acquire these data? How do you envision this first-ever evaluation will be utilized?

2. Create a Logic Model for Westside *Cares'* overall programming. Additionally, create a Logic Model for *one* of the specific programs (i.e., the parenting support group). Ensure that your Logic Model addresses the underlying desired outcomes (vs. the programs).

   How should these Logic Models be integrated into the planning process? Into daily operations? Budgeting? Assessment?

   Will the Logic Model need to be revised for these different uses/audiences or will one size fit all? Justify your decision.

3. After completing your evaluation of Westside Cares, you must present information to both the board of the Westside Settlers and again to the board of Westside Cares. However, you have discovered during your evaluation that six of the Westside Cares board members are overly partial to the day care center, which, based upon your evaluation assessment, has not proved to be contributing to the organization reaching its desired outcome(s).

How will you report your evaluation findings? Please answer for two scenarios: one as an internal evaluator and one as an external evaluator.

Given this situation, what recommendations would you make with regard to Westside Cares' strategic planning process? Would you make any recommendations to Westside Settlers? Justify your decisions.

4. You have been a member of the Westside Settlers for over 5 years and have lived in the Westside community for almost 7 years. You have recently been appointed Program Director for a new to-be-determined Westside Cares' initiative.

What type of information will you seek to learn from the evaluation report and how will you use this information as you begin planning this new initiative?

REFERENCES

Centers for Disease Control and Prevention. (2007). *Developing an evaluation plan.* Retrieved August 20, 2011, from www.cdc.gov/hiv/topics/evaluation/ Health_depts/guidance/supp-handbook/developing.htm#Steps

National Network of Libraries of Medicine. (2006). *Guide 5: Define how a program will work – The logic model.* Retrieved September 11, 2011, from http://nnlm. gov/outreach/community/logicmodel.html

Rasing, M. (2010, March 8). *Organizational development definition.* Retrieved August 20, 2011, from http://ezinearticles.com/?Organizational-Development-Definition&id=3893262

15

Organizing Communities for Public Health Practice–2050: A Futuristic Perspective

Frederick G. Murphy, Rafael Flores, and Lynda Murphy-Freeman

LEARNING OBJECTIVES

What you should learn by studying this chapter:

- To define communities of the future (COF)
- To become aware of the feral city
- To describe the framework for determining healthy and unhealthy communities
- To identify what types of community capital make up a community of the future
- CEOD and COF

This chapter will use the term community leaders (CLs) and public health practitioners (PHPs) interchangeably. It will emphasize just how myopic thinking can be the detriment of any public health progress in cities of the future and will seek to identify and define mandatory methods and strategies the CL and PHP must employ in order to engage, organize, and develop effective public health visions, and to work as broad-based thinkers and planners for public health practice.

It is predicted that 60% of the world's population will live in an urban environment by the year 2030, as opposed to 47% in 2000. Furthermore, the majority of this growth will occur in underdeveloped communities. More than 58 cities will boast populations of more than 5 million people. This report focuses on megacities, cities with more than 10 million inhabitants. However, subsequent research indicated that much smaller cities could also become feral, and so the population threshold was reduced (Brunn, Williams, & Zeigler, 2003).

Communities are highly impacted by a 21st century where urban renewal and rebuilding is rapid and ramped. This urban renewal is accompanied by an aggressive migration of middle class and affluent populations into historically deteriorating inner city areas, which often results in displacing lower income residents whose families have resided there all their lives.

Ironically, this renewal brings with it the increasing interconnection of people and places as a result of advances in environmental reconstruction, transport, e-communication, and other information technologies that cause political, economic, and cultural convergence.

Through policies and structural transformations in city governments—cities such as Atlanta, Baltimore, Boston, Detroit, Chicago, Cleveland, Los Angeles, New Orleans, New York, Philadelphia, Pittsburgh, and many other major U.S. cities—a phenomenon is occurring in which low-cost, physically deteriorated neighborhoods undergo physical renovation and an increase in property values, along with an influx of wealthier residents who may displace the prior residents, many of which are population groups of disparity status. Unfortunately, this process of renewal and revitalization of the inner cities, in most cases results in uprooting of the urban poor by raising rents and taxes and making it impossible for them to stay. Low-income neighborhoods are potentially attractive neighborhoods, with solid housing stock and well laid out streets in close proximity to the city center, and are being discovered by developers, investors, artists, and other professionals. Block-by-block these neighborhoods are rapidly changing as newcomers go about fixing up old buildings. As galleries and cafés open, curb stores and "mom 'n' pop" groceries close. City services improve and the infrastructure is revitalized. In the final phases, wealthier and more educated groups begin to migrate in and dominate the once predominately low-income and African American communities. Thus, the sequence: Reassessments of property values, revision of actuarial tables, and explosive tax bases and insurance premiums all have a coercive impact on the traditional residents of the community. From a strictly economic viewpoint, an increase in the tax base, improvement in site infrastructure, and lowering of crime reflect positively on city officials as property values rise, followed by property taxes and rents (Florida, 2002).

These socioeconomic changes take place in stages, ranging from policy changes to actual displacement, and are viewed by outsiders and the benefiting parties as progressive. But for those who are being displaced and disparaged, they see no benefit; for them the taste is bittersweet.

Some scholars and socioeconomists report that the current trend of upscale population groups moving into poverty-stricken inner city neighborhoods drives comparatively few low-income residents from their homes. They argue that, although some are forced to move by rising costs, there isn't much more displacement in renewal neighborhoods than in nonrenewal ones. Further, they conclude that living in a renewal or renewed neighborhood actually makes a poor resident less likely to move, primarily because of quality-of-life incentives such as more jobs, safer and better maintained streets, better sanitation and utility services, and the like (Freeman, 2005). Still other scholars, who oppose such views, argue that such postulation understates the extent of displacement. However, most agree that in many cases, interesting questions are raised concerning why, in the face of higher living costs, many poor people (low-income African Americans), attempt to stay put. Are they fighting to maintain their traditional sense of family, culture, neighborhood, and community values (Hampson, 2005)?

Key CLs who many times helped to jump-start the neighborhood's comeback, find themselves also having to relocate during the so called renewal and redevelopment process. In numerous instances, these residents are "key CLs," ousted as a result of their own successful efforts to negotiate and bring about renewed and empowered neighborhoods. For such residents, "cultural resilience" is discovered to be nothing more than a conceptual pipe dream, shattered by the loss of traditional community values as well as loss of traditional environmental and territorial boundaries. Further, many communal institutions also suffer as a result of the displacement brought on by radical inner-city change.

The psychology of displacement, as an intricate part of any renewal process, speaks to the usurping of environmental, cultural, and territorial attachment. For decades, in the case of African Americans, community has provided attachments and a sense of identity, familiarity with community, and cultural membership. The disorientation and alienation brought on by displacement leads to adverse psychological, physical, economic, and social effects. The definition of the term "place" is linked to what can be termed the critical three: *attachment, familiarity,* and *identity.* For the African American community, displacement initiates the unraveling of these critical three, precipitating the public health illnesses of territorial and psychological disorientation and alienation. As underlying aspects of displacement, the "critical three" can have a synergistic impact. One only needs to review the public health trauma brought on by relocation during Hurricane Katrina, producing chronic long-term physical and mental illnesses (Fullilove, 1996).

Urban renewal and redevelopment projects are not new phenomena; they are, in most cases, akin to the concept of displacement. For example, Georgia's state flower, the Cherokee Rose, is said to represent the suffering of the Cherokee Indians in the 1880s, who were forcibly removed from their land and marched to reservations in the West. About 4,000 Native Americans died in this dislocation. In more modern times, urban renewal was noted in the 1970s. Motivated by high gasoline prices, suburban sprawl, and a new taste for old architecture, middle-class populations began moving into neighborhoods that had gone out of fashion a generation or two earlier. Such nondiscriminatory negative occurrences may emerge as a result of natural disasters, urban renewal projects, segregation, isolation, and forced territorial settlement.

An historical review of programs, which were developed to rebuild distressed public housing and to address the social and economic needs of the original residents, discovered higher than average disease rates, mostly chronic illness, existing especially among African American women. As national, state, and local leaders of the 21st century attempt to rewrite the relocation process, policies must ensure that displaced individuals, and their families, have access to basic human needs including food, housing, transportation, and access to medical facilities for appropriate health care (Harris & Kaye, 2004).

Such regulatory changes drive lifestyle, behavioral, and cultural patterns such as who lives in the community, how one lives and works there, who buys and sells there, and what artifacts are used to symbolize the community (Form-Based Codes Institute, 2004).

Flores and Morrill highlight this clearly in their work in the City of Seattle, Washington. Unlike cities in which African Americans are significant in number, Seattle—and Washington State—has, by any measure, relatively small minority populations. Indeed, African Americans are not the largest population in Washington by any means. In contrast to the 190,267 African Americans reported by the 2000 Census in a state whose total population (5,894,121) is less than that of the City of Chicago, the census reported the countable number of Latinos in the state of Washington was 441,509, with 29,719 living in Seattle. Gentrification is defined as: *an upward shift in income, house values, education and occupational levels—in other words, in class, which almost always means increasing inequality and a widening gap between the more and the less successful.* This latter consequence is what distinguishes "gentrification" from "revitalization." Revitalization, on the other hand, is defined more positively as: *a renewed pride and investment in a community, mainly on the part of residents, without a big class shift.* These two processes—gentrification and revitalization—often are synchronous and are not necessarily entirely negative processes (Morrill, 2004).

In a real-world gentrification example in a community in Seattle, Flores's (2010) documentary titled *23rd & Union* is the story of an African American young man who murders an Ethiopian restaurant owner because he struggles to cope with the pressures of gentrification and racial profiling in Seattle's Central District. It further highlights and describes the impact gentrification and racial profiling can create, resulting in alienation and increased criminal behavior. The documentary points out that gentrification displaces working-class and middle-class citizens, exacerbating racial profiling and segregation. This displacement particularly alienates men of color and fosters a territorial complex that leads to adverse psychological effects and violent behavior against marginal communities who are part of the gentrifying process.

DEFINING THE FERAL COMMUNITY

Let's imagine for a moment a great metropolis covering hundreds of square miles. Once a vital component in a national economy, this sprawling urban environment is now a vast collection of blighted buildings, an immense Petri dish of both ancient and new diseases, a territory where the rule of law has long been replaced by near anarchy in which the only security available is that which is attained through brute power. The city's social services are all but nonexistent, and the vast majority of the city's occupants have no access to even the most basic health or security assistance. There is no social health safety net. Enter the state of public health in the feral community.

For some countries, especially those facing massive development challenges, accomplishing health equity throughout inner-city communities would be no mean feat. The health care cost would be extremely high, and CEOD for public health practice operation would leave more to be desired than a reclaimed and functioning population center.

Indeed, the majority of threats posed by a feral community would be viewed as both nontraditional and transcommunity. Chief among the nontraditional threats is the potential for pandemics and massive environmental degradation, and the near certainty that feral cities will serve as major transmission points for all manner of illicit diseases and disasters. Although it has been noted, city-born pandemics would not be new. The toxic environment of a feral community potentially would pose uniquely severe threats. A new illness or a strain of an existing disease could easily breed and mutate without detection in a feral community. Since feral communities would not be hermetically sealed, it would be quite easy to envision a deadly and dangerously virulent epidemic originating from such places. For example, the severe acute respiratory syndrome (SARS) outbreak of 2003 seems to offer an example of a city (Guangdong, China) serving as a pathogen incubator and point of origin of an intercontinental epidemic. In the case of SARS, the existence of the disease was rapidly identified, the origin was speedily traced, and a medical offensive was quickly mounted. Had such a disease originated in a feral community or city, it is likely that this process would have been much more complicated and taken a great deal more time. As it is, numerous diseases that had been believed to be under control have recently mutated into much more drug-resistant and virulent forms.

Globally, large communities are already placing significant environmental stress on their local and regional environments. A feral community—with minimal or no sanitation facilities, a complete absence of environmental controls, and a massive population—would be in effect a disease-breeding ground. Yet, this community is still globally connected. It possesses at least a modicum of commercial linkages, and some of its residents have access to the world's most modern communication and computing technologies. It would, in effect, be a "feral city."

The very term "feral city" is both provocative and controversial. Yet, this description has been chosen advisedly. The feral city may be a phenomenon that never takes place, yet its emergence should not be dismissed as impossible. The phrase also suggests, at least faintly, the nature of what may become one of the more difficult security challenges of the new century.

The putative "feral community" is (or would be): *a metropolis with a population of more than a million people in a state, the government of which has lost the ability to maintain the rule of law within the city's boundaries yet remains a functioning actor in the greater international system.*

A feral community experiences massive levels of disease and creates enough pollution to qualify as an international environmental disaster zone. Most feral communities suffer from massive urban hypertrophy, covering vast expanses of land. The community's structures range from great buildings, extravagant new houses, and condominiums, symbolic of wealth, environmental renewal, and gentrification, to ghetto's and massive unemployment. Yet, even under these conditions, these communities continue to grow, and the majority of occupants do not voluntarily leave (Florida, 2002).

Yet, throughout history, major communities have endured massive challenges without "going feral." How could it be determined that a community is at risk of becoming feral? What indicators might give warning? Is a warning system possible? The answer is yes.

Norton et al. (2010) offers such a model, a taxonomy consisting of 12 sets of measurements, grouped into four main categories. In it, measurements representing a healthy community are the color "green," those that would suggest cause for concern are "yellow," and those that indicate danger, a potentially feral condition, "red." In Table 15.1, the upper blocks in each category (column) represent positive or healthy conditions, those at the bottom unhealthy ones.

From this model, we have substituted the term "COF" to give a view from the perspective of the public health practice. Let's take a look at some of key aspects.

Health Leadership

The first category assesses the ability of the state to govern the city. A community "in the green" has a healthy, stable leadership—though not necessarily a democratically elected one. A democratic community leadership is perhaps the most desirable, but some communities governed by authoritarian regimes could be at extremely low risk of becoming feral. City governments "in the green" would be able to enact effective health policies, direct resources, and control events in all parts of the community at all times. A yellow indication would indicate that community health care leadership enjoys such authority only in portions of the community, producing what might be called "patchwork" leadership or "diurnal leadership." Health care authorities would be unable to practice at all equitable public health in a "red" community or would practice in name only. An entity within the community claiming to be

TABLE 15.1   The Health and Unhealthy Communities—A Framework

	GOVERNMENT	ECONOMY
Health ("Green")	Enacts effective legislation, directs resources, controls events in all portions of the community all time. Not corrupt.	Robust, significant foreign investment. Provides goods and services. Possesses stable and adequate tax base.
Marginal ("Yellow")	Exercises only "patchwork" or "diurnal" control. Highly corrupt.	Limited/no foreign investment. Subsidized or decaying industries and growing deficits.
Going Feral ("Red")	At best has negotiated zones of control; at worst does not exist.	Either local subsidence industries or industry based on illegal commerce.

	SERVICES	SECURITY
Health ("Green")	Complete range of services, including educational and cultural, available to all city residents.	Well regulated by professional, ethical police forces. Quick response to wide spectrum of requirements.
Marginal ("Yellow")	Can manage minimal level of public health, hospital access, portable water, and trash disposal.	Little regard for legality/human rights. Police often match/stymied by criminal "peers."
Going Feral ("Red")	Intermittent to nonexistent power and water. Those who can afford to will privately contract.	Nonexistent. Security is attained through private means or paying.

an official representative would simply be another actor competing for resources and power.

Health Economy

The second category involves the community's economy. Communities "in the green" would enjoy a productive mix of outside health resources, service and manufacturing activities, and a robust tax base. Communities afforded a "yellow" rating would have ceased to attract substantial outside health investment, be marked by decaying or growth in disease, and suffer from ever-growing deficits.

Health Service

The third category is focused on community services. Communities with a "green" rating would not only have a complete array of essential services but would provide public education, health service, and cultural facilities to their populations. These services would be available to all sectors of the community without distinction or bias. Communities with a yellow rating, while lacking many opportunities, would be able to maintain minimal services such as of public health and sanitation. Trash pickup, ambulance service, and access to hospitals would all exist. Such a community's water supply would pass minimum safety standards. In contrast, communities in the "red" zone would be unable to supply little more than intermittent power and water, and some not even that.

Security and Emergency Service

Security is the subject of the fourth category. "Green" communities, while obviously not crime free, would be well regulated by professional, ethical police emergency service, able to respond quickly to a wide spectrum of threats. "Yellow" cities would be marked by extremely high inequity crime rates, disregard of whole families of "minor crimes" due to lack of police resources, and criminal elements capable of serious confrontations. A "yellow" community's police emergency service would have little regard for individual rights or legal constraints. In a "red" community, the police force has failed altogether or has become merely another health service group seeking power and wealth. Citizens must provide for their own protection, perhaps by hiring independent security health care personnel or by paying protection to criminal organizations.

Corruption

A special, overarching consideration is corruption. Communities "in the green" are relatively corruption free. Scandals are rare enough to be newsworthy, and when corruption is uncovered, self-policing mechanisms effectively deal with it. Corruption in communities "in the yellow" would be much worse, extending to every level of the city administration. In yellow communities, "patchwork" patterns might reflect which portions of the community were able to buy security and health services and which were not. As for "red" communities, it would be less useful to speak of leadership corruption than of criminal and individual opportunism, which would be unconstrained.

Further—and it should come as no surprise—massive communities in the developing world are at far greater risk of becoming feral than those in more developed communities. Not only are support networks in such regions much less robust, but as a potentially feral city grows, it consumes progressively more resources. Efforts to meet its growing needs often in succeed maintaining the status quo or, more often, merely slowing the rate of decay of government control and essential services. All this, in turn, reduces the resources that can be applied to other portions of the community, and it may well increase the speed of urban hypertrophy.

Feral cities, as and if they emerge, will be something new on the international landscape. Cities have descended into savagery in the past, usually

as a result of war or civil conflict, and armed resistance groups have operated out of urban centers before. But feral cities, as such, will be a new
phenomenon and will pose security health threats on a scale hitherto not
encountered. It is questionable whether the tools, resources, and strategies that would be required to deal with these threats exist at present.
The feral community/city may be a phenomenon that never takes place,
yet its emergence should not be dismissed as impossible. The phrase
also suggests, at least faintly, the nature of what may become one of the
more difficult public health challenges of the new century. However,
given the indications of the imminent emergence of feral cities, it is time
to begin creating the means for addressing public health inequities in an
effective way.

CEOD AND COF

In a global sense, as mentioned in the section above, many of the challenges and opportunities that are coming to define the early part of the
21st century are at their most visible in the communities in which a growing proportion of the world's population now lives.

The question(s) then become: What are the principal challenges and
trends that are influencing PHPs of all disciplines, and what are strategies for delivering an effective public health environment for citizens of
all classes? What are the key elements of any inner-city community that
is divided into a number of different and important components? What
forms the basis for developing a strategic public health agenda that will
take a community forward? These questions focus on key elements and
cover people, knowledge, natural resources, technical infrastructure,
finances, political aspects, and cultural values that a community embod-
ies. Using these elements, then, let us examine how, in future decades,
PHPs of all stripes can engage, organize, and assist community residents
to organize and develop their understanding of each element. Further, let
us see how they can ensure that they engage and develop communities to
make the best use of the resources they possess, and develop those which
may be in shorter supply, for the public health good of the community.

There are six different, but key, types of resources or capital that COFs
will have, more or less, that should be organized, studied, and cultivated
by the PHP in the CEOD process. These include the following.

Intellectual and Social Capital

The CLs and the PHPs must identify the key people, knowledge, and skill
levels of the community targeted.

Intellectual capital is identified by the community leadership as one of
if not the most, important assets a community possess. In the knowledge
economy, it is the people in the community—their skills, capabilities, and

knowledge—that can make a critical difference in the community's ability to successfully adopt health initiatives.

How do communities measure and map their intellectual capital? Measuring intangible assets is very difficult and the evidence suggests that, to date, very few communities have specific initiatives in place to do so. However, it is clear that in the future many CLs will be trying to develop policies that will make their communities attractive to the skilled and entrepreneurial people that will help their communities to succeed in the economic uncertainties of the 21st century (see section on Gentrification). One of the key drivers of a community's attractiveness is the extent to which people feel connected to one another, in other words, the degree of social capital that exists. This simply means ensuring that the appropriate people, skills, and capabilities are developed, with the community leadership demonstrating that they understand how these qualities can be captured and allowed to prosper.

Social capital is difficult to define but expresses itself in the quality of informal and formal relationships that characterize communities. The degree of social capital in communities is linked closely to low levels of crime, to educational achievement, and to physical and mental health. In COF, PHPs and CLs will face the challenge of ensuring that divisions and segregation are not allowed to develop between rich and poor and between different cultures. Engaging all residents equitably therefore is a major challenge for COF.

Inclusive Capital

One positive means the PHP can use to develop opportunities for participation and consultation is through the development of community coalition boards, which can become an essential component for building inclusiveness. This inclusiveness would call for tapping into: community residents, elected officials, business persons, educators, health professionals, and any other individuals that could serve as assets to the communities public health process. Each of these individual resources would work for the betterment of the community's health and would be accountable and transparent in their dialogue with other CLs. All would work to achieve the commitment of the whole community on its journey into the future improvement of the community's health status. In COF, the public health professional will need to develop new partnerships with different stakeholders, and engage in new forms of partnership that go beyond simply listening to the views of others. Community residents become more than just voters or customers—they are engaged as coproducers in the policies that will shape the community's health initiatives and, subsequently, its future health status.

Channels for "real-time" interaction in COF will also expand significantly through various forms of social media. More than simply providing information, social media provides a platform for genuine dialogue between communities and community residents in a way that traditional channels could not easily accommodate.

Inclusiveness also calls for communities to develop accountability, which will be a key aspect of the strategies that COF adopt to engage their residents and partners. They must do this by disclosing their own targets and recording their performance against them, and by creating collaborative forums with specific interest groups (e.g., business) and by arranging their community services around the needs and priorities of their residents.

Cultural Capital

The CLs and the PHPs must seek to identify cultural values, behaviors, and public expressions. The competition within and among COF will be strong. A community will comprise a complex array of attributes that provide it with a unique identity. Communities that succeed in attracting visitors, residents, and businesses do so by creating a "brand" that encapsulates the qualities that only that community offers, and generates powerful and memorable positive associations.

In building a brand, a community has to be aware of how it is seen by the outside world. What are the culture qualities it is seen to have? What is the lifestyle associated with the community? A PHP seeking to design and implement health initiatives may very well need to understand, and to address, what cultural capital needs are in the community, how they are presently viewed and, from that understanding, develop the steps needed to move their health initiatives forward.

There is one single plan for creating a successful community brand. However, there are many existing strategies available that can help a community draw attention to their qualities. Therefore, community leadership of the future, wishing to embark on this journey, would need to ask critical questions. For example, they need to consider what will attract the attention of the world to their community and, more importantly, what will keep it there.

Environmental Capital

The CLs and the PHPs must identify natural/environmental resources in the targeted community. Environmental issues are near the top of all agendas for COF, especially as quality of life becomes an important source of competitive advantage. Community leadership will always focus on providing a clean and safe environment for their residents, therefore, the quality of life that a community offers is a fundamental aspect of its ability to prosper and improve its overall public health status. Offering its residents a clean, green, safe, and attractive environment will be high on the list of priorities for leadership.

Balancing economic development with environmental impact will be a significant challenge for all COF. Pollution, in all its forms, is a major problem for most communities, and so leadership must seek to have policies developed that incorporate economic and environmental consideration.

Pursuing and developing sustainability necessitates a joined-up approach to decision making. This means that environmental considerations must be an integral part of policy development across the spectrum of the community. Planning, transport, finance, and economic policies all need to reflect the environmental health goals. The pace and extent of change that COF will have to cope with requires them to become particularly adept at program and project involvement and management. To do so effectively means they will need to take on the right skills that can guide and support change within their communities. It means they will have to influence environmental health policies and be encouraged to take responsibility for the quality of the environment in which they live. Engaged residents become a prerequisite for success in developing sustainable environmental improvements.

Technical Capital

The CLs and the PHPs must identify, establish, and rely on social media, man-made capital, and existing community infrastructure.

The enormous complexity of communities in the future means that the demands on their infrastructure will be relentlessly challenging. Not only will the "basic" needs of a transport, housing, water, and energy be under strain, but new demands for effective methods of communication will make the supply of, for example, broadband and electronic networks an increasingly important element of infrastructure provision. To cope with these challenges, COF will need to adopt an integrated approach to their public health planning. Rather than planning for the separate provision of health-intervention programs and clinical medical care, for example, a more holistic view will need to be adopted that seeks to measure the combined impacts of different types of health education, medical education, and primary care treatment. This integrated approach also means that COF will need to look to establish partnerships and new forms of collaboration that allow them to deliver infrastructure requirements in new ways. Public–private partnerships to deliver a public health infrastructure must become a common feature of many COF, allowing them to share the health community's vision, and provisions, with partners from all sectors.

The pressure on COF to operate more efficiently and, at the same time, improve their services to residents must be increasingly responded to by the adoption of technological solutions. Improving processes and work-flows within the community's administration itself will be a key focus for COF. Using new technology to improve communications and the flow of data within a COF will be made possible through the application of e-information solutions that can connect across the traditional boundaries to allow more effective collaboration, resulting in better service for its community residents (see the chapter on CEOD and social media).

Financial Capital

The PHP must identify money and other assets necessary for community CEOD. Growing demands, combined with diminishing revenue bases, will mean that COF will need to be creative and flexible in their financial strategies and increase partnerships with the private sector.

The COF face a number of common financial challenges. Budgets will be under intense pressure from a host of competing demands. At the same time, community residents will continue to demand better services but will be reluctant to pay more for them. The familiar dilemma of having to do more with less is one that all COF will face. In order to respond to this challenge, COF will have to be innovative in how they establish accounting policies and analyze their financial position. They will need to become more sophisticated in this area, learning skills by themselves while also partnering with skilled professionals that can introduce them to financial disciplines and performance management methodologies. Further, they will need to adopt entrepreneurial approaches to the way that they finance and provide services. They will need to understand the true costs of the services and products that they supply in order to evaluate whether alternative provision (such as shared services) may be more efficient. Some COF may be more effective in certain areas than others. Thus, they should seek opportunities to "trade" or "barter" with other communities—selling those services that they perform most efficiently and buying into those where it makes financial sense to do so.

Again, new forms of partnership will be critical. Many CLs will discover the advantages of working with the private sector to fund the provision of services and infrastructure in innovative ways. Taken together, the demands on COF finances will call for planning that sets out to achieve the health-related goals and tasks that are realistic, and establishes how the funding and investment they require can be most effectively put in place. By consulting and examining the experience of others, they will be able to begin developing the financial structures that will allow them to meet their present and future needs.

Organizing all of this capital together requires strong leadership. The PHP as a leader, will need to develop a style of leadership that is both highly consultative and yet directional. They will need to inspire and fulfill the dreams and visions of the COF in order to help share with the people and organizations that their health efforts are targeting. A value-based approach is one that COF leaders will be increasingly seeking to adopt. Therefore, this value-based leadership will need to operate on the basis of a number of specifics including shared values that are communicated clearly throughout the community, along with those that reflect positively on the institutions and organizations from which the PHP leadership originates. The agendas of these agencies will, primarily, guide the daily thoughts and actions of PHP because they are in fact who pays the PHP salary!

In the CEOD process, identifying and organizing these key elements effectively means taking a holistic approach into COF, since each one these elements depends on the other. So then, the necessity of taking a holistic approach becomes an essential component of the overall CEOD process. PHPs involved in the CEOD process should first project their planning for the future and do some forecasting to see just how their methods and strategies can adapt to these six dynamics existing in their target communities.

This process is one of community health navigation into the community's future. To make sure that communities reach their intended health destination, both the practitioner and community residents need to be aware of their starting position. This requires the PHP to facilitate by asking some important strategic questions, identifying community strengths, and working toward eliminating areas of weakness. Once the PHP has identified *where they are*, they will need to decide *where they want to be* with the community health initiative they seek to launch. And to do this, they will need to understand the significant trends that will influence the direction in which the community's future unfolds. In addition to understanding these trends, the PHP will need to identify the significant challenges that lie ahead when creating the strategic plan for the community health initiative.

These COF will be highly complex units. The PHP will need to respond to the ever-increasing demands of many different groups (i.e., financially, culturally, educationally, socially, etc.) and work within and manage the allocation of resources needed to address the differences, and often competing, health-related claims.

Developing the capabilities to ensure that COF manage their capitals effectively means engaging with the people, helping to organize the community processes, and identifying resources, skills, and property that are needed to manage and achieve their overall community health goals. Without effective organization and performance management, COF will not be able to create a culture of continuous disparity reduction and health improvement.

STRATEGIC SOCIAL ANALYSIS

When navigating into the future with community residents, the PHP requires an open mind and leadership. A cynical attitude among some experienced leaders is that the future is simply a recycling of old ideas and concepts under different and new names. The "old wine in new bottles" adage! This philosophy and approach says that the future is behind us. There is nothing new to come, and no expectation of real change in the future. But, change is real and the demands of the future are pressing on all, and leaders, such as the PHP, must have the vision and the dreams that will empower and inspire community residents about improving their health status and their overall quality of life.

Rapidly changing modern societies are creating a need for strategic development that offers constant innovation and renewal of processes and people's attitudes. It is important that leaders of COF are able to see things in a new way, incorporating the good ideas of the past with new and innovative methods appropriate for the future. Strategic social analysis (SSA) can be defined as: *the gleaning of intelligence learned from the past but, most importantly, understanding the likely direction of the future.* The SSA intelligence is an area of vital importance related to what we call "intelligent communities (ICs)."

An IC has to be able to see what happens through time, that is: it (1) *analyzes*, (2) *reaches conclusions*, and (3) *defines its present reality*. ICs learn to develop their strengths and eliminate their weaknesses. It is through these three processes that vision, ideas, and strategy are created. Consequently, this is how the IC will create and prepare for the future. It is essential that COF have the power to work through and implement all of these three processes. Some communities, for example, will remain in the analytical phase and never move on to formulating and implementing their visions and dreams.

PHPs, in many instances, will be like the navigators of a ship. In this way, PHPs have been assigned to *knowledgably navigate* the waters, and have taken on the leadership role of the community health initiative. The crew and passengers include *community residents, employees,* and *other consumers.* For the PHP, the first concern is strategic positioning of: *where are we right now?* The next consideration is destination: *where are we going?* Then: *what are our health visions* or dreams for the community? Finally, there is route and speed: how quickly and by which path will we reach our destination? To create a vision and a dream takes time, but there is no time, however, in most health initiatives; time is of the essence. The reality in most health initiatives—whether it be community health-intervention programs, community-based research, or primary care services—is that time sensitivity is a real life factor. The PHPs' navigation process demands they consider today, now, both their position as professionals and the communities they serve. They must quickly analyze what kind of approach will be used to reach the future vision of community, while simultaneously meeting the goals and objectives set forth in the grant application or the research protocol or primary care regimen. Following are four different factors a PHP can consider when navigating in relation to the community to be served.

Inactive: No interpretation of trends, ignoring all present and future trends

Reactive: Responding to the agenda of others as set by the community, institution, or agency for which they are employed

Proactive: Making detailed plans for the future and setting trends based on exiting knowledge, incorporating community needs, and institutional agendas

Interactive: Shaping and responding to changing trends over time

The PHP leaders of tomorrow need the right approach to the journey as they try to understand and adapt their course according to trends forecast for the future. When conditions change, leaders will need to respond immediately. They may have to sail against the wind for a while, but then change again. During this process, the leader needs to develop a "mental GPS" based on intelligence gathered from a wide variety of sources. This introduces another term for the PHP, coined "knowledge navigation (KN)" that is a relevant term in this context. This KN is a way of working, and is only an option, if there is a clear-cut appreciation of the direction to take—which, in turn, requires a strong vision linked to both committed leadership and a well-managed institutional organization. To achieve this, leaders have to analyze both from the outside in (global trends and tendencies) and from the inside out (visions for the communities and its organization).

DEFINING MEGA TRENDS

A mega trend (MT), in it broadest sense, can be defined as: *any event or occurrence that affects the majority of areas of civil, business, and public life*. It creates consequences everywhere and for everyone, not least for communities themselves. Some examples of MTs include the following.

Globalization or Glocalization

The global economy is becoming truly integrated. Today's simultaneous global and local focuses create a new framework of ideas and opportunities. Global companies and economies work in local competition within global structures. This is sometimes called "glocalization." When a big company either arrives or leaves a community, it affects many areas of life for that community and its residents. New international networks and cooperation among communities can create significant strategic advantages.

Individualism

Individualism has become an increasingly important social trend. We see it in marketing, with developments like "one-to-one" and relationship marketing instead of strategies that focus on groups. Persons of the future will be known as the "I generation," which means they will be people who are individualistic, informal, informed, interactive, and yet international in their thinking and behavior. This phenomenon will have an important impact on the dialogue between COF and their demanding residents. Community leadership will need to think of their citizens as "consumers," and ensure that public health and social services match the standards of the very best in the private sector.

Merging

Many areas of life in COF will merge together in new ways, similar to what is taking place between larger communities such as countries and nations (e.g., European Union); between technologies like Hi-Tec, Bio-Tec, and medicine; between cultures and values; between work and leisure; and between the public and private sectors in public–private partnerships (PPP). The COF will begin to redraw boundaries through redistricting, sharing, and separate use of utilities and services, causing shifts in voting power and other resources available.

Accelerated Communication and Social Media

Speed is increasing in all areas of life. This is often driven by information and communication technology (ICT) and the search for growth. The COF will want online access to all public and private services, and the "democratic dialogue" will increasingly demand rapid exchange of information. Access to high-speed information will have direct implications for the delivery of all services including administration, education, health care, transportation, and more. In the COF there will be more and more of the science and technology in the delivery of health care, regardless of health sector.

Urbanization

The United Nations Habitat Report 2004 predicted that by 2030 around 60% of the world's population will live in the inner city, thus, the term "metropolitanization." This term refers to the growing influence of large cities on the economic health and prosperity of wider regions and, in some cases, entire nations.

Migration

Urbanization is also linked to increased global migration. There is no doubt that increased migration in COF will present major challenges around social cohesion, integration, health promotion, and employment. However, it also presents great opportunities as COF seek to capitalize on "knowledge migration." One negative aspect of knowledge migration is the expertise and experience that is lost when companies relocate or outsource parts of their businesses. A positive aspect to be considered is how knowledge and skills of immigrant communities can be harnessed to improve COF. Often migrants bring a wealth of skills to their new communities, but sometimes their qualifications and training are not recognized by their destination country. For example, they may not be eligible to work in their profession or sector without certain licensure or retraining. As a consequence, many high-skilled immigrants often end up in low-paid jobs in their new communities. Migration patterns and trends in COF will impact on employment rates, and also on issues of health and social cohesion and inclusiveness. While migration issues have been ongoing for many centuries, in COF, this issue will intensify. This will mean that the strategic health and social agendas of tomorrow will call for a unique interpretation of these trends and, subsequently, their impact on the community in practical terms.

In COF, these issues will be highly complex and changes will occur rapidly. The following are examples of some of the challenges that will have a significant impact on COF:

- *Aging population* will cause increased financial burdens on health and welfare systems
- *Economic restructuring* will bring increased unemployment, and the end of "lifelong" working
- *Disasters* including natural catastrophes, terrorism, and epidemics (HIV/AIDS, Avian Flu)
- *Crime* (not least economic), safety and security
- *Migration and immigration* (people and knowledge)
- *Segregation, disparity, inequality, and poverty*
- *Social cohesion and equality*
- *Sustainable* development and economic growth from both the local and global perspective

The COF will recognize the challenges in ensuring that they can attract and foster the people, skills, and capabilities they need to prosper in the knowledge economy. These leaders must become facilitators of change. Each community will learn from its past and historical heritage. However, lessons available from other successful communities will be studied and adopted as well (Radovanovic, 2003).

For the visionary "Dream Communities," one of the most important aspects for the future is organizing and building community coalitions and boards. An IC will need to create the context and forums where knowledge individuals can exchange their ideas and engage their creativity (Figure 15.1).

Community leadership and PHP will need to be oriented toward the future, to sense and analyze what will be most important tomorrow. To find out what to expect in the future, they will need to gather data that enable them to create scenarios and estimate future trends. Every community will need to engage leadership to motivate its citizens and create a spirit, with as many persons as possible becoming contributors, and taking

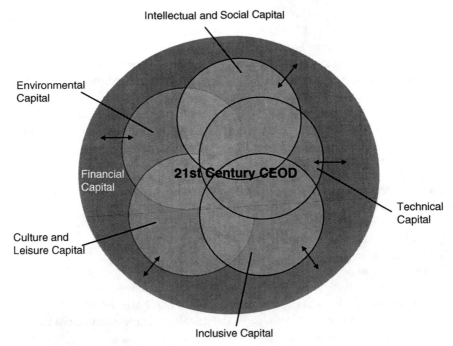

FIGURE 15.1   Intelligent communities (ICs) of the future.

"ownership" of the community. Intelligent leadership will seek to engage community residents for them to take on specific development roles. The trick is to join them together, foster collaboration, and assist them in creating a corporate identity.

The well-known military leader General Von Klausewitz defined strategy as the "art of knowing how to win a war" and so communities will need to have visions and dreams before they try to implement initiatives. Therefore, the COF will need to develop it Unique Selling or Strategic Points (USP) for achieving its goals and objectives.

FUTURE TRENDS IN CEOD

One key to the success for COF is the ability of PHPs to create public trust and enhance their accountability, while simultaneously encouraging dialogue between residents and leadership, and finding new forums for collaboration between CLs, community residents, and health care providers and their respective institutions.

The problem with good ideas and strong vision is that in order to fully realize them involves a lot of hard work. The PHPs and CLs alike must turn vision into reality. Thus, action is critical. Vision without action is meaningless. They will need to provide the circumstances in which residents can fulfill their potential. Further, they must create visions that show "multimutual benefit(s)," where both they and the community eventually receive benefits. These benefits need to be communicated to residents in such a way that inspires all to take ownership in what the community can achieve. Examples of multimutual benefits for strong visions in a community could include (1) *motivating people by giving hope and belief for the future,* (2) *providing both the PHP and the community with direction;* (3) *developing inspiration for new challenges,* (4) *agreeing on a common description of a desirable future,* and (4) *providing a strategic position in marketing, communicating, and branding the community.*

Further, three *major trends* are emerging that, taken together, provide the tools to bring all the players together and the mutual benefits for COF. These trends include:

1. *Transparency*
2. *Including new forms of participants*
3. *Development of partnership*

Let's examine how these identified trends can help the PHP to fortify some of the public health initiatives they seek to implement in communities they target (Figure 15.2).

Trend 1: Transparency

The push for transparency comes from a number of different sources. The "Information Age" or "Social Media Age" powered by the Internet has created unparalleled access to information about almost everything and, increasingly, transparency is a vital building block of trust and relationship building between community individuals and organizations. Trust and accountability are inextricably linked and so the creation and maintenance of trust is a key challenge for CLs that want to be accountable to their residents, the economy, and society. Transparency is dependent on two-way communication that flows between PHP leaders and the people who live and work in communities to be served. Trust-based relationships are more effective and efficient. To create trust, the PHP leader must provide community residents and other stakeholders with information about financial results, and also about how plans, goals, and decisions are made and results achieved—good as well as bad. Accountable leadership reports regularly to community members about performance.

The two-way communication that strongly supports the trust-based relationship process permits the PHP to more fully engage with community members, and enables them to present their views and listen to the views of community residents.

More than simply providing information, PHPs as CLs should use technology to enhance their accountability by giving residents direct access

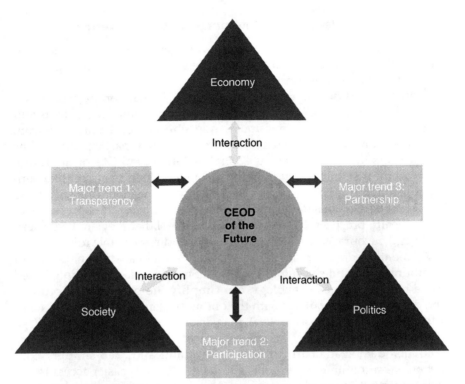

FIGURE 15.2 Interactions among politics, society, and economy with the three major trends to optimize CEOD capital.

and creating ready dialogue with them. This accountable state reflects and accommodates residents' needs and concerns by using methods such as e-communication-based complaint management and opinion research methods and surveys. However, dialogue with citizens is not enough: PHP leaders must be responsive to residents' input. They must accept a new relationship that sees information flowing from them to residents and then back again to reinforce their leadership role. Rather than being organized from the point of view of the administration and its requirements, community residents and their needs become the organizing principle for services and information. Resident-centricity is a key trend in the development of transparent and accountable community trust. It is a trend that COFs all over the world will respond to.

Freedom of information is also an important basis for creating community empowerment and for helping to facilitate transparency. Thus, the accountability state takes community empowerment seriously. It informs community residents about overall performance comparing its original plans to the actual results achieved. In the accountable state, transparency is a fundamental element of building trust.

Trend 2: Participation Interaction and Empowerment

Whenever major community residents' issues are at stake, concerned citizens should be able to participate formally and informally through what is called deliberative assemblies.

Deliberative assembles create constructive interaction opportunities, which allow the PHP to interact more fully with community residents and subsequently gain a more grassroots understanding of the problem from "on-the-ground level." Residents are seen as active participants and as coproducers in decision making. Therefore, successful CLs of the future must promote public policies that regard its residents as more than simply consumers of public services. They must view residents holistically, as important participants in the implementation and realization processes of public health practices. In this way, residents feel that they are taken seriously and encouraged to play a more active and responsible role.

As mentioned earlier, the Internet has ushered in a whole new way of communicating and sharing information. Smart e-communication, based on advanced Internet technology, can simplify the participation process. The digitalization of politics with the online presence of parties and institutions (e.g., national assemblies), and discussions with politicians (e.g., candidate domains), play an important role in enhancing community residents' democratic participation. E-communication can simplify contact between community residents and the PHP, create easier access to relevant information, promote transparency, and speed-up access to health information.

The COF will routinely seek to engage the communication platform—such as mobile telephones—to increase community residents' participation and engagement. This allows residents to participate in debates and policy decisions via their mobile phones and to interact with administrators and CL through the use of SMS and MMS messaging. The benefits of social media participation through the Internet and so on include the permanent availability of information, the possibility of visualization and interactivity, fast updating and feedback, and low-access barriers.

However, the PHP must be aware that in some disparity and underprivileged communities, e-participation can become a disadvantage, because of little or no access to Internet services. In order to avoid such individuals from becoming even further disadvantaged by the digital divide, the PHP needs to take steps and make investments to provide e-literacy skills training and create means for technology access to community residents. Thus, in some cases, where disparity, depravity, and inequity are at high rates, use of e-commerce may slow public health innovation, so the planned use of various forms of communication should be assessed thoroughly and utilized prudently and carefully based on access within the prevailing cultural context. Community residents need to have an effective voice within their communities. They should also be empowered with sufficient autonomy to make their own decisions, take ownership, and be entitled to participate adequately in the decision-making processes at all levels.

Let's take a brief look at some basic guidelines and how each can be used by a PHP to ensure that community residents have access to and can participate in community-based health initiatives.

Interaction: The declining attractiveness of traditional forms of community participation needs to be addressed with new and active forms of interaction. For example, the PHP should seek to combine representative inclusion with forms of direct participation. Balancing and calibrating the different forms of participation is a key success factor for optimizing participation and ownership.

More is not always better or effective participation: Participation should be made more effective through a focus on higher quality and less quantity, with residents getting maximum benefit from a minimal input of their time. Residents have a right to understand the health issues facing their communities and to have an ongoing voice in helping to decide how those issues are dealt with by the PHP. Through partnerships, community residents can have input into the decisions about important questions that affect them where they live.

Empowerment: Communities should be empowered with sufficient competencies and resources to fulfill their tasks and should have the ability to participate in and influence the decision-making process at all levels of public health planning and implementation.

Trend 3: Partnerships

In COF, increased demands on public health services caused by, among other things, an aging population, coupled with decreasing revenues as the tax base declines, mean that communities will need to have direct input into fulfillment of all their public health service obligations. Dwindling resources and more demanding residents, who take an increasingly consumerist attitude to the health services their community provides, means that new ways of financing and providing public health services must be found. The COF will have to look beyond their traditional role and develop collaboration and partnerships with the private sector and with other community groups. Community leadership and PHPs have to find ways to attract people and businesses that will allow their cities to compete in the global economy. A thriving local economy benefits everyone who lives and works in the community, and so the community leadership must have a direct interest in finding ways to work with the private sector and city government to achieve mutually beneficial outcomes. This will call for innovative/new forms of partnership in which the community, public, and private sectors find new ways to work together. To create these new forms of working is an imperative for all communities in the future. Figure 15.3 describes the variables that

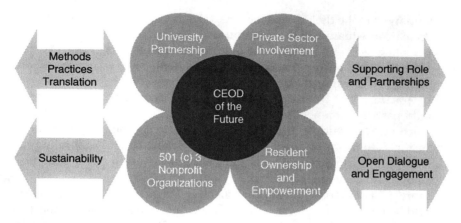

FIGURE 15.3   Practices, values, and attitudes underpinning successful CEOD partnerships.

must overlap in order for meaningful partnerships to occur in the CEOD model for COF.

A modern community will need a renewal of "civic pride," a vital element in COF. This means that community residents will have to be mobilized in the common interest and will have to be motivated to engage in activities that generate wide sociohealth benefits. As COF become more fragmented as a result of greater mobility (i.e., gentrification, etc.), the PHP has a role to play to encourage residents to participate in the public interest. Community residents must seek formal and informal partnerships in order to improve their own situations. They must seek partnerships that focus on improving their environment and the health status of their community, all the while learning to formulate goals and proposals of their own, which can be discussed in detail at joint meetings attended by local politicians and other leaders.

Initiatives to create new forms of partnership like these introduce a broader view to aspects of future community life and are often capable of reaching innovative and creative solutions. By empowering community residents to get involved in the resolution of social and public health issues, these initiatives encourage self-reliance and responsibility. Of course, these partnerships have to be piloted with professionalism and suitable caution. Risks have to be managed and efficiency and effectiveness of the arrangements evaluated carefully, especially in projects that demand large investments of both time and money. However, many cases prove that investments in new forms of partnership can provide "value for money" and tangible benefits. Partnerships between players from the public, the private sector, and the communities can enhance the success of COF. Let's now take a look at some of the criteria needed to determine meaningful community partnerships.

Efficiency: Cooperation with social groups facilitates the implementation of policy.

Legitimacy: The involvement and backing of community residents and leadership create broad agreement and backing for decisions.

Addressing complexity: Through partnerships with different community, economic, and social groups, problems can be viewed holistically and futuristically.

Motivation: The motivation for traditional political participation has declined. Partnerships, however, offer strong incentives to benefit COF and also to influence political health-related decision making.

Political engagement: Democracy is strengthened by the PHP and COF cooperating with the different interest groups.

Innovation: Innovation is also a key to responding to community resident concerns about new forms of partnerships.

Many different models have emerged around the world and intelligent capital is strengthened when PHP leaders work with community residents to find the right model for their circumstances.

SUMMARY

How can these major trends (transparency, participation, and partnership) best be promoted? They need to be communicated within the society, the economy, and the politics of the community. Tasks and responsibilities need to be allocated to the community at large and at diverse levels. Broad discussion of their impact on each major set of stakeholders will help to entrench and foster the development of bilateral and trilateral relationships. In order to engage all three elements in the pursuit of transparency, participation, and partnership, it is important to show the benefits that each will receive. The PHP and community leadership needs to ask themselves how transparent they are now, and what potential they see for greater transparency? They need to ask if communication flows are truly two-way or if they are dominated by an outflow that smothers the input from or listening to the voices of community residents. Community residents and the PHP need to develop their understanding of different forms of democratic participation and see how they might work in the specific context of the communities served or to be served. New and innovative platforms for engagement and dialogue—such as the social media—also need to be examined and made to work in the unique conditions and context of each individual community.

The infrastructure of COF will exceed the simple provision of transport and utilities—although they will still represent a considerable challenge in their own right. Infrastructure will also include information transfer, technology, and communications that link COF with institutions, health care services, other communities and businesses. The COF will expect fast, responsive services, and will want to be able to transact their dealings online, efficiently and effectively. In combination, these pressures will mean that COF will have to find new ways to develop their infrastructure in an integrated manner. They will have to develop new partnerships, collaborations, and ways of working that can help them to deliver infrastructure solutions that are efficient, environmentally sustainable, and cost effective.

Case Study Exercises

Individually, or as a group, review the following case studies and respond to the questions posed at the end of the study, as appropriate. Be sure to focus on the why, how, and what emphasized in each question. Your professor/instructor will provide you with specific guidance on how you are to report your findings for the class.

Case Study 15.1: Exploring a Healthy COF

Review the description and scenarios provided below for COF and develop responses to the questions listed at the end of the study.

Based on the discussion of healthy and unhealthy communities in the chapter picture a community that emerges as a mosaic, and like an artist's mosaic it can be expected to contain more than one color. Some healthy communities function with remarkable degrees of corruption. Others, robust and vital in many ways, suffer from appalling levels of criminal activity. Even a community with multiple "red" categories is not necessarily feral—yet. It is the overall pattern and whether that pattern is improving or deteriorating over time that gives the overall diagnosis.

It is important to remember a diagnostic tool such as this merely produces a "snapshot" and is therefore of limited utility unless supported by trend analysis. Remember, situations can exist in all the categories. For example, an urban center with an overall red rating—that is, a feral city— might boast a tiny enclave where "green" conditions prevail. On the other hand, quite healthy communities could experience both cycles of decline and improvement. For this exercise, here are some specific examples of green, yellow, and red communities:

Healthy Community: Tax Base: New York. To some it would seem that New York is an odd example of a "green" community. One hears and recalls stories of corruption, police brutality, gentrification, crime, pollution, neighborhoods that resemble war zones, and the like. Yet, by objective indicators (and certainly in the opinion of the majority of its citizens), New York is a healthy community and in no risk of "going feral." Its health care system is highly reputable and of high quality, its police force is well regulated, well educated, and responsive. The community is a hub of national and international investment. It generates substantial revenues and has a stable scope of health care services, including a wide range of educational and cultural opportunities. Does this favorable evaluation mean that the rich are not treated differently from the poor, that services and infrastructure are uniformly well maintained, or that there are no inequities or disparities in economic opportunity or race issues? Absolutely not. Yet, despite such problems, New York remains a viable municipality.

The Yellow Zone: Mexico City. This sprawling megalopolis of more than 20 million continues to increase in size and population every year. It is one of the largest urban concentrations in the world. As the seat of the Mexican government, it receives a great deal of state attention. However, Mexico City is now described as an urban nightmare.

Mexico City's air is so polluted that it is routinely rated medically as unfit to breathe. There are square miles of slums, often without sewage or running water. Law and order is breaking down at an accelerating rate. Serious crime has doubled over the past 3 to 4 years; it is estimated that 15.5 million assaults now occur every year in Mexico City. Car-jacking and taxi-jacking have reached such epidemic proportions that visitors are now officially warned not to use the cabs. The Mexico City police department has 91,000 officers—more men than the Canadian army—but graft and corruption on the force are rampant and on the rise. According to the Mexican senator, Adolfo Zinser, police officers themselves directly contribute to the city's crime statistics: "In the morning they are policeman. In the afternoon they're crooks." The city's judicial system is equally corrupt. Not surprisingly, these aspects of life in Mexico City have reduced the willingness of foreign investors to send money or representatives there.

Johannesburg: As in many South African communities, police in Johannesburg are waging a desperate war for control and it is not clear whether they will win. Though relatively small in size with only 2.9 million official residents, Johannesburg nevertheless experiences more than 5,000 murders a year and at least twice as many rapes. Over the last several years investors and major industry have fled the city. Many of the major buildings of the Central Business District have been abandoned and are now home to squatters. The South African National Stock Exchange has been removed to Sandton—a safer northern suburb. Police forces admit they do not control large areas of the city; official advisories warn against driving on certain thoroughfares. At night, residents are advised to remain in their homes. Tourism has dried up, and conventions, once an important source of revenue, are now hosted elsewhere in the country.

The city also suffers from high rates of air pollution, primarily from vehicle exhaust but also from the use of open fires and coal for cooking and heating. Johannesburg's two rivers are also considered unsafe, primarily because of untreated human waste and chemicals leaching from piles of mining dross. Mining has also contaminated much of the soil in the vicinity.

Like those of many states and cities in Africa, Johannesburg's problems are exacerbated by the AIDS epidemic. Nationally, it is feared that the number of infected persons may reach as high as 20% of the population. All sectors of the economy have been affected adversely by the epidemic, including Johannesburg.

Study Questions

1. Determine what kind of cultural community of the future you envision for your community? Thoughts: Can you imagine the kind of cultural community you want to live or work in?
2. How will our country be unified as a cohesive whole, if people separate into many different cultural groups?
3. In order to be a part of the American dream, must I assimilate?
4. Are there structural problems in our government or economic system that serve to divide cultural groups? How can they be changed?
5. Should I put my community building and civic energies into my own cultural community, rather than the mainstream culture? Where can I have the biggest influence?
6. Can oppression be stopped by legislation, or does each person have to overcome their individual prejudice, or both?
7. Why do immigrants have to hold onto their own cultures and languages when they come to the United States?
8. If my group is excluded from the American dream, what can I do?
9. How do I protect my children from being targeted by racism or sexism and other forms of discrimination if I live in a diverse society? Shall I send them to an Afrocentric school, or a female-only school, or another appropriate school?
10. What do you think about these questions? Which issues do you struggle with? What other issues are important to you or your cultural group?
11. What other issues do you think are important to consider? What are your next steps?

Case Study 15.2: Gentrification of COFs: Fact or Fiction

This case study is based on research conducted to develop the real-life documentary and short film entitled: *23rd & Union*. This film explores the events behind the murder of an Ethiopian restaurant owner at the hands of a young African American who was struggling to cope with the pressures of gentrification and racial profiling in Seattle's Central District. The film's premise is based on the idea that gentrification and racial profiling can produce displacement, mental illness, disorientation, and alienation. Accordingly, the film suggests that, in extreme cases, alienation can lead young men of color to commit hate crimes against immigrants and gays.

Social media is a tool that scholars and social activists have been increasingly utilizing in an attempt to survey the community and try to bridge the gap between cultures, academia, and the general public. The role that *23rd & Union* has played in promoting public dialogue about gentrification in Seattle and its various ramifications is a useful case study to approach the discussion about the potential advantages that social media offers for promoting community engagement and planning public health practices in the future.

Since its premiere in 2011, "23rd & Union" has commanded considerable interest and attention. For one, it has been the subject of various radio, newspaper, and blog discussions. In addition, it has won several awards at various film festivals and has also toured the United States, Lesotho, Mozambique, Swaziland, and South Africa—places where the social issues portrayed in the film have prevailed in similar forms. More recently, it has been featured on the University of Washington's TV channel. The exposure that the film has received is significant, considering that it was made with a shoestring budget; it has been marketed as an independent academic tool and has no major distribution deal.

One of the primary tools the director used to increase both community engagement and the marketing potential of such an academically oriented social media project was the creation of a soundtrack that bridged the gap between independent artists in Seattle's music scene and the local film industry. Another approach to community engagement the director utilized was a grassroots campaign staffed by volunteers that canvassed the city and passed out flyers announcing the initial community screening. Finally, the Internet and all related social media outlets (Facebook, MySpace, and Twitter) were among most effective tools to enhance community engagement and augment public participation.

For this case study the director of *23rd & Union* speaks about (1) the production techniques and strategies he adopted to make the film, and (2) the obstacles he encountered when engaging the community. After reflecting on the director's remarks, design a short social media project that you can utilize to expose the general population to relevant information and public health practices, thereby enhancing academia's engagement with the community. When designing the project, remember to consider the various emerging forms and strategies of social media that can increase the appeal of these issues to the public, attract individuals to participate in a larger social forum, and connect local issues to a global dialogue.

Study Questions

As a group discuss and respond in writing to the questions listed below. Identify problems, arguments, and solutions that address the concepts of feral cities and gentrification. Discuss the degree to which they reflect, or not, on the public health of the community and the role of the PHP.

1. How can racial profiling become a function of gentrified areas?
2. Is the alienation produced by gentrification a public health concern?
3. Can alienation and disorientation produced by displacement be alleviated? If so, how?
4. Does municipal legislation directly impact the needs of displaced families?
5. Do lending companies discriminate against African American families?
6. How are small businesses affected by or contribute to the effects of gentrification?
7. What can be done to combat the negative effects of gentrification?
8. How do you think it feels to live in a gentrified community?
9. Is gentrification only a class issue?
10. Is gentrification of communities a bad practice?
11. Why could there be tension among immigrants, gays, and African Americans in gentrified areas?
12. How can "cultural differences" contribute to the alienating effects of gentrification?
13. How can senior citizens and young men of color be affected by gentrification?

REFERENCES

Brunn, S. D., Williams, J. P., & Zeigler, D. J. (2003). *Cities of the world: World regional urban development*. Lanham, MD: Rowman & Littlefield

Flores, R. (2010). *23rd & Union*. Retrieved from www.greeneyedmedia.com/reviews-interviews/University of Washington's TV interview with Rafael Flores

Florida, R. (2002). *The rise of the creative class: And how it's transforming work, leisure, community and everyday life*. Washington, DC: Washington Monthly.

Form-Based Codes and Methods. (2004). Chicago, IL: Driehaus Estate, Lake Geneva, WI.

Freeman, L. (2005). Displacement or succession? Residential mobility in gentrifying neighborhoods. *Urban Affairs Review, 40*(4), 463–491.

Fullilove, M. J. (1996). Psychiatric implications of displacement: Contributions from the psychology of place. *American Journal of Psychiatry, 153*, 1516–1523.

Hampson, R. (2005). Studies: gentrification a boost for everyone. *USA Today*, April 20, pp. 13A–14A.

Harris, L. E., & Kaye, D. E. (2004): *How are Hope VI families faring?* Health, Metropolitan Housing and Communities Center, Brief No. 5. Washington, DC: The Urban Institute.

Morrill, R. (2004, Spring). *Gentrification in Seattle*, 55 Central Puget Sound Real Estate Research Report 81.

Norton, R. J. (2010). Feral cities – The new strategic environment. *Naval War College Review, LVI*, 97–105.

Radovanovic Dragana (2003) Intelligence and Lund, Sweden, University of Lund. Taken from: Cities of the Future, Global Competition and Leadership; Price Waterhouse Coopers (2005): Global Competition and Leadership.

BIBLIOGRAPHY

Bettcher, D., & Wipfli, H. (2001). Towards a more sustainable globalization: The role of the public health community. *Journal of Epidemiology and Community Health, 55*(9), 617–618.

Eliot, T. S. (1972). The Wasteland. In Helen Gardner (Ed.), *The new oxford book of English verses: 1250–1950* (p. 881). New York, NY: Oxford University Press.

Miskel, J. F., & Norton, R. J. (1997). Spotting trouble: Identifying faltering and failing states. *Naval War College Review, 50*(2), 79–91.

Murphy, F. G., Bond, T. M., Warren, R. C., & Maclin, S. C. (2008). Globalization in the twenty-first century: Impact of gentrification on community health. *American Journal of Health Studies, 23,* 66–73.

News in Science. (2003, April 7). China criticized for dragging feet on outbreak, p. 1.

Pricewaterhouse Cooper. (2005). *Cities of the future: Global competition, local leadership.* United Nations Environmental Program, Global Environmental Outlook—2000. London: Earthscan, 2001.

Index

ethnicity, 33–34, 39, 51, 90, 95, 99, 100, 103, 143, 195–197, 212, 232. *See also* race/racism
etiquette, 16
Evaluation Logic Model, 306, 307. *See also* Logic Model
evaluator, 301–303
excess deaths, 196–197
expert, positioning yourself as, 261

Facebook, 248, 249, 252, 254, 260, 263–264, 343
face-to-face interviews, 15
faith, 134–135
  -based community, 131–151
  horizontal, 132, 140, 150–151
  vertical, 132, 140, 150–151
familiarity, and "place," 317
Federal Communications Commission, 253
Federal Emergency Management Agency (FEMA), 294
Federally Qualified Health Centers (FQHCs), 126
feral community, 318–320
financial capital, 327–328
flash photography, 259
Flickr, 254
framing, 257–259
Franklin County Health Department, 25–26
freedom of information, 335
funders, responsibility of, 68
fundraising, 24

gender distribution, 33
gentrification, 318
  of COEs, 342–344
globalization, 330
glocalization, 330
grant funding, 24
Grey's Anatomy, 255
grossly unethical behavior, 67
group identification, 143
group survey administration, 16. *See also* surveys

Hamilton County Child Fatality Review Team (CFRT), 230

"Harry and Louise" campaign, 251–252, 265
Hart-Cellar Act of 1965, 92
health
  defined, 52, 131, 142, 193
  disparities, 196–197, 212–213
    eliminating, 232
  economy, 321
  education for, 141–142
  inequalities, 35
  insurance, 98. *See also* Medicaid; Medicare
  leadership, 320–321
  policy, 211, 213
  poor health, causal factors for, 35
  service, 321–322
health belief model (HBM), 167–168
health care divide, bridging, 158–159
health care reform, role of media in, 250–263
health equity, advancing, 227–239
  background, 229
  communities, empowering and mobilizing, 237–238
  data for decisions, using, 237
  feedback, monitoring, evaluating and providing, 238
  health and development connection, facilitating, 238
  health disparities, eliminating, 232
  Infant Vitality Surveillance Network, role of, 233–236
  obstacles to, 238
  problem description, 229–230
  public health policy, role of, 230–232
  shared priorities, identifying, 238
  social policies, evaluation of, 236
Health Insurance Association of America (HIAA), 251, 252, 265
Health Reform Law of 2010, 98
Health Security Act, 251
Heckler Report on Minority Health, 232
heroes, 79
holistic wellness approach, 289